Prostate Cancer

Prostate Cancer
Prevention and Cure

by Lee Nelson, M.D.

HUNTINGTON PRESS
LAS VEGAS, NEVADA

Prostate Cancer Prevention and Cure

Published by
    Huntington Press
    3687 South Procyon Avenue
    Las Vegas, Nevada 89103
    telephone: (702) 252-0655
    facsimile: (702) 252-0675
    email: books@huntingtonpress.com

ISBN: 0-929712-14-5

Cover design by: Laurie Shaw
Interior design & production: Laurie Shaw

In this text, the author has tried to provide the most comprehensive, up-to-date information about prostate cancer prevention and treatment. Neither he, nor the publisher, makes any claims, however, that the information presented here will cure prostate cancer or prevent it from developing. The information in this book is intended only as a guide to improve your chances of success. The author strongly advises every reader to consult closely with his team of prostate cancer specialists in devising a treatment plan.

*This book is dedicated to my recently deceased mother,
who died of lung cancer. This is for you, Mom.
Your graciousness and peerless sense of humor
will always be a beacon for me.
And to my namesakes, Uncle Nelson and Aunt Lee.*

Acknowledgments

Many people have made significant contributions to this book. Without their input, this project would have been impossible.

First, I thank Dr. Howard Soule and the staff of the Prostate Cancer Foundation (formerly CaP CURE) for reading the manuscripts, providing invaluable introductions to the most knowledgable professionals in the field of prostate cancer, and inviting me to the CaP CURE retreats. Without Dr. Soule's boundless support and encouragement, this book would never have gotten off the ground.

I'm confident I speak for all prostate cancer survivors in thanking the Prostate Cancer Foundation/CaP CURE for its prodigious effort in helping to find treatments for prostate cancer and in the search for a cure.

I thank Michael Milken for consenting to the highly instructive personal interview and Jeff Moore for editing it.

I'm very grateful to Dr. Anthony D'Amico, Dr. Snuffy Myers, and Dr. William Grant for all their e-mail correspondence, which helped me to sort out complex issues, both personally and for this book.

I deeply appreciate the doctors, all of whom graciously consented to interviews or chats: Howard Scher, M.D.; Paul Lange, M.D.; Edward Giovannucci, M.D.; Chris Logothetis, M.D.; Moshe Shike, M.D.; David Heber, M.D., Ph.D.; Celestia

Higano, M.D.; Mathew Smith, M.D., Ph.D.; June Chan, Sc.D.; Dan Petrylak, M.D.; Stuart Holden, M.D.; Steven Strum, M.D.; Mack Roach, M.D.; Eric Small, M.D.; John Kurhanewicz, Ph.D.; Ken Pienta, M.D.; Avigdor Scherz, Ph.D.; Carl Rossi, M.D.; David Agus, M.D.; Ken Russell, M.D.

I'm also indebted to my excellent group of personal physicians: Dr. Howard Scher, Medical Oncologist; Dr. Stuart Holden, Urologist; Dr. Ken Russell, Radiation Oncologist; Dr. John Mathews, Radiation Oncologist; Dr. Erica Lauder, General Practice.

I thank Beth Ginsberg for the fabulous recipes that keep me healthy and happy.

I thank Barbara Byczek for her tireless efforts to pin down Dr. Scher so that I could talk with him.

Two people deserve special mention. My editor, Deke Castleman, who believed in this project, was there every time I needed him, and worked his schedule around to accommodate mine. Thank you, Deke. You're a fine editor and a good friend. And my lovely wife typed the manuscript and supported me during periods of frustration.

I thank Harry Schultz, author of the renown international HSL financial newsletter, for his support and for sending me pertinent articles. You're a good friend, Harry.

To all these wonderful and caring people, I express my heartfelt gratitude.

Contents

Introduction

At age 55, I underwent a routine PSA (prostate-specific antigen) blood test. I'd spent the previous five years living in remote parts of Asia where this screening test for prostate disease was unavailable. A visiting doctor friend of mine (general practitioner) had done a digital rectal exam (the dreaded "finger wave") three years prior, and he found that my prostate was generally enlarged, but there were no areas of hardness. The prostate border was smooth and regular. I'd had minor urinary symptoms for years, getting up two to three times each night to urinate. This was compatible with my age and the moderately enlarged prostate my doctor friend felt when he examined me, but it was certainly no cause for concern. Benign prostatic hypertrophy (BPH), as this condition is called, is quite common in men over 50 and usually responds to medicinal treatment.

I started taking a remedy containing saw palmetto oil to shrink the prostate gland. I also started taking a new over-the-counter "wonder drug" called DHEA. I really liked the effects of DHEA. I felt much more energetic and focused. As you'll read later, however, DHEA and prostate cancer don't mix.

When my PSA (prostate specific antigen) came back at 11.2 (normal is less than 4.0), I was shocked, to put it mildly. I had been extremely health conscious since graduating from medical school nearly 30 years earlier. I ate very little red meat, used only "good" oils, exercised regularly, and took antioxidant-rich vitamin supplements. Surely this was a lab error. I repeated the test and the result was the same. From my medical training, I knew that at my age a PSA of this magnitude meant that the probability of prostate cancer was high.

I sought out a top-notch urologist who did another digital rectal exam (DRE). Unlike the one three years earlier, this test revealed an area of hardness in the right base of the prostate. A few more blood tests and a prostate biopsy later and the diagnosis was confirmed—prostate cancer.

I felt scared and confused. What to do? As I had done so often in medical school, I decided to find out as much as possible about this disease and its treatment. What I discovered was one of the most muddled areas in modern medicine.

Recognized experts in the field diametrically disagreed with each other as to the preferred treatment. To be sure, there were many options, but none was a clear-cut magic bullet. And there were many nasty potential side-effects to consider. Despite my medical training, given my level of confusion, I found it hard to imagine how someone who was not a doctor could successfully navigate the maze of options.

Indeed, most don't. They simply put themselves in the hands of their local urologist, do what he says, and hope for the best.

My purpose in writing *Prostate Cancer—Prevention and Cure* is to familiarize as many readers as possible with the current state of the art in the diagnosis and treatment of prostate cancer. This book is not only for someone who's been diagnosed with prostate cancer, but also for anyone who's a potential candidate for it—in other words, all men. It's also for women whose partners are either prostate cancer patients or who simply want to understand the disease in the event that it enters their lives.

In writing this book I reviewed more than 2,000 papers

in the medical literature. Armed with this background information, I then spoke with many of the top doctors in the field of prostate cancer—urologists, medical oncologists, and radiation oncologists. Each expert has his own view of the disease: which treatment to use, how to evaluate side-effects, and an overall approach, or philosophy, for dealing with prostate cancer at different stages.

However, this book has been written with the best interests of the patient as the overriding paradigm. I've tried to demystify the way doctors think in order to provide you with clearer insights, allowing you to take control of your illness. Then, once you've gotten rid of the cancer cells, I teach you the most optimal course for staying healthy.

The fact is, there's only one person whom you can rely upon to significantly improve your chances of cure from prostate cancer: You! Your active involvement in managing your disease is likely to increase your chances of success.

From this book and other sources, learn all you can. Ask questions, even if you think they might be dumb or embarrassing (such as those that concern sexual implications, incontinence, or bowel problems). Do not blindly accept medical pronouncements.

Optimistic and informed action is likely to improve your overall health and outlook.

Cancer is usually a defining event in someone's life. It can be viewed as a curse or a wake-up call. If you choose to behave as a passive victim, you are less likely to survive, and the quality of your life may erode. However, if you choose to view it as a catalyst for change in lifestyle and thinking, it can become a blessing in disguise. The course you set now will shape the balance of your life. It's up to you.

SECTION I:

WHAT IS
PROSTATE CANCER?

Prostate Cancer Basics

In the year 2000, roughly 500,000 American men died of cancer. If you're between the ages of 45 and 64 your chances of dying from cancer are greater than from any other cause; if you are older than 65, cancer deaths are surpassed only by deaths from heart disease.

The two most common cancers for men are skin cancer and prostate cancer. Cancer of the prostate is second only to lung cancer as the leading cause of male cancer deaths. According to the American Cancer Society, in 1998 about 184,000 American men were newly diagnosed with prostate cancer and 39,000 died from it. In 2002, new cases were estimated to be 189,000, with 30,200 deaths. While new cases have increased slightly during the past four years, deaths from prostate cancer have decreased by about 23%. This dramatic decrease in death rate is probably attributable to both earlier detection and better treatment. If you're over 50, statistically you have a 50% chance of getting prostate cancer at some point in your life.

The prostate (not prostrate) gland is about the size and shape of a plump chestnut. The gland is surrounded by a protective sheath called the prostate capsule. The gland/capsule is located in the space between the bladder and the rectum. The urethra, through which both urine and semen flow, passes through the middle of the prostate. When the size of the prostate increases due to either benign or malignant growth, it can compress the urethra, producing symptoms. These symptoms may include frequent urination, especially at night, start-and-stop urination, difficulty in starting the stream of urine, and reduction in the rate of flow.

The prostate is an expendable gland. You can live quite nicely without it. Its limited functions include providing fluid that may help transport sperm and protecting the urinary system against bacterial infections. It's not required for erections or fertility. As men age, the prostate becomes a liability.

Most aging men are well aware of the annoying symptoms of an enlarged prostate, which is caused by cell proliferation, whether benign (non-cancerous) or malignant. Benign prostatic hypertrophy (BPH), as it's called, is a common problem. Fortunately, the symptoms of BPH can usually be controlled by medicines or herbal formulas.

Another common prostate problem is prostatitis, or inflammation of the prostate. It's usually caused by bacteria. Often the invading bacteria are difficult to identify. Symptoms of prostatitis can mimic those of BPH or prostate cancer. Prostatitis can also dramatically raise blood levels of PSA (prostate specific antigen). Measuring the PSA is a screening test for prostate cancer (see "Screening and Diagnosis"). Prostatitis can sometimes be mistaken for prostate cancer; when the two occur together, prostatitis can make the cancer seem more advanced than it really is.

Prostate cancer may produce symptoms identical to BPH or prostatitis. But it can also grow for years without causing any symptoms at all. The cause of prostate cancer is unknown. About 9%-15% of the cases are hereditary. Inflammation from hit-and-run infections, hormone levels, and lifestyle factors like diet and exercise are thought to play a role in the development, growth, and spread of prostate cancer.

What all these possible causes have in common is that

they damage the DNA, or the genetic blueprint, of prostate cells. The DNA of our cells is perpetually being damaged by internal and external factors, and our cells are constantly repairing DNA damage. A delicate balance exists between factors that stimulate cell growth and agents that trigger cell death. This balance is controlled by proteins. The production of these proteins is controlled by the DNA of genes. One gene produces one specific protein.

Some of these proteins turn cells "on," some turn cells "off." If the DNA in particular genes is damaged, this fine on-off balance is disrupted. Genes that stimulate prostate cell growth may act unimpeded by genes that suppress cell growth, if these "suppressor" genes have been damaged (see "Risk Factors: Age").

For example, some genes control a built-in suicide program in cells. In due course they program cells to die. This process of programmed cell death is called "apoptosis." You will see this term often when you read about prostate cancer. When genes that control apoptosis are damaged, cells continue to live longer than normal. Much longer. New cells continue to be formed, but old cells don't die. This leads to clumps of cells growing out of control: cancer.

As these clumps of aberrant cells continue to grow, they require more nutrients. When a clump of cancer cells reaches no more than one cubic millimeter, about the size of the head of a pencil, it requires new blood vessels to provide nutrients for continued growth. The cancer cells secrete proteins that stimulate cells lining small adjacent blood vessels to grow, thereby creating new minute vessels. This process is called "angiogenesis" (blood-vessel development). It's important to understand that no cancer, no matter which kind, can grow without new blood vessels. In fact, one of the most fertile fields of anti-cancer research is the development of "anti-angiogenesis" agents, drugs that interfere with the ability of cancer cells to form new blood vessels. Prostate cancer is no exception. Anti-angiogenesis is discussed in detail in the chapter titled "New and Future Developments."

As prostate cancer cells continue to grow, cells can break off from the clump and be carried away in either the blood or lymph systems. Most of these cells are killed by the body's immune system. Special lymphocytes (white blood cells) called T-cells, and other lymphocytes called natural killer (NK) cells, attack and kill these circulating cancer cells. But as their number increases, some cancer cells may slip through the body's defenses. They may wind up establishing themselves far away from their original source. Here they grow, forming new clumps and stimulating the formation of new blood vessels. These distant groups of cancer cells are called "metastases." These cells grow faster than the surrounding normal cells and don't die. Like weeds in a garden, they eventually crowd out the cells in the organs where they settle, compromising their function.

Prostate cancer has a particular affinity for bone. Most prostate cancer cells that break off of a clump wind up in the bone or bone marrow. In fact, the cause of death for most men who die from prostate cancer is complications from bone metastases. One of the most important goals in the treatment of prostate cancer, as you will read in the chapter on bisphosphonates, is to prevent it from getting established in bones. Accomplishing this goes a long way toward improving your chances of recovery.

Prostate cancer is not a single disease. In other words, it exhibits different characteristics in different individuals. This makes intuitive sense, since there are undoubtedly multiple causes. It's not surprising, therefore, that some men have very slow growing cancers and other men have aggressive cancers. Actually, the two are probably different diseases entirely. As such, it makes sense to treat them differently. We will discuss treatment options later. For now, suffice it to say that men who have slow-growing cancers have more treatment options and generally less disease than men with aggressive cancers. Determining whether you're dealing with a tortoise or a hare is a major role of the tests your doctor will order for you.

Prostate cancer usually develops in more than one location in the gland (multi-focal). By age 90, virtually all men have microscopic pockets of prostate cancer. This has been confirmed by autopsy results. But most men die with their prostate cancer, rather than from their cancer. As you will read, there are things you can do, steps totally within your control, to delay the development and growth of this cancer. Understanding the risk factors and lifestyle factors that affect your chances is a good start.

1

RISK FACTORS

Who gets prostate cancer? Who's at risk? Some risk factors, like age, race, and family history, are well-established. Recent studies also present strong evidence for dietary factors, hormonal influences, lack of exposure to sunlight, and environmental contaminants as significant influences on the incidence of prostate cancer. Some medical conditions, like diabetes and obesity, appear to predispose men to prostate cancer. Other potential risk factors, including vasectomy, baldness, and body type, are more controversial.

If you have known risk factors, you can increase your level of vigilance to reduce your risk. Annual PSA blood testing and digital rectal exam (DRE) from as early as age 40 can help in early detection and treatment of prostate cancer. Dietary and lifestyle changes may slow a developing cancer. Thus, there are steps you can take if you are at increased risk. Let's look at each risk factor.

Age

Not much you can do about this one. The older you are, the greater your risk of getting prostate cancer. You may have heard this truism: "All men will die from prostate cancer if they don't die of something else first." This indicates how common prostate cancer is in aging men. And it *is* common. Upwards of 20% of all American men will get clinically significant prostate cancer sometime in their lives. Many more will have microscopic pockets of prostate cancer found at autopsy that caused them no trouble in life. In fact, virtually 100% of men lucky enough to make it to 90 have evidence of cancer in their prostate tissue. No other cancer is so prevalent. Yet most men die from other causes.

It's generally believed that these microscopic cancer foci are precursors (forerunners) of clinical prostate cancer. Interestingly, these small pockets of cancer occur pan-culturally—Japanese, Chinese, and Thai men are just as likely to harbor them as Swedes, Frenchmen, or African-Americans. But *clinical* prostate cancer is a far different matter. Here, other factors seem to come into play changing insignificant microscopic lesions into a potentially life-threatening disease. Both hereditary and environmental forces may influence this unwanted metamorphosis.

That brings us back to age. The chance of a man 39 years old or younger developing this active clinical form of prostate cancer is less than 1 in 10,000. From 40 to 59 the odds dramatically plummet, to 1 in 78. Between 60 and 79 they drop again, to 1 in 6!

Why does age make such a difference? A big part of the reason seems to be the increased tendency for DNA to be damaged over time. DNA controls all cell processes. It's the stuff that genes are made of—the building blocks of life. Destructive environmental forces, such as radiation, pesticides, heavy metals, and free radicals, damage DNA. As we've seen, our bodies are constantly repairing damaged DNA. But if destructive elements overwhelm our ability to mend DNA, cells become abnormal. Over time, this can lead to cancer. As we age, it appears, there may be a build-up of damaged DNA. Our bodies may not be as efficient repairmen.

One class of genes that's pivotal in keeping prostate cancer at bay is the tumor suppressors briefly mentioned earlier. There are at least several of these. As the mysteries of the human genome are unraveled (the complete genome has now been mapped), more of these tumor-suppressing genes are likely to be discovered. The proteins produced by these genes are a large family of natural proteins that block numerous pathways involved in progression to malignancy.

One key suppressor gene is called p53; this gene is crucial for DNA repair. When it's altered, damaged DNA can't be mended. About half of the men with advanced prostate cancer have mutations (alterations) in p53. By special testing, changes in p53 can be detected in a prostate biopsy specimen. If p53 has mutated, the chance of the cancer recurring after treatment is higher. For this reason, some oncologists (cancer specialists) will treat patients who have altered p53 at the time of diagnosis more aggressively. So it may be worthwhile requesting this test when you have a biopsy that shows prostate cancer.

It's likely that advancing age increases the chances of gene mutations. A probable example of this phenomenon comes from a potential risk factor reported in the *American Journal of Epidemiology* in late 1999. Investigators from Boston University Medical School found that a father's age (not the mother's) at the time of *conception* affected the chances of his sons developing prostate cancer. Men who have male children early in life impart far less risk of prostate cancer to their offspring than men who reproduce later in life. Men aged 38 or more had about a 70% greater chance of having an affected son than men under age 27. Fathers between 27 and 38 had less risk of having an affected son than older men, but their risk was still 20%-30% higher than men whose age was less than 27 years old. The researchers postulated that the reason for this previously undiscovered risk factor might be genetic changes (mutations) to sperm cells due to advancing age.

Age may also predict the ability to cure prostate cancer. A recent study out of Johns Hopkins University discovered that older men who underwent radical prostatectomy (removal of the prostate by surgery) had less chance than younger men of being cured of their disease. In fact, the researchers were surprised to discover that age was a better predictor of disease outcome than the highly informative PSA levels. PSA is the global blood test used to screen men for prostate cancer. Although controversial, it's generally agreed that PSA levels above 4.0 nanograms per milliliter (ng/ml) are abnormal. In men with prostate cancer aged 40 to 50 with PSA levels greater than 10 ng/ml and who had no detectable lump in the prostate on rectal examination, the chance of surgical cure was 73%. This compared with only a 49% chance of cure in men 61 to 73 years of age with comparable PSA levels, rectal exam status, and identical surgery. So advancing age seems not only to predispose men to the development of clinically significant prostate cancer, it also appears to reduce the chances of cure.

Key References

Carter H and Coffey D. The prostate: an increasing medical problem. *Prostate* 1990; 16: 39-48.

Zhang Y et al. Father's age affects prostate cancer risk. *Am J Epidemiol* 1999; 150: 1208-1212 (from Reuters medical news service).

Carter H, Epstein J, and Partin A. Influence of age and prostate-specific antigen on the chance of curable prostate cancer among men with nonpalpable disease. *Urology* 1999; 53: 126-130.

Race

Race significantly influences the incidence of prostate cancer. Asians have very low rates, Caucasians intermediate rates, and African-Americans very high rates of prostate cancer development. The difference in death rates between African-Americans and American whites is surprisingly large. As a report from the National Institute for Health (NIH) puts it, "The disparity in mortality rates from prostate cancer is greater between white and black men than for any other type of cancer in the U.S. and possibly the world." Several studies confirm that African-Americans have a 35% higher chance of developing prostate cancer, and a more than 220% chance of dying from it, than white men.

If the gap between African-Americans and western Caucasians is large, the disparity between African-Americans and Asians is cavernous. African-Americans are between 50 and 200 times as likely to die of prostate cancer than their various Asian counterparts.

Meanwhile, Asian men living in the United States have more chance of getting prostate cancer than men who remain in Asia. Put it all together and it's highly probable that both environmental and hereditary forces are at work in determining the racial make-up of who gets prostate cancer and who doesn't.

Why are African-Americans more prone to develop prostate cancer and much more likely to die from it than American whites? This is a hotly debated topic in the corridors of a number of centers for prostate cancer. The definitive answer remains elusive. A combination of factors seems to be involved.

One element that has received a lot of attention in medical publications of late is that African-Americans are less likely to be screened for prostate cancer. This may be due both to a lack of awareness and a lack of access to PSA blood testing and digital rectal exams. Without proper screening, black men often have significantly more advanced and aggressive disease at the time they first seek medical attention. Often they will have troublesome symptoms that lead them to seek medical help.

One multi-institutional study from North Carolina showed a statistically significant inverse correlation between income level and health-insurance status and advanced prostate cancer in black men. The study found that black men with lower income levels and/or no health insurance were more likely to have advanced cancer than those with higher income and health insurance. No such correlation was observed in white men in North Carolina.

Another study showed significantly lower levels of literacy in black men showing up at the doctor's office with prostate cancer than in whites. In a study of 212 lower-income-level men diagnosed with prostate cancer in Louisiana and Illinois, only 48% of African-Americans possessed at least a sixth-grade literacy level; 91% of Caucasian men of comparable income had achieved at least sixth-grade literacy. Interestingly, in this study, when adjustments were made for literacy, age, and geographic location, race was no longer a predictor of advanced disease. The authors postulate that low literacy rates in African-Americans may lower their awareness to the availability of screening. They suggest that literature designed specifically to literacy level might go a long way toward rectifying the increased risk among black men.

Although screening is getting the lion's share of racial attention lately, it's unlikely to be the whole story. For one thing, African-Americans had higher incidence and mortality before screening became popular. Also, researchers at Wayne State University's Harper Hospital led by Dr. Powell found that black men have a greater risk of recurrent cancer than white men if the cancer has spread beyond the prostate. These investigators observed that African-American men and Caucasians develop prostate cancer at similar ages. But across all age groups, black men have metastatic cancer much more often than whites. They concluded that the reason black men have worse outcomes is due to more aggressive cancers in black men under 70 years of age. Why? See below.

These findings were confirmed by research from the Southwest Oncology Group (SWOG). At the May 2000 meeting of the American Urological Association (AUA), Dr. Thompson revealed that in the SWOG data black men had more extensive disease and more bone pain than whites. Additionally, race independently predicted survival outcome when variables like age, bone pain, etc. were factored out.

Besides race, other considerations that might affect risk in African-American men include diet, hormonal influence, infections, and response to sunlight.

There is now considerable evidence, though not yet conclusive, that consuming fat may stimulate changes from dormant to active prostate cancer. Some investigators have noted that African-Americans have more fat in their diets than whites. Similarly, whites take in more fat than Asians. Mortality from prostate cancer correlates with fat intake.

Not only the amount of fat in a man's diet may predispose him to prostate cancer, but how much its cooked also seems to make a difference. Cancer-causing compounds, called heterocyclic amines (HAs), are formed when meat is cooked. According to a recent study, meat type, intake rate, cooking method, and meat doneness all influence the amount of carcinogenic HAs that are formed. Pan-fried meats produce the most HAs. Surprisingly, chicken (with skin) is the largest source of HAs among the different types of meat.

This study showed that African-American men over age 30 consume about three times as much HAs as whites. A national survey showed a preference amongst African-American men for well-done meat, which increases the HA content. About ⅔ of HA content is comprised of a compound that causes prostate DNA to mutate and induces prostate cancer in rats.

A recent study by the National Cancer Institute (NCI) showed that increased amounts of animal-fat intake doubled the risk of blacks getting prostate cancer, but did not significantly increase the risk in whites. This lends support to the idea that cooking with its increased HA content is a significant risk for prostate cancer and predominately affects black men.

The risk of prostate cancer progressing to advanced disease is also increased by animal-fat intake, but in this case both blacks and whites with comparable fat intake are equally affected. Since HAs have been implicated in the initiation of prostate cancer and the amount of animal fat consumed has been associated with the cancer progressing and spreading, this NCI finding makes sense.

Young black men have been found to have a higher level of circulating testosterone than white men of equivalent age— about 15% higher. Testosterone levels also appear to decrease more slowly in aging black men. Although these hormonal differences may account for some of the black-white difference, this has not been proven.

African-American men have a higher incidence of a known prostate cancer risk factor called prostatic intra-epithelial hyperplasia (PIN). Thought to be a precursor to cancer, PIN is an area of inflammation and cellular growth within the prostate. It may be part of a process that starts with an infection in the prostate and becomes an area of smoldering inflammation. Then, under hormonal influences primarily from DHT and estrogens, DNA changes may occur. A study by Dr. Sakr at Wayne State University noted that blacks had more areas of PIN in their prostates and that the PIN tended to be of higher grade (more abnormal) than in a comparable group of white men. This difference started when men were in their twenties.

The researchers compared the prostates of black and white men in several ways. At autopsy they found that extensive higher-grade PIN was present in 7% (25/364) of black men less than 50 years of age compared to 2% (4/208) of white men. When they examined prostates removed surgically in a group of 1,200 men, they consistently found more extensive and higher grade PIN in African-Americans, especially in those under 50. In men with disease discovered by PSA testing and no evidence of cancer upon digital rectal exam, 33% of blacks had extensive high-grade PIN compared with only 12% of whites, a highly significant difference.

Dr. Sakr concludes: "Our findings suggest an important role for high-grade PIN in the development of clinically significant, potentially aggressive prostate cancer in African-American men."

Yet another ingredient that may influence African-American susceptibility is response to sunlight. Here, there is some conflicting data. While blacks seem to have reduced ability to convert sunlight into vitamin D, recent data show that vitamin D levels are equivalent in black men whether or not they have prostate cancer. Vitamin D is thought to play a protective role in halting the growth of prostate cancer. What significance, if any, it has in relation to the higher death rate from prostate cancer in African-Americans is unclear. It seems prudent, however, for all men with prostate cancer to periodically check their vitamin D blood levels. If low, whether the man is black or white, he'll probably benefit from supplemental vitamin D. The active form of vitamin D, known as calcitriol (Rocaltrol), is available only by prescription and must be taken under doctor's care (see "Sun Exposure" later in this chapter and the section on vitamin D in the "Nutrition" chapter).

A great deal of work is being done to reduce the risk of death from prostate cancer in African-American men. One technique that shows great promise is interactive screening. Dr. Myers and colleagues report in a recent issue of the journal *Cancer* that understandable printed material, combined with telephone follow-up, lead to a far greater turnout for a screening examination and PSA blood test when compared with men who only received a letter inviting them to be screened. Undoubtedly better screening will help close the gap between black and white men.

Key References

NCI's Risk, Burdens, and Outcomes Science. http: //www.nih.gov/prostateplan8.html

Bennett CL et al. Relation between literacy, race, and stage of presentation among low-income patients with prostate cancer. *J Clin Oncology* 1998; 16: 3101-3104.

Pienta KJ and Esper P. Risk factors for prostate cancer. *Ann Intern Med* 1993; 118: 793-803.

Wingo P et al. Cancer statistics for African-Americans 1996. *CA Cancer J Clin* 46: 113: 126.

Conlisk E et al. Prostate cancer: demographic and behavioral correlates of stage at diagnosis among blacks and whites in North Carolina. *Urology* 1999; 53: 1194-1199.

Powell I et al. Prostate cancer biochemical recurrence stage for stage is more frequent among African-American than white men with locally advanced but not organ-confined disease. *Urology* 2000; 55: 246-251.

Powell I et al. Prostate cancer is biologically more aggressive among African-

Americans than Caucasian men under age 70; hypotheses supported by autopsy and SEER data. Program and abstracts from the American Urological Association 95th Annual Meeting; April 29-May 4, 2000; Atlanta, Georgia. *Abstract 243.*

Thompson I et al. African-American ethnic background is independent predictor of survival in metastatic prostate cancer. Program and abstracts from the American Urological Association 95th Annual Meeting; April 29-May 4, 2000; Atlanta, Georgia. *Abstract 242.*

Whittemore A, Kolonel L, et al. Prostate cancer in relation to diet, physical activity, and body size in blacks, whites, and Asians in the United States and Canada. *J Natl Cancer Instit* 1995; 87: 652-661.

Myers R et al. Adherence of African-American men to prostate cancer education and early detection. *Cancer* 1999; 86: 88-104.

Roach M. Finally, good news about prostate carcinoma in African-American men. *Cancer* 1999; 86: 1-2.

Sakr W. Prostatic intraepithelial neoplasia: A marker for high-risk groups and potential target for chemoprevention. *Eur Urol* 1999; 35: 474-478.

Pienta KJ, Goodson JA, and Esper PS. Epidemiology of prostate cancer: molecular and environmental clues. www.cancer.med.umich.edu

Bogen, KT et al. U.S. dietary exposures to hetero-cyclic amines. *Journal of Exposure Analysis and Environmental Epidemiology* 2001; 11: 155-168.

Grover, PL and Martin, FL. The initiation of breast and prostate cancer. *Carcinogenesis* 2002; 7: 1095-1102.

Hayes RB et al. Dietary factors and risks for prostate cancer among blacks and whites in the United States. *Cancer Epidemiol Biomarkers Prev* 1999; 8: 25-34. (NCI study)

Heredity

Regardless of race, the risk of prostate cancer escalates for a man when his immediate male relatives (father, son, or brother) are diagnosed with this disease. If your father (or son) is affected, your risk doubles. If your brother is affected, your risk triples. One study reported that if your brother or father got prostate cancer at 50 or younger and another first-degree relative (brother, father, son) is also diagnosed, your chances of developing prostate cancer increase seven-fold!

Overall genetic factors are believed to account for about 9%-15% of all cases of prostate cancer. However, for men under age 55, the chance of genetically determined disease skyrockets. In this group 43% of all instances of prostate cancer are thought to be due to genetic factors.

Due to the increased risk, for men in families with known

prostate cancer, especially when the onset in a close relative occurs early in life (age 50 or less) or if more than one first-degree relative is involved, initial screening for prostate cancer should begin at age 35. Normally, screening is not recommended until age 50.

Generally, although hereditary prostate cancer starts earlier than non-hereditary prostate cancer, it does not appear to differ significantly in its characteristics or survival patterns.

Key References

Gronberg H et al. Age-specific risk of familial prostate carcinoma. *Cancer* 1999; 86: 477-483.

Carter B et al. Hereditary prostate cancer: epidemiologic and clinical features. *J Urology* 1993; 150: 797-802.

Whittemore A et al. Family history and prostate cancer risk in black, white, and Asian men in the United States and Canada. *Am J Epidemiol* 1995; 141: 732-740.

Giovannucci E. How is individual risk of prostate cancer assessed? *Hematol Oncol Clin North Am* 1996; 10: 537-548.

Bratt O et al. Hereditary Prostate Cancer: clinical characteristics and survival. *J Urology* 2002; 2423-2426.

Obesity and Fat Consumption

Besides being at greater risk for heart disease and diabetes, obese men appear to be more vulnerable to aggressive prostate cancer than men who are overweight, or of normal weight. Dr. Amling and associates reported at the AUA meeting in May 2000 that 20% of a group of 860 men who had surgery for prostate cancer were obese. These men had significantly more aggressive prostate cancers on average, they got cancer much earlier in life, and they had more advanced cancer than slimmer men. Dietary factors are an obvious place to begin in accounting for these differences.

Obese men have high levels of insulin-like growth factor-1, a hormone that has been associated with markedly increased chances of developing prostate cancer (discussed in depth later in this section). If the increased risks of heart disease, diabetes, and other debilitating conditions are not persuasive enough to compel obese men to lose weight, perhaps the increased risk of dying from prostate cancer added to the list will help provide sufficient motivation.

One popular theory floating around the halls of prostate cancer academic centers is that various kinds of fat might stimulate the change of dormant prostate cancer to the more dangerous clinically significant form. Since microscopic prostate cancer is essentially equally prevalent for all cultures, diet, specifically fat consumption, is one element that might make a difference. A 2002 study from the Fred Hutchison Cancer Research Institute in Seattle, Washington, shows an association between fat intake and total caloric intake, not with the initiation of prostate cancer, but rather with its spread (see "Nutrition").

Fat intake is discussed in detail in the chapter "Nutrition." Suffice it to say here that animal fat (saturated fat) and polyunsaturated oils containing either linoleic acid (corn oil, soybean oil, safflower oil, etc.) or linolenic acid (flax oil) are potential contributors to the promotion of prostate cancer. Char-broiling or frying animal or fish fat produces cancer-causing substances known as heterocyclic amines that cling to the surface of fat molecules. Heavy ingestion of these carcinogens may increase risk.

> **HELPFUL HINT**
>
> Avoid eating animal fat. If you eat fish, eat it raw (sushi and sashimi), steamed, or poached, to minimize heterocyclic amines consumption.

In addition, nutrients that have medical evidence to support a protective effect against damage from fat ingestion include selenium, vitamin E, soy protein (but not soybean oil), green tea, cruciferous vegetables and sprouts, silymarin, and curcumin (see "Nutrition"). Olive oil and oil from fish appear to be helpful. However, since olive oil is high in calories, it's probably best to use only the necessary amounts for cooking and salad dressing. Olive oil should be the predominant oil consumed. Other beneficial oils are macadamia nut, avocado, and walnut oils.

Key References

Amling C et al. The impact of obesity on pathologic variables and surgical complications undergoing radical prostatectomy. Program and abstracts from the American Urological Association 95th Annual Meeting; April 29–May 4, 2000; Atlanta, Georgia, *Abstract 254.*

McCarthy MF. Vegan proteins may reduce risk of cancer, obesity, and cardiovascular disease by promoting increased glucagon activity. *Med Hypotheses* 1999; 53: 459-485.

Giovannucci E. Nutritional factors in human cancers. *Adv Exp Med Biol* 1999; 472: 29-42.

Environmental Hazards

More and more evidence is now coming out on the link between environmental contaminants and cancer. In mid-2000, the *Washington Post* published a summary of a report yet to be released from the Environmental Protection Agency (EPA) on dioxin. Dioxin is a bi-product of waste incineration, as well as paper-pulp production and other industrial sources. You may be aware that Agent Orange, the defoliant used in the Vietnam War, has been shown to significantly increase the risk of a variety of cancers. Dioxin is the prime active ingredient of Agent Orange. The EPA now concedes, according to the *Post*, that dioxin is a "human carcinogen."

Accumulating in animal fats, fish fats, and dairy products, dioxin is ubiquitous—people worldwide have measurable blood-dioxin levels. This toxin accumulates over time and the effects are cumulative. The EPA now estimates the risk of cancer from dioxin consumption to be 10 times as high as previous estimates. Cancer of the lung and lymphoma are increased by dioxin exposure. Since toxin exposure is usually not organ-specific, it's likely that dioxin increases the chances of getting a variety of cancers. I would not be at all surprised to ultimately discover that prostate cancer is one of these.

Another risk factor for cancer is traffic pollution. Two

recent Scandinavian studies showed a clear-cut increase in lung cancer in people exposed to prolonged periods of heavy traffic. In a Swedish study, 30-year exposure resulted in a 40% increase in the chances of getting lung cancer for both smokers and non-smokers. Ten years of exposure increased lung cancer probabilities by 20%.

One contaminant in auto-exhaust fumes is cadmium, a heavy metal. Although cadmium in polluted air has not been directly linked to prostate cancer, prostate cancer is an occupational hazard for workers exposed to cadmium in battery manufacturing. Other substances that increase the risk of prostate cancer are pesticides, metallic dust, liquid fuels, lubricating grease and oil, and aromatic hydrocarbons. Dr. Kristan Aronson found that in Montreal, Canada, men working in aircraft manufacture, gas and water utilities, and around jet fuels had an increased risk of prostate cancer. Farmers regularly exposed to pesticides and herbicides also appear to be more vulnerable. Dr. Aronson estimates that about 10% of prostate cancer cases are due to occupational hazards, primarily exposure to environmental toxins.

Lack of Exposure to Sunlight

As you'll read in the Nutrition chapter, there is considerable evidence that vitamin D may retard the growth and spread of prostate cancer. Vitamin D production depends upon the skin's exposure to sunlight—specifically UV-B rays, according to Dr. William Grant. Demographically, the incidence of prostate can-

> **HELPFUL HINTS**
>
> Avoid walking or jogging in areas with heavy traffic. Select organic produce whenever possible to reduce pesticide ingestion. Thoroughly soak all fruits and vegetables in water before eating. Peel apples, pears, persimmons, and peaches, if not organically grown. Buy organic strawberries whenever possible. Strawberries, although rich in a nutrient associated with a reduction in prostate cancer, are one of the most highly sprayed fruits.

cer in the United States increases incrementally as you head south to north. The farther north you live, the greater your chances of getting prostate cancer. This may be due to a deficiency of vitamin D.

Although most studies of cancer and sunlight use average yearly amounts, Dr. Grant believes that lack of winter sun is the key variable. The long northern winter may deprive men of UV-B rays, impairing their ability to make vitamin D. This may account for increases in prostate cancer occurrence in northern areas. By the way, according to Dr. Grant, winter UV-B exposure also reduces the risk of colon and breast cancer. It appears that those winter vacations to sunny destinations may have even greater benefits than mere stress reduction.

2

SCREENING

More than 10 million Americans who have had cancer are living today. I'm amused when people I know come up to me, look searchingly into my eyes, and ask, "Are you all right?" The clear implication is that they believe, since I have prostate cancer, I must be dying. A female friend who hadn't seen me in more than a year became wide-eyed and blurted out, "Lee, you still have hair!"

Cancer is not a death sentence. The earlier it's discovered, the greater your chances of cure. A simple blood test (PSA) and an annual digital rectal exam (DRE) can pick up most prostate cancers while they're still imminently curable. As you'll read in the "Treatment" section, men with tumors caught early do well regardless of which treatment they select; men with more advanced cancers at the time of diagnosis have fewer treatment choices and tend to do more poorly.

PSA

The PSA blood test has revolutionized the evaluation and treatment of prostate cancer. PSA stands for prostate specific antigen. For practical purposes, significant amounts of PSA are produced only by prostate cells. The antigen's main purpose is thought to be in helping to dissolve a gel that forms after ejaculation (from a little leftover semen). In a normal prostate, PSA goes directly into seminal fluid, not blood. But small amounts "leak" out and diffuse into the circulation. These minute amounts can be measured by sensitive assays in nanograms per milliliter (ng/ml). When prostate cells become cancerous, however, their normal orientation and structure change. Instead of "leaking" into circulation, cancer cells actively release PSA into the fluid that surrounds them. The result is that cancer cells elevate blood PSA levels 30 times more than normal cells!

PSA blood tests to screen men for prostate cancer started being used in the mid-1980s. Even today, there is considerable debate in the medical literature as to whether PSA screening is worthwhile. Against PSA screening are the following arguments:

• PSA may be elevated by diseases other than prostate cancer: specifically, BPH and prostatitis. Elevated PSA levels may lead to unwarranted prostate biopsies, causing patients needless anxiety and discomfort.

• Even if an elevated PSA results in the ultimate discovery of prostate cancer, unnecessary treatment with potentially serious side effects may be inflicted on a man who has no symptoms. This may seriously, and unnecessarily, compromise his quality of life.

Although there is some credence to these positions, they are overwhelmed, in my opinion and in the opinion of most top prostate academicians, by the fact that PSA testing *saves lives*. Although screening impugners argue that this has not been firmly established, I disagree. I believe the evidence is far too strong to be denied. Consider this:

• After consistently rising for 20 years, the death rate from prostate cancer has been falling since the early 1990s. The National Cancer Institute reported a reduction in the number of deaths from prostate cancer from 25 per 100,000 men in 1990 to 17 per 100,000 men in 1995. This dovetails perfectly with the effects of PSA testing. During this five-year period, death rates in younger Caucasian males declined nearly 12%. Although the decline in death rate was not as dramatic in African-Americans, it still went down along the entire age spectrum. The smallest decrease in mortality rate was seen in eld-erly black men—a 3% decrease.

- Deaths from prostate cancer continue to fall. From 1997 to 2002 they fell by an additional 27% in American men, according to the American Cancer Society.

- A massive study of 65,123 men was conducted in Tyrol, Austria. Here it's standard operating procedure to aggres-sively treat virtually all men diagnosed with prostate cancer. Ninety-six percent of the men with prostate cancer had a radical prostatectomy (prostate removed by surgery). In a study begun in 1993 Dr. Bartsch and associates compared the death rate of Tyrolean men who had been screened (and treated) with mortality statistics from the rest of Austria. They found a 48% decrease in deaths from prostate cancer in the men from Tyrol.

- In the area around the Mayo Clinic in Rochester, Minn., where testing is prevalent, death rates have also dropped con-siderably more than the national average.

- A Finnish study randomized men in two groups. One received screening, the other didn't. Of the men in the group to be screened, about 10,300 men took a PSA test, while 23,400 men didn't. The investigators found that 86% of can-cers found in the screened group were confined to the pros-tate at the time of diagnosis. This compared with only 67% in the unscreened group, a highly significant difference. What this study strongly shows is that *screening allows prostate cancer to be picked up at an earlier, less dangerous stage in the screened group*.

Estimates from prostate cancer experts are that PSA test-ing allows prostate cancer to be picked up as much as five years earlier than by standard examination (DRE).

Decreasing death rates in all age groups and races in the United States sharply reduced death rates in screened men in Tyrol, Austria, and clinically less advanced prostate can-cer in PSA-screened men in Finland—all potent evidence in support of screening.

It now appears that there are three different forms of

prostate cancer: those that are aggressive, fast-growing, and potentially lethal; those that are very slow-growing and far less likely to be fatal; and those in between whose behavior may mimic either fast- or slow-growing types. This intermediate type is often lumped in with aggressive tumors.

One of the most important aspects of screening is that aggressive cancers can be picked up while they're still curable in men with 20-30 years of life left. In my case, for example, I had a moderately aggressive cancer that showed signs it was about to spread, if it hadn't already done so. I had no symptoms. The PSA test was part of a routine checkup. Had I waited even one more year, my cancer would almost surely have spread. The PSA screening test probably saved my life.

And I'm not alone. There are more, many more, men I know personally, all with one thing in common. They were in great health, but a routine PSA showed they had prostate cancer that was at a very dangerous stage. There is no doubt that, left undiscovered, many of these cancers would likely have been fatal.

Twenty-five percent of all prostate cancers are found in men under age 65. It's in this group, men who have 20 or more years to live, that PSA testing is most beneficial. Make no mistake. *PSA testing saves lives.* If you're 50 years of age or older, you should have an annual PSA blood test and a DRE. (As you'll read shortly, less frequent testing may be possible if your PSA is 2.0 or less.) If you have a brother or father who has prostate cancer, you should start annual screening at age 40. African-Americans should also consider starting screening at age 40. An initial PSA test at age 35 for men at very high risk (like a father and brother with prostate cancer) is probably warranted. If less than 1.0, it would not need to be repeated for five years.

At the May 2002 annual meeting of the American Society of Clinical Oncology (ASCO), Dr. E. David Crawford of the University of Colorado made a provocative presentation.

He and his associates reviewed the medical records of

27,863 men between the ages of 55 and 74 who had annual PSA tests. Fifty-five percent of these men had initial PSAs of 2.0 or less. The generally accepted upper limit of normal for PSA testing is 4.0.

In the nearly 15,000 men whose first PSA was 2.0 or less, Dr. Crawford's group found the following:

• 98.8% of men whose initial PSA was 1.0, or less, had a PSA less than 4.0 five years later.

• 98.8% of those whose initial PSA was 1.0 to 2.0 had a PSA less than 4.0 two years later.

Based on these findings, Dr. Crawford recommends that men with PSAs of less than 1.0 be tested every five years; men with PSAs 1.0 to 2.0 be tested every two years; men with PSAs higher than 2.0 be tested annually.

If these recommendations are accepted and the American Cancer Society is giving them a hard look, it would save the health system $500 million to $1 billion annually in PSA testing costs, according to Dr. Crawford.

Key Reference
Proceedings of the 38th Annual American Society of Clinical Oncology meeting notes. May 18-21, 2002.

Why is the issue of PSA testing still hotly debated? First, medical insurers are still trying to determine the economics of screening. And second, the results of a prospective, randomized study, the sine qua non of indisputable proof in the medical world, are not yet in. Dr. Crawford's findings, if accepted as standard, may help bridge these gaps.

The National Cancer Institute (NCI) mounted just

> **HELPFUL HINT**
>
> PSA screening has been shown to help detect prostate cancer at an earlier stage when it's still confined to the prostate. Prostate-confined tumors have very high cure rates. PSA screening saves lives.

such a study in 1994. But it could take another 10 years before the definitive results are fully known. This issue has such wide-ranging ramifications that it's rumored the NCI may take a look at the accumulated results as early as next year. While we wait for the definitive answer, I strongly urge you to get tested.

DRE (Digital Rectal Exam)

Part of the screening process for prostate cancer involves a DRE. Although not the most pleasant experience for most of us, it's generally more embarrassing than uncomfortable. It should be done by a urologist, a doctor who specializes in diseases of the urinary system (including the prostate gland). The doctor inserts a single, gloved, well-lubricated finger (digit) into your rectum. Then gently (some are more gentle than others) he, or she, will thoroughly examine your prostate. The prostate should feel soft, with a regular outline. Both sides of the gland should be about equal in size and shape. Areas of hardness, irregularity, or asymmetry are warning signs that often point to cancer.

Dr. Jacobsen and his associates studied a large group of men in Minnesota, comparing those who had screening with DREs with those who hadn't. They found that having a DRE during the prior 10 years reduced a man's chance of dying from prostate cancer by 50%. In men who had no symptoms that caused them to seek medical attention, but were in for a DRE as a precaution, the results were even more dramatic. In this group a screening DRE reduced the risk of death from prostate cancer by a whopping 69%!

In the PSA era, the majority of prostate cancers are not identified by the DRE. This is a positive event. I have a close friend who was diagnosed with a moderately aggressive cancer and had a PSA of 22.0. His urologist could not feel any sign of the cancer in this man's prostate. Although generally a PSA of 22 might be considered too high for surgery, my friend "wanted the damn thing out." At surgery, his disease was totally confined to his prostate and his outlook is excellent.

A DRE is an important part of the prostate cancer workup, especially the process called "staging," which helps determine risk level. Grin and bare it.

Elevated PSA—Now What?

The "official" normal range for PSA is 0.0 ng/ml to 4.0 ng/ml. For men under 60, PSA readings of between 2.5 and 4.0 are also suspect, especially for younger men. Some urologists do not believe men over 75 should be screened because, even if they have prostate cancer, treatment may not be advisable. Many men of this age will die of other causes long before their prostate cancer kills them. Whether a 75-plus-year-old man should be screened, in my mind, should depend on his overall health. If he is in generally poor health with a myriad of medical problems, I agree that checking for prostate cancer may not be warranted. But if he's healthy, I think he should be tested. Since people are now living longer, he could have 15-20 years left. (With genetic medicine just around the corner, it could be even longer.) He may want to be treated, although surgery might not be his treatment of choice.

Within the "normal" PSA range of 0.0-4.0, there can be big differences in the chances of contracting prostate cancer. Dr. Gann and colleagues found that men with PSAs between 2.01 and 4.0 were five to eight times as likely to develop aggressive prostate cancer over a 10-year period than men with PSAs of less than 1.0.

For this reason, some top urologists, such as Dr. Catalona at Washington University Medical School in St. Louis, believe that all men with PSAs above 2.5 ng/ml should be further evaluated. Twenty-two percent of these men have been found to have cancer when biopsied, and 14% of these were considered to be aggressive cancers (Gleason score of 7 or higher—see "Staging"). Since 81% were found to be contained within the prostate at the time of surgery, Dr. Catalona argues that lowering the upper limit of the screening threshold from 4.0 to 2.6 ng/ml may cure more cancers, by catching them before they spread. At surgery, men with PSAs of 4.0 or less have about an 83% chance of having the tumor limited to the prostate. This compares to about 70% organ-confined cancers for PSAs 4.0-10.0, and 53% for PSAs above 10.0.

In any event, if your PSA is above 4.0 (or 2.5 to play it safer), additional tests should be done. Often these will show that the increased PSA is not due to cancer. Remember, an elevated PSA can come from benign causes, like BPH and prostatitis. Even with a PSA as high as 10.0 ng/ml, there is only a 50% chance of cancer; with PSAs between 4.0 and 10.0, 70% will be traced to benign causes.

But how do you distinguish between benign and malignant etiologies? The most definitive way is by biopsy (a surgical procedure by which bits of living prostate tissue are removed from different areas of the prostate gland and examined by a pathologist, a doctor trained to identify normal and abnormal cells). But since much of the time biopsies don't turn up any cancer, researchers have (mercifully) looked for less invasive tests that help distinguish between benign disease and cancer.

Just such a test has now been developed that spares men from needless biopsies. The *free PSA test* is especially useful in the PSA 2.6-10.0 group. Men with PSAs above 10 have such a high risk of cancer that virtually all are biopsied. But PSAs between 2.6 and 10.0 are in a gray area.

PSA travels in the blood either in free form or bound to protein. With prostate cancer the percentage of free PSA tends to be lower than with BPH. The higher the percentage of free PSA, the less likely you are to have cancer.

A number of studies have been done to determine a reasonable cutoff point that will detect the most cancers, while sparing as many men as possible the unpleasantness of a biopsy. A recent (June 2000) study from the University of Washington in Seattle demonstrated that not doing biopsies on men with free PSA percentages of 26.4% or more in men with total PSAs of 4.0-10.0 would have detected 96% of cancers, while eliminating 27% of the biopsies. By lowering the cutoff point for biopsy to 20% free PSA, Dr. Gann and his group, using a database of 15,000 men from the Physicians' Health Study, determined that 50% of unnecessary biopsies would be avoided, although a few more cancers (11% vs. 4%) would be missed. Like Dr. Catalona, Dr. Gann believes that if free PSA levels are used as a guideline for biopsy, men with PSAs of 3.0 ng/ml and above should be tested. This is not much different from Dr. Catalona's 2.6 ng/ml level. Of note is this fact: *25% of all prostate cancers have PSAs of less than 4.0.*

Dr. Roehl, Dr. Catalona, and their colleagues found that out of 132 men who had surgery for prostate cancer at Washington University in St. Louis and whose PSAs were 2.6 ng/ml to 4.0 ng/ml, 80% had no sign of cancer beyond the removed prostate. Yet they determined that in their view, most of the removed cancers were clinically significant and 14% were considered to be aggressive.

What happens if this combination of tests misses a cancer? All is not lost. Since the PSA is already elevated, it will be closely monitored. Dr. Gann observed in his study that cancers missed by combined PSA and free PSA testing probably developed more slowly than detected cancers and were likely to be diagnosed later with the cancer still confined to the prostate. In other words, the missed cancers were unlikely to be the aggressive type.

If the PSA continues rising, a biopsy will undoubtedly be suggested. If you're in this position, you should be aware that free PSA testing is only now starting to become more widely used. If your doctor is not associated with an academic center, he may not be familiar with this test. If you have a PSA of less than 10.0 and your doctor is unfamiliar with a free PSA and wants to do a biopsy, I suggest you educate him. Failing this, it might behoove you to seek help at a university cancer center.

Key References

Catalona W et al. Detection of organ-confined prostate cancer is increased through prostate-specific antigen-based screening. *JAMA* 1993; 270: 948-954.

Roehl K et al. Robustness of free prostate specific antigen measurements to reduce unnecessary biopsies in the 2.6-4.0 ng/ml range. *J Urology* 2002; 168: 922-925.

Perrotti M et al. Early prostate cancer detection and potential for surgical cure in men with poorly differentiated tumors. *Urology* 1998; 52: 106-110.

Stenman et al. Prostate-specific antigen. *Can Biol* 1999; 9: 83-93.

Polascik T et. al. Prostate specific antigen. A decade of discovery—what we have learned and where we are going. *J Urology* 1999; 162: 293.

Bartsch G et al. Decrease in prostate cancer mortality following introduction of prostate specific antigen (PSA) screening in the federal state of Tyrol, Austria. Abstract from the AUA 95th Annual Meeting. April 29-May 4, 2000; Atlanta, Georgia. *Abstract 387.*

Makinen T et al. Detection of clinical organ-confined prostate cancer is increased in the Finnish screening trial. Abstract from the AUA 95th Annual Meeting. April 29-May 4, 2000 Atlanta, Georgia. *Abstract 385.*

Catalona W et al. Lowering PSA cutoffs to enhance detection of curable prostate cancer. *Urology* 2000; 55: 791-795.

Vessella R et al. Probability of prostate cancer detection based on results of a multicenter study using toe AxSYM free PSA and total PSA assays. *Urology* 2000; 55: 909-914.

Trinkler F et al. Free/total prostate-specific antigen ratio can prevent unnecessary prostate biopsies. *J Clin Oncol* 1998; 52: 479-486.

Gann PH et al. Strategies combining total and percent free prostate specific antigen for detecting prostate cancer: a prospective study. *J Urology* 2002; 167: 2427-2434.

3

DIAGNOSIS

Prostate Biopsy

Let's say your PSA is 6.0 (too high) and your free PSA comes back at 15% (too low). What's next? Since your free PSA is less than 20%, it's prudent to have a biopsy. This is usually done in the urologist's office. The procedure involves the insertion of an ultrasound device, a plastic instrument about one inch in diameter, into the rectum. The perineum, the area between the scrotum and the anus, is then anesthetized with a local anesthetic. Under guidance from the ultrasound, a special needle is inserted through the now-deadened perineum. The needle has a small nipper attached that can take a snip of the prostate. If done properly, at least six snips from six separate areas should be taken (known as a "sextant" biopsy). Some urologists recommend up to 11 snips (the upper snip limit) from different parts of the prostate. Doctors from M.D. Anderson Cancer Center in Houston, Texas, claim that a greater number of samples is more likely to find cancer, if any is there. I recommend insisting on at least a sextant biopsy. Current thinking is that eight snips is optimal. Biopsies aren't fun, so they should be done correctly the first time.

The reason that an 8-snip biopsy is probably best is revealed by the results of two studies reported in the June 2002 edition of the *Journal of Urology*, both from excellent academic institutions. The first, from Dr. Catalona's group at Washington University in St. Louis, Missouri, showed that in 2,526 volunteers who underwent prostate biopsy at this institution using either a 4-snip biopsy (prior to May 1, 1995) or a 6-snip biopsy thereafter, only 75% of cancers were discovered on the first biopsy. Ninety-one percent were uncovered by two biopsies; 97% by three biopsies; 99% by four biopsies. Note that 73% of cancers missed by the first biopsy were discovered by a second 6-snip (sextant) biopsy.

A group at Stanford University studied 185 men whose cancer was missed on the first biopsy using an 8-snip biopsy for the repeat, rather than a sextant biopsy. The 8-core biopsy detected 95% of all prostate cancers, compared to only 73% with 6-cores. Had the 8-snip biopsy been done originally, many of these men would not have to have been subjected to a second biopsy.

How much pain is involved? Depends who you ask. Most urologists will tell you, "It's a little uncomfortable." But when I asked a nurse who had observed many of them, she vouchsafed, "They look pretty bad to me." I decided I didn't want to find out, so I insisted on intravenous Versed, a fast-acting drug similar in effect to Valium. With Versed you don't remember a thing. However, I came out of it a little early—just in time to get the full flavor of the last snip. I practically jumped off the table! The pain was quite sharp; thankfully, it only lasted a couple of seconds. Personally, I wouldn't have wanted to have to endure six bites without good drugs. But some men I talk to say it's no big deal.

This may depend on age. Men over age 65, one study reports, seem to experience less pain than younger men. Whether this is because younger men are more squeamish or the nerve plexus in the area is more sensitive in younger men remains to be established. Whatever the reason, it does seem that, in general, younger men have more discomfort from biopsies.

Dr. Mark Soloway from the University of Miami Medical

School has come up with an elegant solution. In the January 2000 issue of the *Journal of Urology*, he concedes that many men complain of pain during prostate biopsies. He then details a procedure using local anesthesia to deaden the nerves in the area surrounding the prostate, much as a dentist uses a nerve block to deaden your mouth before drilling. Dr. Soloway concludes: "Many patients have pain during transrectal ultrasound-guided biopsies of the prostate and few clinicians provide a periprostatic nerve block before this procedure. A periprostatic nerve block administered before the biopsies dramatically decreases discomfort. We urge all urologists to attempt this procedure, and we are confident they will adopt it as part of their practice." Amen, Dr. Soloway!

Nitrous oxide (laughing gas) provides another effective form of pain relief during prostate biopsies. In a British study of 110 patients that was randomized, double-blind, and placebo-controlled, men who received nitrous oxide gas instead of air reported a highly significant reduction in pain. In a double-blind study, neither the patient nor the doctor knows which treatment is being administered. Nitrous oxide is safe and seems effective for pain relief from a prostate biopsy.

Forty-nine out of the 51 men who received nitrous oxide said they would have a repeat biopsy (with nitrous oxide) if needed. Of the 45 men who got the air placebo, 2 had to withdraw from the biopsy due to pain; 19 would prefer more anesthesia if the procedure had to be repeated, and two men would prefer general anesthesia.

The study's authors recommend that use of nitrous oxide be widely adopted by others and that it should become the "analgesia (pain reliever) of choice for this procedure."

Key References

Roehl KA et al. Serial biopsy results in prostate cancer screening study. *J Urology* 2002; 167: 2435-2439.

Chon CH et al. Use of extended systematic sampling in patients with a prior negative prostate needle biopsy. *J Urology* 2002; 167: 2457-2460.

Soloway M and Obek C. Periprostatic local anesthesia before ultrasound-guided prostate biopsy. *J Urology* 2000; 163: 172.

Masood N et al. Nitrous oxide (Entonox) inhaltation and tolerance of transrectal ultrasound guided prostate biopsy: a double-blind randomized controlled study. *J Urology* 2002; 168: 116-120.

Evaluating The Biopsy

It's extremely important that a skilled pathologist examine the prostate biopsy. If the results come back positive for cancer, a second expert opinion is probably warranted. You'll be making consequential decisions based on the biopsy, so you want to be certain of its accuracy. Although I'm sure there are a number of highly competent pathologists at local hospitals across the country (I personally know several), I recommend that you choose a "pathological prostate specialist" for this task. Fortunately, this is easier than it sounds.

Two labs routinely evaluate biopsy specimens from urologists all over the country: UroCor, Inc. in Oklahoma City, Okla., and Dianon Laboratories in Boston, Massachusetts. Either of these is an excellent place to send your biopsy specimens. To accomplish this, simply instruct your urologist on where you want your biopsy sent. Although he may argue that the pathologists at his hospital are "just as good," I think it's better to go with a "known dog." If you insist, your urologist will comply. After all, you're the one paying the bill.

If the diagnosis comes back cancer, a second opinion should be sought from one of these expert pathologists:

Jon Epstein at Johns Hopkins Medical School in Baltimore, Maryland.

David Bostwick at University of Virginia Medical School.

John McNeal at Stanford University Medical School, Palo Alto, California.

Michael Becich at University of Pittsburgh Medical School, Pittsburgh, Pennsylvania.

What Can Be Learned From The Biopsy

Several items of information include the Gleason score, the PIN grade, perineural invasion, p53 and bcl-2, and the number of positive cores. Let's examine them one at a time.

The Gleason Score

The biopsy can provide some very useful information that will help determine the probable extent of your disease and thus the treatment options. First, it will "grade" the cancer. This helps determine how aggressive it's likely to be. Grading uses a scoring system known as the "Gleason score." Named after its creator, Dr. Gleason at Johns Hopkins, the Gleason score determines the extent to which the cancer cells are differentiated (in other words, how close they are to normal cells) and how well the borders of the tumor are defined. The more the differentiation and margin definition, the less aggressive the cancer; the poorer the differentiation and less distinct the cancer margins, the more aggressive the tumor.

In determining the Gleason score, both a primary and a secondary cancer pattern are determined by the pathologist. The Gleason score is expressed as a single number, which is determined by adding the primary pattern and secondary pattern scores together. Tumors are graded from 1 to 5: 1 is the most differentiated (best), 5 the least differentiated (worst). The higher the Gleason score, the worse the prognosis. The best Gleason score possible is a primary pattern of 1 and a secondary pattern of 1. This results in a Gleason score of 2 (1+1). The worst possible Gleason score is 10 (5+5).

A Gleason score of 6 (3+3) or less is a favorable sign. The majority of newly diagnosed cases in the PSA era fall into this category. A Gleason score of 6 or less on biopsy, combined with a PSA of 10 or less and a DRE where the doctor could either not feel a lump or feels a lump comprising half or less of only one side of the prostate, is considered to be low-risk prostate cancer. Men with this profile have about an 80% chance of being cured by either surgery, radiation, or radioactive seed implants. In fact, these types of cancers are generally so slow growing that some experts are now beginning to recommend significant life-style changes as treatment for men willing to commit to changing their eating habits, exercise programs, and stress levels, while closely monitoring their PSA. A conservative approach like this may be particularly suited for men with normal-feeling prostates on digital rectal exam (see "Watchful Waiting"), in whom the size of the tumor is likely to be small.

Not only is the total Gleason score an important prognostic indicator, but the primary and secondary patterns are also significant. This important point is often overlooked by both patient and clinician. A Gleason score of 3+4 and 4+3 are both Gleason 7s, but the probable outcomes are different. The chances of cure for a man with a Gleason 3+4 is greater than for a man with Gleason 4+3, even though they are both classified as Gleason 7s.

Dr. Anthony D'Amico, a brilliant researcher, and his colleagues at Harvard Medical School, have studied this difference. They found that in a group of men with PSAs of 10 or less who had radical prostatectomies (surgery), men with Gleason 3+4 in their biopsies had a better outlook than men with Gleason 4+3. Estimates of the five-year outcome without a rise in PSA were about the same for the 3+4 group as for men with biopsy Gleason scores of 2 to 6. About 80% of both groups were free from cancer five years out, as determined by PSA testing. But only 62% of men with Gleason 4+3 were biochemically free from disease (no measurable PSA) after 5 years. Additionally, at the time of surgery 17% of men with Gleason 4+3 had cancer in their seminal vesicles; only 4% of the 3+4 group had seminal vesicle invasion. (Cancer in the seminal vesicles significantly increases the chance of recurrence.) If you have a Gleason 7 tumor, be sure to ask your doctor whether it's a Gleason 3+4 or a Gleason 4+3.

Another top group of doctors from Stanford University

Medical School, led by urologist Dr. Stamey and pathologist Dr. McNeal, made an interesting related discovery. They found that measuring the actual percentage of Gleason grade 4 or 5 in the tumor removed at surgery was highly predictive of outcome—another indication that the amount of grade 4 (or 5) in the tumor makes a difference. Obviously, 4+3, where 4 is the primary pattern, has a higher percentage of grade 4 than does 3+4.

Another study, this one from Johns Hopkins Hospital, showed that even small percentages of grade 4 or 5 patterns in prostate cancer removed by surgery significantly raised the odds of the cancer returning. In a large number of patients, this team found small pockets of Gleason grade 4 or 5 in tumors from men with Gleason scores of 6 or less. Though these pockets generally comprised less than 5% of the total tumor (designated as "tertiary" patterns), the consequences of this finding was sufficiently significant for the investigators to suggest a modification in the Gleason scoring system, which recognizes primary and secondary, but not tertiary, patterns. Since this research group includes acclaimed doctors like urologist Alan Partin (of Partin tables fame; see "Prognosis") and first-rate pathologist Jon Epstein, there's a good chance this recommendation may be heeded.

The authors of this study noticed that some men have a tiny tertiary (third most common) tumor pattern of Gleason grade 4 or 5. If a man has a total Gleason score of 5 (3+2 or 2+3), or 6 (3+3), but has a small area of grade 4 as well, even though this grade-4 tumor is not a primary or secondary pattern, in this study it still has prognostic significance. Men with this tertiary grade 4 pattern did not ultimately fare as well as a group, compared to the pure Gleason 5s and 6s. They did better, however, than the Gleason 7s. So they formed a group that was intermediate in its outcome prediction between Gleason 5-6 and Gleason 7.

Men with Gleason 7 tumors who had small tertiary pockets of Gleason grade 5 in their tumors also had significantly higher rates of cancer progression than men with Gleason 7s and no tertiary grade 5 areas. In fact, just this small amount of grade 5 made their predicted outcome statistically no different from men with Gleason 8 cancers. Based on Dr. D'Amico's work, these Gleason 7 tumors that behave much like Gleason 8s are more likely to be 4+3 than 3+4. Researchers at Johns Hopkins confirm that men with Gleason 4+3 tumors tend to have more extensive disease than men with Gleason 3+4 at the time of surgery.

In fact, Dr. Partin, who participated in this study, subsequently changed the Partin tables to reflect the difference in Gleason 7 cancers. The latest edition divides Gleason 7s into two groups: those whose primary tumor pattern is 3 and those whose primary pattern is 4.

Keep in mind that after surgery, the pathologist re-examines the surgical specimen and re-evaluates the Gleason score. The scores sometimes differ; perhaps the tumor changed between the time of the biopsy and surgery, or the biopsy didn't tell the whole story. The Gleason score based on the pathologist's examination of the removed prostate after surgery is used from this point forward in evaluating risk, as it is the most current and accurate information available. Of course, for men selecting radiation or seeds, the biopsy Gleason score is used to determine risk.

Note that Dr. D'Amico, a radiation oncologist, used biopsy Gleason score in his study, while the Hopkins surgeons used post-surgical (tertiary) findings to fine-tune prognosis. Though not specifically stated, the tertiary findings would be less frequently identified in biopsy specimens, if at all.

You may be wondering why I'm spending so much time on this subject. The reason is that these pathological subtleties play a huge role in determining the appropriate treatment. The higher the risk the cancer will come back, the more aggressive the treatment choice. Selecting the treatment that offers the best chance of cure starts with the pathology report from the biopsy. This is why it's critical to have your biopsy slides reviewed by a highly experienced pathologist whose special area of interest is the prostate. What he finds, or doesn't find, is likely to have significant impact on your approach to this cancer (see Appendix II).

Want a practical example? Okay. Let's look at the difference as described above between a Gleason 7 (3+4) and a Gleason 7 (4+3). In Dr. D'Amico's recent paper he concludes, "Patients with biopsy Gleason 3+4 disease and PSA less than or equal to 10 ng/ml may be suitable candidates for radiation therapy directed at the prostate only." Men with 4+3 disease would likely be treated more aggressively with wider field radiation and hormonal therapy.

Key References

D'Amico A et al. The impact of the biopsy Gleason score on PSA outcome for prostate cancer patients with PSA < or =10 ng/ml, and T1c, T2a: implications for patient selection for prostate-only therapy. *Int J Radiat Oncol Biol Phys* 1999; 45: 847-851.

Stamey T, McNeal J, et al. Biological determinants of cancer progression in men with prostate cancer. *JAMA* 1999; 281: 1395-1400.

Pan C, Potter S, Partin A, and Epstein J. The prognostic significance of tertiary Gleason patterns of higher grade in radical prostatectomy specimens: a proposal to modify the Gleason grading system. *Am J Surg Pathol* 2000; 24: 563-569.

Makarov D et al. Gleason score 7 prostate cancer on needle biopsy: is the prognostic difference in Gleason scores 4+3 and 3+4 independent of the number of cores involved? *J Urology* 2002; 167: 2440-2442.

Prostatic Intra-Epithelial Hyperplasia (PIN)

This medical mouthful is thought to be a "pre-cancerous" condition. Commonly seen in biopsy specimens, it consists of areas of proliferation (growth) and changes in the shape of prostate cells. These areas are not "normal," but they're also not cancerous (at least not yet). There are three grades of PIN. The one called "high-grade PIN" is the one that should concern you. High-grade PIN is the only form of PIN believed to be able to develop into cancer. PIN is not an indication for aggressive therapy, but it must be closely monitored. I recommend PSA testing every six months and an annual DRE. The presence of PIN, especially the high-grade variety, is also an excellent time to initiate lifestyle changes, such as nutrition and exercise.

Clinical Staging

Once cancer has been diagnosed in the prostate biopsy, the next step is to establish its stage, or how far it has progressed. Everyone undergoes the first staging, called "clinical staging," prior to treatment. Men who have surgery reap the benefits of a second staging, called "pathologic staging." This is done by a pathologist with surgically removed specimens of cancerous prostate glands.

The system by far most widely used for clinical staging is called "TNM," short for "tumor, lymph node, and metastasis." The first piece of staging evidence comes from the DRE. Can the tumor be felt by a DRE? If so, is it located on one side of the prostate or both? If localized to one side, does it comprise more or less than half the volume? An ultrasound is used to assist in making the "T" rating. Newer techniques improve accuracy: erMRI (endorectal magnetic resonance imaging) and spectroscopic MRI (magnetic resonance imaging). These new tests were not available when the original TNM system was devised.

The "N" or lymph-node portion of the clinical staging has been classically evaluated by CT-scan and MRI, but both have low sensitivity for picking up involved (cancerous) nodes. A recent development, the ProstaScint Scan, has improved sensitivity. It's limited to some extent, by false positives.

The "M" stands for metastasis to bone. The test used to determine this is the bone scan.

If cancer is present, but the urologist can't feel it upon rectal examination, the stage is said to be T1c. In the current era of PSA screening, this is the most common stage.

If the urologist finds an area of hardness, or a nodule, this is T2 disease. If the area of hardness is only on one side of the prostate and comprises up to half the volume, this is called T2a; if more than 50% of one side is involved, it's a T2b. If both sides of the prostate are involved, it's a T2c.

If the cancer has spread beyond the prostate, its clinical stage is referred to as T3 (for complete TNM staging, see "Appendix I").

Even though the tumor may appear to be well-defined within the prostate on DRE (stage T2), the cancer may be more extensive. This has been repeatedly shown at surgery.

As mentioned, in men who elect to have surgery a "re-staging," or pathologic staging, will be done by a pathologist on a specimen of the removed prostate. There is no guess-work here. This is the true stage of the disease. If the patho-logical stage is worse than the clinical stage, there will be an "up-staging" done to reflect this.

When you read medical articles that refer to staging, try to determine if the authors are talking about clinical or patho-logic staging. Remember that clinical staging may be under staged. Even men who have no palpable tumor on DRE can have cancer that has spread beyond the prostate, but this may not become known prior to surgery.

Tests to Help Determine Stage

A number of tests are used to help doctors distinguish between organ-confined disease and cancer that has escaped beyond the prostate. Here are some of the most used and most useful.

Prostatic Acid Phosphatase (PAP)

A simple blood test, the PAP should be a part of every prostate cancer work-up. If the PAP is elevated, concerted effort should be made attempting to find metastatic disease. Even when metastases are too small to be found by imaging techniques, such as those described below, the PAP may pick-up "micro-metastatic" disease. In most men when the PAP is elevated, systemic therapy, like hormones, is added to local therapy (surgery or radiation). Systemic therapy goes all over the body. It's designed to kill cancer cells that may have escaped the prostate. Hormonal therapy and chemotherapy are examples of systemic treatments.

CAT Scan and MRI

I'm not going to spend a lot of time on these frequently prescribed tests. I think they're generally overrated and overused. Their purpose is to try to ascertain whether the cancer has spread to the lymph nodes. The problem is that when lymph-node metastases are known to have occurred (found at surgery), these two tests pick them up only 20% of the time. In my opinion, they're often not worth the time, money, discomfort, and anxiety. This is especially true for men with Gleason scores of 6 or less, clinical stage T2a or less, and PSAs of 10 or less. Men with this profile have a mere 2%-3% chance of having lymph-node involvement. Combining the low 20% identification rate with the low 2%-3% chance, CAT scans and MRIs reveal lymph-node metastases, on average, in one out of every 200 men tested.

In a study of 861 men with newly diagnosed prostate cancer, only 13 (1.5%) had a positive scan and all 13 had PSAs higher than 20 ng/ml. This is a solid indication that CAT scans are often being used unnecessarily. I should know. I had one and didn't need it. I could have spared myself the unwanted radiation and expense.

Unless the PAP is elevated, using MRI and/or CAT scans in this group is unwarranted. However, in men with an elevated PAP, regardless of PSA, Gleason, and clinical-staging status, an MRI and/or CAT scan should be considered. As you now know, an elevated PAP shifts the odds in favor of metastatic disease. In this case, I think all the stops should be pulled out in an effort to discover cancer that has spread.

Key References
Levran A et al. Are pelvic-computed tomography, bone scan, and pelvic lymphadenectomy necessary in the staging of prostate cancer? *Brit J Urology* 1995; 75: 778.

Kindrick A et. al. Use of imaging tests for staging newly diagnosed prostate cancer: trends from the CaP SURE database. *J Urology* 1998; 160: 2102-2106.

Endorectal MRI (erMRI)

As overused as the MRI and CAT scan appear to be, that's how underused is the erMRI. This is a superb test to help determine if the tumor is organ-confined. Unfortunately, this test is not yet widely available. Perhaps by the time you read this book, it will be available in your area. On the west coast it's available at the University of California Hospital in San Francisco. On the east coast this test is available at Sloan Kettering in New York and Dana Farber in Boston. If it's not available in your area, you might try one of these.

> **HELPFUL HINT**
>
> To get an accurate fix on whether your disease is organ-confined, have the endorectal MRI done *before* starting hormones. Hormones are likely to shrink the tumor, making it difficult to determine whether it has penetrated the prostate capsule.

This test involves the insertion of a small coil into the rectum adjacent to the prostate. You are then placed inside a long plastic cylinder that contains powerful magnets. The combination of the wave emissions from the coil and the magnetic fields allows the prostate to be clearly viewed on radiographic film. The radiologist can distinguish normal prostate tissue from cancer.

More importantly, this test can distinguish cancer contained within the prostate from cancer that has penetrated the prostate capsule, the thin sheath that encloses and protects the gland. When the cancer penetrates the capsule, it has now, by definition, "escaped" from the prostate, even if only by a few millimeters; this is known as "extracapsular extension." From this point, the cancer may spread into the soft tissue and fat that surrounds the prostate gland. Once in the surrounding tissues, the cancer has a tendency toward faster growth and metastasis. This is important in selecting the appropriate treatment. Surgery, for example, is not generally the treatment of choice if capsular penetration is confirmed. Capsular penetration appears as a blurred, or irregular, margin on the film. The erMRI is far and away the best test for helping to determine this critical variable. According to a French group that has considerable experience with erMRI, it can predict spread to the surrounding tissues with 95% accuracy.

Another use of the erMRI is in helping to detect prostate cancer in men who have had negative prostate biopsies, but the doctor still suspects undetected cancer. In a pilot study, Perrotti and his colleagues found cancer in five of seven men with highly suspicious erMRIs by repeating the biopsy in the area that appeared suspicious on the erMRI. I think an erMRI can be very useful in helping to locate tumors in men where prostate cancer is strongly suspected, but prior biopsies were normal.

Dr. D'Amico at Harvard has come up with an ingenious way of using the erMRI to help determine whether a tumor is prostate-confined. He found that after an initial erMRI, if the patient is given a complete hormone treatment, the response of the tumor helps predict organ confinement. In a 1998 pilot study of 21 men, Dr. D'Amico and colleagues found that hormones shrunk the overall size of the prostates of all 21 men. However, only 10 of 21 (48%) had a reduction in their tumor volume as determined by erMRI, after hormone treatment for an average of three months. These 10 men were far more likely to have organ-confined disease than men whose tumor volume remained unchanged after hormones.

If confirmed in a larger study still in progress as this book is being written, quantifying tumor volume has practical value. In men considering surgery versus radiation, if the tumor volume shrinks in response to hormones (as seen in an erMRI), increasing the likelihood that the disease has not escaped the prostate, surgery may be the way to go. But if the tumor volume doesn't shrink in response to hormones on erMRI, radiation might be the wiser choice. (See the "Treatment" section for a complete description of both.)

Key References

Perrotti M et al. Prospective evaluation of endorectal magnetic resonance imaging to detect tumor foci in men with prior negative biopsy: a pilot study. *J Urology* 1999; 162: 1314-1317.

D'Amico A et al. Assessment of prostate cancer volume using endorectal coil magnetic resonance imaging: a new predictor of tumor response to neoadjuvant androgen suppression therapy. *Urology* 1998; 51: 287-292.

Cornud F and Oyen R. Role of imaging in detecting and staging of prostate cancer. *J Radiology* 2002; 83: 863-880.

ProstaScint Scan

While the erMRI can often identify cancer that extends immediately beyond the prostate capsule, the ProstaScint scan is used to help determine if prostate cancer has spread to lymph nodes. Although this test is not always accurate, it's the best test currently available for identifying lymph-node metastases.

Here's how it's done. There is a substance on the surface of prostate cancer cells called prostate specific membrane antigen (PSMA). The test uses an antibody to PSMA that has a radioactive isotope attached. This PSMA antibody, injected via IV, now travels through the bloodstream. If it encounters its complementary antigen, PSMA, on a prostate cancer cell, it attaches to it. Then, the radiologic image (like an x-ray image) is taken with a ProstaScint scan and these antigen-antibody combinations become visible (the attached radioactive marker leaves bright spots on the radiographic film).

The ProstaScint scan identifies up to 80% of lymph-node metastases. Unfortunately, 20%-30% of the time, this test indicates cancer in the lymph nodes when none exists. This is called a "false-positive" result. It can cause needless added anxiety in men already on pins and needles, worrying if their cancer has spread.

For this reason, I think it's helpful to discuss the risk of a potential false positive with men before they get this test. Then a positive reading won't automatically be interpreted as disastrous. Factors that support a positive reading are PSAs over 20 ng/ml, elevated PAP blood test, and high Gleason scores (7-10). If one or more of these factors are present and the scan indicates cancer cells in the pelvic nodes, or nodes along the aorta where prostate cancer is most likely to spread, further tests, such as a biopsy of the suspected lymph nodes, should be done.

An interesting innovation has recently been developed by a group at the University Hospitals of Cleveland, the hospital associated with Western Reserve University. By combining the ProstaScint scan with a CT-scan, they've developed a technique to fuse the images from these two tests to more clearly view the location of the cancer within the prostate gland. This new technology dramatically improves the clarity of the imaging, giving a far clearer view of the location of the cancer.

This novel imaging technique can be quite helpful in guiding the urologist doing a prostate biopsy by identifying the areas where the biopsy needle is likely to find cancer. It can also help show whether the cancer has spread to the seminal vesicles.

This innovation allows for better targeting when radioactive seeds or external beam radiation is used, insuring that adequate treatment is delivered to areas of the prostate likely to be affected with cancer. If you have intermediate or high-risk prostate cancer and can get to Cleveland, I think it's well worth the trip. Don't have a CT-scan before going; get it done there. Hopefully, this technology will become more widespread.

Key References

Seaward S et al. Improved freedom from PSA failure with whole pelvic irradiation for high-risk prostate cancer. *Int J Radiat Oncol Biol Phys* 1998; 42: 1055-1062.

Ellis R J et al. Radioimmunoguided imaging of prostate cancer foci with histopathological correlation. *Int J Radiat Oncol Biol Phys* 2001; 49: 1281-1286.

Ellis RJ et al. Feasibility and acute toxicities of radioimmunoguided prostate brachytherapy. *Int J Radiat Oncol Biol Phys* 2000; 48: 683-687.

Sodee D et al. Prostate cancer and prostate bed SPECT imaging with ProstaScint: semiquantiative correlation with prostatic biopsy results. *Prostate* 1998; 37: 140-148.

If the ProstaScint scan, along with PAP, PSA, and Gleason score, indicate a significant risk of lymph-node metastases, the nodes that appear to be involved should be removed and examined by a pathologist to determine if they harbor cancer.

Recently, a surgical procedure has been developed to remove suspicious lymph nodes with minimal invasiveness. Using a technique known as laparoscopy, the surgeon is able to view the nodes through a tube. This tube is inserted through a very small incision in the skin. Although it does require general anesthesia (being put to sleep), it results in little postoperative pain. As Dr. Charles (Snuffy) Myers at the American Institute for Diseases of the Prostate in Charlottsville, Virginia, who had 25 lymph nodes removed by this procedure, put it: "I didn't even need to take the Tylenol!"

Like so many of the new procedures in prostate cancer, laporoscopic lymphadenectomy (lymph-node removal through a tube) must be done by a skilled hand. Dr. Myers used Dr. Kavoussi at Johns Hopkins, who has authored scores of papers on all sorts of laparoscopic procedures. He is an acknowledged expert in the field of laparoscopic surgery. Once again, choosing the best person you can find pays dividends.

Besides being helpful in detecting lymph-node involvement in the initial prostate cancer evaluation, the ProstaScint scan has also proved useful in locating cancer in men when the cancer recurs after surgery or radiation (see "Advanced Disease").

HELPFUL HINT

A laparoscopic lymphadenectomy is only indicated if the ProstaScint scan shows suspicious nodes and a man is at high risk for lymph-node metastases (Gleason 7 or more, or PSA 20 or more), or has an elevated PAP blood test.

Key References

   Manyak M and Javitt M. The role of computerized tomography, magnetic resonance imaging, bone scan, and monoclonal antibody nuclear scan for prognosis prediction in prostate cancer. *Semin Urol Oncol* 1998; 16: 145-152.

   Kava B et al. Results of laparoscopic pelvic lymphadenectomy in patients at high risk for nodal metastases from prostate cancer. *Ann Surg Oncol* 1998; 173-180.

   Cadeddu J et al. Effect of laparoscopic pelvic lymph node dissection on the natural history of D1 (T1-3, N1-3, M0) prostate cancer. *Urology* 1997; 50: 391-394.

Spectroscopic MRI

Another high-tech, state-of-the-art, staging test is the spectroscopic MRI. Developed by Dr. Kurhanewicz at the University of California-San Francisco, this test greatly enhances the accuracy of the erMRI. Used together they make a dynamite diagnostic combination, providing a highly accurate assessment of the location, extent, and aggressiveness of the tumor. Studies have consistently attested to their accuracy, and proven that they're considerably more powerful when used in tandem than when used separately.

At the time of this writing, the only institutions I know of that use both of these fine tests are the University of California-San Francisco and Sloan Kettering in New York. In the South, try M.D. Anderson in Houston. If you can't find a hospital that offers both these tests, San Francisco is a lovely city to visit. But beware. Both tests are expensive and may not be covered by insurance. You'll want to check if your insurance covers them before jumping on a plane. But if you can arrange to have both these tests, you'll have the best tests currently available for determining tumor location and capsular penetration.

Spectroscopic MRI is currently being evaluated as a way to get more accurate seed placement for brachytherapy, and as a guide for the new intensity-modulated radiation therapy, IMRT. (see "Radiation").

Key References

Kurhanewicz J et al. The prostate: MR imaging and spectroscopy. Present and future. *Radiol Clin North Am* 2000; 38: 115-138.

Scheidler J et al. Prostate cancer: localization with three-dimensional proton MR spectroscopic imaging — clinicopathologic study. *Radiology* 1999; 213: 473-480.

Bone Scan

One of the most important items to determine on the prostate cancer agenda is whether the cancer has spread to bone. Fortunately, now that PSA testing is becoming progressively more common, bone metsatases in newly diagnosed men are becoming rarer.

In the event that a test is necessary, the one used to pick up prostate cancer in bone is the bone scan. In this test, a radioactive substance is injected into the bloodstream, then tumor cells in bone pick up this marker and "light up," forming small bright spots on the x-ray film where cancer has lodged. Injuries and arthritis will also light up, but these are usually readily distinguishable from tumor. Questions about whether an area of activity on the scan is tumor-related can be answered with an MRI of the area in question.

Like the CAT scan, the bone scan is overused by many doctors. In one study, in men with an initial PSA of less than 20, the chances of the bone scan being normal was 99.7%. Only one out of 306 men with PSAs in this range had a positive bone scan. Yet many good doctors still prescribe bone scans for men with far lower PSAs, "just to be sure."

In my case, I had a bone scan, with a starting PSA of 11.2. Like my CAT scan and standard MRI, the bone test showed nothing, was expensive, and exposed me to needless radiation, discomfort, and anxiety. But you know more now than I did then. If diagnosed today, I'd skip the CAT, MRI, and bone scan, but would definitely have a PAP blood test, endorectal MRI, and spectroscopic MRI. If I lived in the Midwest, I'd go to Cleveland for the CT-scan-ProstaScint diagnostic tandem. (Note: The terms CAT scan and CT-scan are identical.) If either the erMRI/spectroscopic MRI combo or the CT-scan-ProstaScint tandem were inconclusive, I'd have the other done. This way I'd learn far more about the extent of my cancer than I knew at the time I had to make a treatment decision. This information is vital for men faced with treatment decisions for intermediate or high-risk prostate cancer. For low-risk cases, the inconvenience and expense of these sophisticated tests are probably unnecessary.

4

PROGNOSIS

How to Quantify Risk

The burning question in the minds of most men with prostate cancer is, "Has it spread?" Even if all the sophisticated tests indicate that the cancer is well-contained within the prostate, there's still a chance that it has escaped. It may not have grown large enough to be detected. But prostate surgery has taught us that when the surgeon gets in there, he frequently finds more extensive disease than the tests have indicated.

Dr. Alan Partin, a urologist at Johns Hopkins, observed the surgical findings in more than 700 patients. Although the clinical tests estimate the severity of the tumor, the actual surgical findings provide an exact measure. After noting the surgical findings, Dr. Partin went back and looked at the PSAs, Gleason scores, and clinical stages for these men, and correlated them with what he found from surgery. He then prepared a set of tables that predicts the risk of extension of the tumor past the capsule of the prostate, seminal vesicle involvement, and lymph-node metastases.

The Partin Tables, as these risk tabulations are called, provide men with critical information. They can be of great help in determining the choice of treatment. For example, in my own case, with PSA 11, Gleason 7, and stage T2a, my chance of organ-confined disease was only 36% according to the Partin Tables. In other words, there was a 64% chance that the prostate capsule had already been penetrated by invading cancer.

Delving deeper into the tables, I was able to determine that the chance of seminal vesicle involvement in my case was 19%, and the chance of the cancer having spread to my lymph nodes was 9%. I also had another poor prognostic sign from the biopsy that I'll discuss later in this section, referred to as "perineural invasion." For now, let's just say that this biopsy finding increased my chances of capsular penetration from 64% to 77%. That means there were roughly three chances out of four that my tumor had escaped the confines of the prostate. There were also significant risks of seminal vesicle and/or lymph-node metastases.

Knowing these risks, I shied away from surgery, which might not have been able to get all of the tumor. I opted for hormones combined with external beam radiation. Without the Partin Tables I would not have been able to clearly understand these risks and would have had a far more difficult time making an intelligent treatment decision.

The Partin Tables were updated in 2002 to include initial PSA ranges starting with 0.0-2.5 and separating Gleason 7 tumors into two groups (3+4; 4+3). See "Appendix II" for Web site details.

Number of Positive Biopsy Cores Predicts Outcome

Dr. Anthony D'Amico and his group at Harvard found that the percentage of positive biopsy cores, as each snip in a prostate biopsy is called, made a highly significant difference in predicting progression of cancer after surgery. He also found that erMRI was also independently useful in predicting outcome.

He studied 977 men with T2 disease (positive DRE) and found that men with the following profiles were at high risk of having their cancer recur after surgery.

• Men with erMRI that shows T3 (instead of T2 by DRE), three of six or more positive cores on biopsy, Gleason score 6 or higher, and a pre-surgery PSA of more than 10 but less than 20 ng/ml.

• Any Gleason score when the pre-surgery PSA is over 20, and erMRI shows T3 disease.

• ErMRI shows T2 disease, but three out of six biopsy cores have cancer, while the Gleason score is 8 or higher and the pre-surgery PSA is greater than 20 ng/ml.

Men in these high-risk categories should strongly consider adjuvant androgen blockade (hormones), combined with either surgery or radiation.

The importance of the percentage of positive biopsy cores has been confirmed by at least three other high-powered groups: Johns Hopkins, the Mayo Clinic, and the University of California Medical School in San Francisco. In the Hopkins study, researchers compared pre-surgical data like Gleason score, PSA, number of positive cores, and a slew of other variables. Their objective was to evaluate the significance of these factors in predicting whether or not the tumor would be organ-confined at surgery. They found that of all the variables they looked at, the two that were most predictive of organ-confined disease were the number of positive cores and the Gleason score. Here are the interesting results of 113 sextant (six core) biopsies, after which all men had a radical prostatectomy.

• Gleason score 6 or less and two or fewer positive cores and PSA 0-4ng/ml: Chance of tumor being confined to the prostate proven by surgery, 89%.

• Gleason score 6 or less and with two positive cores on one side of prostate only (unilateral): Chance of tumor being confined to the prostate, 87%. (Note that PSA was not considered in this calculation.)

• Gleason score of 7 or more and more than one positive core: Chance of tumor being confined to the prostate, 10%. (Note: I had two positive cores and a Gleason score of 7. Combining this risk assessment with other data, the chance that my disease had already escaped the prostate capsule was 80%-90%.)

The third and most recent study on the predictive value of the percentage of biopsy cores that show cancer (positive biopsy cores) comes from the evaluation of 1,265 men, all of whom had surgery for their prostate cancer. Investigators led by Dr. Gary Grossfeld determined the risk of recurrence in this group of men. They asked this seminal question: Does the risk of cancer coming back increase as the percentage of positive cores found at the time of prostate biopsy increases? If so, how can this information be used to help make an optimal treatment decision?

They divided the men into three groups:

• Low risk: PSA at diagnosis of 10 or less *and* biopsy Gleason score of 6 or less *and* clinical staging of T1-c or T2-a (note: need all three).

• Intermediate risk: PSA at diagnosis of 10.1 to 20.0 *or* biopsy Gleason score of 7 *or* stage T2b.

• High risk: PSA greater than 20 *or* biopsy Gleason score 8-10, *or* clinical stage T2-c or T-3.

These men had a median follow-up period of 3.3 years from the time of surgery. As groups, without considering the number of positive biopsy cores, these investigators calculated the probability of recurrence at five years to be:

Low risk: 18%

Intermediate risk: 28%

High risk: 36%

The number of cancer-effected biopsy cores was then taken into account. They were stratified into three groups: 0%-33% positive biopsy cores; 34%-66% positive cores; 67% and higher positive cores.

The percentage of positive biopsies proved to be a significant predictor of recurrence in all three risk categories.

For low-risk patients the risk of recurrence 5 years after surgery more than doubled when the percentage of positive cores increased to 34% to 66%. Only 12% of low-risk men who had 0% to 33% positive cores had a recurrence within five years; 28% of patients with 34% to 66% positive cores had a return of their cancer. Only seven out of 427 men at low-risk had greater than 66%, too few to draw accurate conclusions.

For men at intermediate risk, the probability of disease recurrence five years after surgery varies widely depending on the percentage of positive biopsy cores:

0% to 33%: 17%

34% to 66%: 37%

above 66%: 47%

Again, the risk of recurrence more than doubles when the percentage of positive biopsy cores increases to 34%-66%, as opposed to 0%-33%, and nearly triples in the greater than 66% group.

For high-risk men, the relevant 5-year recurrence risks were:

0% to 33%: 24%

34% to 66%: 34%

above 66%: 59%

As you can see, the percentage of positive biopsy cores makes a big difference when considering the risk of the cancer returning after surgery. The researchers believe that this is especially important for the intermediate-and high-risk groups. Local therapy, either surgery or radiation, is probably enough for men with 0% to 33% positive cores; men with a greater percentage of positive cores than this will probably do better if they add a systemic therapy, like hormones, to their treatment plan (see Chapter 11). Additionally, these men would be well-advised to consider making significant changes regarding diet, exercise, and stress-reduction.

Accurately assessing risk prior to selecting a treatment plan will provide you with an objective basis for making a tough decision. Don't be surprised if your doctor doesn't

---

HELPFUL HINT

Establish whether your prostate cancer is low-risk, intermediate-risk, or high-risk. Then take the percentage of positive biopsy cores into account to further assess your risk of recurrence when working with your doctors to obtain optimal treatment.

try to establish this kind of rational risk assessment. Few private practitioners do. Most make treatment recommendations by "feel" or "experience." For me, knowing the probabilities of treatment failure formed a foundation to discuss treatment options with my doctors in a meaningful way. The facts are always friendly.

A number of university medical centers are now setting up comprehensive multi-discipline cancer centers. At these, you're more likely to get a better handle on both the risks and treatment options.

Key References

Partin A et al. The use of prostate specific antigen, clinical stage, and Gleason score to predict pathological stage in men with localized prostate cancer. *J Urology* 1993; 150: 110-114.

Grossfeld G et al. Predicting disease recurrence in intermediate and high-risk patients undergoing radical prostatectomy using percent positive biopsies: results from Capsure. *Urology* 2002; 59: 560-565.

Other Prognostic Factors in a Nutshell

Perineural Invasion (PNI)—At biopsy, when the cancer is seen to be spreading along nerves, it's a poor prognostic sign. Studies show that when PNI is present in the biopsy specimen, 77% of prostates removed by radical prostatectomy have cancer that has penetrated the prostate capsule. In addition, 51% of these cases had positive margins, microscopic evidence of cancer right up to the edge of surgically removed prostate, another poor prognostic sign, according to a Johns Hopkins study; a third had either seminal-vesicle or lymph-node involvement. It seems that prostate cancer spreads faster along nerve sheaths. I had PNI present in my biopsy—another reason I chose radiation and hormones over surgery.

Just because the cancer has penetrated the prostate capsule doesn't mean that it will recur after treatment. As you'll read later, quite often the penetration is only by a few millimeters and the cancer can still be completely removed by surgery or killed by radiation or radioactive palladium seeds.

Two studies done after my radiation treatment showed that PNI does not significantly increase the risks of recurrence.

Key References:

Alexandre de la Taille et al. Can perineural invasion on prostate needle biopsy predict prostate specific antigen recurrence after radical prostatectomy? *J Urology* 1999; 162: 103.

Nelson CP et al. Preoperative parameters for predicting early prostate cancer recurrence after radical prostatectomy. *Urology* 2002; 59: 740-746.

O'Malley K et al. Influence of biopsy perineural invasion on long-term biochemical disease-free survival after radical prostatectomy. *Urology* 2002; 59: 85-90.

D'Amico A et al. Combination of the preoperative PSA level, biopsy Gleason score, percentage of positive biopsies, and MRI T-stage to predict early PSA failure in men with clinically localized prostate cancer. *Urology* 2000; 55: 572-577.

Wills M et al. Ability of sextant biopsies to predict radical prostatectomy stage. *Urology* 1998; 51: 759-764.

Sebo T et al. The percent of cores positive for cancer in prostate needle biopsy specimens is strongly predictive of tumor stage and volume at radical prostatectomy. *J Urology* 2000; 163: 174.

Holmes GF et al. Excision of the neurovascular bundle at radical prostatectomy in cases with perineural invasion on needle biopsy. *Urology* 1999; 53: 752-756.

Ploidy Status—Ploidy status refers to the microscopic appearance of the cancer cells. Diploid is considered the most favorable, because it's closer in appearance to normal prostate cells; aneuploid is considered to be the least favorable configuration. Although it's debatable whether ploidy status is an independent predictor of outcome, if your tumor is diploid, this should be considered as a plus. Diploid tumors are generally slower growing and less aggressive.

p53 Mutations—As previously discussed, p53 is a cancer-suppressing gene. When it mutates, it loses its ability to inhibit cancer growth. A number of studies have shown a strong correlation between p53 mutations and advanced prostate cancer. A recent study released from the Mayo Clinic showed that if 10% or more of the cells of specimens removed by radical prostatectomy stain positive for mutated p53, the chance of cancer recurrence triples. p53 status can be tested in the biopsy. I advise you to do so. If more than 10% of the cells in the biopsy show altered p53 genes, you might want to consider being more aggressive in treatment.

Key References

Quinn D et al. Prognostic significance of p53 nuclear accumulation in localized prostate cancer treated with radical prostatectomy. *Cancer Res* 2000; 60: 1585-1594.

Leibovich BC et al. Outcome prediction with p53 immunostaining after radical prostatectomy in patients with locally advanced prostate cancer. *J Urology* 2000; 163: 1756-60.

Bcl-2—This is an oncogene (cancer-causing gene) for prostate cancer. The prostate biopsy can test for it. Positive bcl-2 testing is a poor prognostic indicator. The combination of a p53 abnormality and bcl-2 positivity is a particularly bad prognostic sign. Most men with this profile will eventually have a recurrence.

Formula for Estimating the Probability of Lymph Node Involvement

Dr. Roach at the University of California Medical Center in San Francisco, California, has come up with a formula to give a rough approximation of the risk of lymph-node metastases. Here is the formula. It's not as complicated as it may appear at first glance:

2/3 x initial PSA + 10 (Gleason score—6) = risk of lymph-node metastases.

In my case, the initial PSA was 11.2 and the Gleason score 7. Using Dr. Roach's formula: 2/3 x 11.2 + 10 (7-6) = 17.5%. According to the Partin Table, my chance of lymph-node involvement was 9%. Combining the two, I rate my chance at about 13%.

SECTION II:

TREATMENT

5

SELECTING YOUR DOCTORS

One of the most important decisions you'll have to make if you have prostate cancer is selecting physicians. How can you make the proper choice in this regard?

The usual course of events is for your family physician, or internist, to order a routine PSA. If it's significantly elevated, he will refer you to a urologist. Urologists are surgeons. A good portion of their income comes from removing prostate glands. Your primary-care physician may select a particular urologist for various reasons:

• The urologist may be conveniently located nearby.

• They may have gone to medical school together.

• They may have an informal arrangement to share referrals with each other.

• Your doctor has researched the top urologists in a wide area (West Coast, Midwest, East Coast) and gives you a list of highly skilled surgeons.

Of these reasons for se-

HELPFUL HINT

There are no randomized studies that show the superiority of one treatment over another for the treatment of localized prostate cancer. Several trials are currently underway.

Only one randomized trial has been done comparing surgery with watchful waiting (expectant management under a physicians care). Although this study did show that surgery reduces the chances of dying from prostate cancer, the overall death rate, when all causes were considered, was not significantly different.

lecting a urologist for referral, only the last one has significant value for you. However, even if you're now in the hands of a top-notch surgeon, you should not, in my opinion, base your decision exclusively on his advice. He should do the work-up on you, including the prostate biopsy. But if it turns out that you have cancer, my advice is that you seek additional medical help.

Why do I make such a strong recommendation? Because if you acquiesce, as the majority of men do, to the family doctor-urologist connection, nine times out of ten you'll find yourself in the operating room. Although this may be the best choice for many men, it's far from the only choice. To make a proper decision, you need to have all the options objectively laid out for you. In most cases, there are options available to you other than surgery.

Unfortunately, many urologists will not present you with an objective picture of your alternatives. In a recent article in the *Journal of the American Medical Association*, 91% of more than 500 urologists surveyed favored surgery for a hypothetical 65-year-old patient whose disease had not spread. Before you judge the urologists too harshly, 91% of more than 500 radiation oncologists also surveyed recommended radiation for the same hypothetical patient!

Again, not to condemn the urologists, when most of them push you toward surgery, it's not exclusively a matter of financial self-interest. They genuinely believe that surgery is the best choice for most men who are in a reasonable state of general health. Their belief is supported by studies that show that surgery is at least as effective as the newer 3-D conformal beam radiation therapy, or brachytherapy (seeds). In addition, since surgery has been around longer, they can reassure patients (and themselves) of its long-term benefits. So far, so good.

Where some surgeons fail patients, in my opinion, is by not objectively presenting other viable options that are currently available. Even if your urologist genuinely believes that his treatment is best, he's not the one who has cancer.

You are. And the urologist can't possibly begin to understand your needs, fears, time availability, or tolerance to a variety of possible side effects from treatment without thoroughly exploring all options with you. Regrettably, although there are some notable exceptions, few urologists are dispassionate enough about surgery and willing to take the required time to adequately explore other avenues. The same can be said about radiation oncologists.

In point of fact, at the time of this writing there has been no reported randomized prospective study comparing the effectiveness of surgery versus radiation, although currently a study is in progress. Moreover, and this will probably surprise you, there is no conclusive proof that surgery increases overall life expectancy, although a study that came out just prior to going to press showed that surgery reduces the chance of dying from prostate cancer specifically (see "Watchful Waiting"). This new Scandinavian study failed to show an increase in life expectancy for men who had surgery over men who remained untreated when all causes of death were considered.

So, what to do? First, don't take the urologist's opinion as gospel. Seek additional consultation. My advice is to select a medical oncologist from the list provided later in this chapter. An oncologist is a cancer specialist. The list provided here is limited to experts in prostate cancer. Why are medical oncologists an effective counter-balance to urologists and radiation oncologists? They have no ax to grind, no inherent conflict of interest. If you ultimately select surgery, your medical oncologist is not the one who will perform the operation. If you choose radiation or seeds, he's not the one who will design your treatment plan or perform the procedure. A good medical oncologist is a well-informed unbiased consultant who will generally take the

---

HELPFUL HINT

Consult a medical oncologist subspecializing in prostate cancer to assist you in the decision-making process.

required time to understand your concerns and fully answer all your questions.

Often there are several treatment choices that are likely to be equally effective. Your choice might depend on which side effects are most palatable. Fully understanding the side effects of each treatment option is the purview of the medical oncologist.

Unfortunately, there are far too few medical oncologists in the country whose sub-specialty is prostate cancer. Although the list provided here is not exhaustive, it includes the vast majority of this select group. I have tried to list those connected with a major hospital where you'll be able to consult not only a medical oncologist, but also a radiation oncologist, a urologist (if you want a second opinion from a surgeon), and, perhaps, a nutritionist. If you're coming from out of state, several consultations can usually be scheduled on the same day. Each is likely to provide you with useful information that may help you in making the difficult decision about what to do.

> **HELPFUL HINT**
>
> Don't be pushed into making a decision by doctors, family, or friends. You should feel satisfied that you have the necessary information to make an informed decision.

If, for any reason, you're not satisfied with the information you have received, I suggest you seek additional counsel. Keep plugging away until you're completely satisfied that you have the necessary information to make an informed decision. Don't panic. Avoid feeling compelled to make a quick decision based on incomplete information or pressure from anyone. You have time to make the right choice. It's important to your overall success that you feel confident that you have selected the best course for yourself. As you'll see, the best course for me may not necessarily be best for you.

Medical Oncologists Specializing In Prostate Cancer

East Coast

Nancy Dawson	University of Maryland	Baltimore, MD
Mario Eisenberger	Johns Hopkins University	Baltimore, MD
Anna Ferrari	Mt. Sinai Hospital	New York, NY
Marc Garnick	Beth Israel Hospital	Boston, MA
Gary Hudes	Fox Chase Cancer Center	Philadelphia, PA
Phil Kantoff	Harvard University	Boston, MA
Dan Petrylak	Columbia University	New York, NY
Bruce Roth	Fox Chase Cancer Cnt	Philadelphia, PA
Howard Scher	Sloan Kettering Memorial Hospital	New York, NY
Donald L. Trump	Roswell Park Med. Center	Rochester, NY

South

Chris Logothetis	M.D. Anderson Hosp.	Houston, TX
Charles Myers	American Institute for Diseases of the Prostate	Charlottsville, VA
Oliver Sartor	Stanley Scott Cancer Cnt	New Orleans, LA

Midwest

Michael Glode	University of Colorado	Denver, CO
Maha Hussain	University of Michigan	Ann Arbor, MI
Ken Pienta	University of Michigan	Ann Arbor, MI
George Wilding	University of Wisconsin	Madison, WI
Nicholas Vogelzang	University of Chicago	Chicago, IL

West Coast

Celestia Higano	Univ. of WA Hospital	Seattle, WA
Derek Raghavan	Norris Cancer Center, Univ. of So. California	Los Angeles, CA
Eric Small	Univ. of CA Hospital	San Francisco, CA

Qualities To Look For In Your Doctors

Okay. You've selected a medical oncologist from the above list based on location or availability or some other factor. You're sitting in his or her office. How can you tell if this oncologist really knows what he or she is talking about? I've noticed a few traits that the best doctors in this field have in common.

Here are the lists of those qualities:

Confidence Without Arrogance

Doctors who are truly gifted in an area convey their expertise without making pronouncements or acting like demigods.

Concern for Your Needs

The best oncologists (and doctors in general) are usually not committed to any one approach. They're good listeners and want to fully understand how you think and what's important to you. This is especially true when it comes to side effects. Since all treatments have potential side effects, the better physicians will thoroughly explain these to you and help you to understand and evaluate those that represent an acceptable risk in your case, and those that don't. This evaluation is of critical importance. For men whose prostate cancer has been detected by a routine PSA, and the level is 10 ng/ml or less, and the Gleason score is 6 or less with a clinical stage of T1 or T2a (low-risk prostate cancer) surgery, external beam radiation, and seed implantation are considered to be about equally effective. Lifestyle changes combined with close medical follow-up and PSA monitoring may also be an option for some men in the low-risk group (see

---

HELPFUL HINT

For many men with newly diagnosed prostate cancer, the choice of treatment may come down to which potential side effects are most acceptable.

"Watchful Waiting"). It's, therefore, reasonable to choose a treatment based on the most acceptable side-effect profile. Acceptability varies from person to person. The best clinicians will make sure to help you understand the advantages and disadvantages of each treatment. They realize that the final decision can be made by only one person. You!

Patient and Thorough

The best doctors in this field are incredibly busy. You may have to schedule your consultation a month or more in advance. A proper evaluation may take as long as two hours. This should include a thorough history and physical, including a digital rectal exam (DRE). The doctor will review all of your lab results, including the PSA, pathology report of your prostate biopsy, and radiologic tests (erMRI, bone scan, etc.). He or she should carefully and thoroughly explain the various treatment alternatives available, then provide detailed answers to all your questions.

Do not be afraid to ask any questions you might have. Some men refrain from asking questions that are important to them, because they're afraid they may sound "stupid." In this realm, there are no stupid questions! For you to be truly comfortable with the difficult decision you're about to make, you must air all your concerns. Don't hold back. Questions about sexual issues, incontinence, diarrhea, and the like are germane. Your doctor will not be put off by questions, no matter how intimate. Should the physician be female, and a number of very fine ones are, she will be every bit as comfortable in responding to intimate questions as her male counterparts. So inquire about everything that's on your mind.

Involves You in the Decision-Making Process

The best clinicians understand the importance of your involvement, and that of your wife or partner, in the decision-making process. Be wary of the doctor who states, "You must have surgery; it's the only reasonable choice," or any

similar dogmatic proclama-
tions. The expert's role is to
present you with accurate information, not to make decisions for you. Men who are
involved in the decision-
making process tend to have
a better outcome. They know
what to expect, because

> **HELPFUL HINT**
>
> Men involved in the decision-
> making process and in the overall
> management of their disease
> generally have a better outcome
> and feel better than uninvolved
> men.

they've asked pertinent questions and received satisfactory
answers. Top clinicians are compassionate facilitators who
assist you in determining what's right for you.

Still, you're likely to be left with choices. When considering among several options, the way you relate to the doctor
who'll be treating you is an important variable. It's often
useful to meet with each of the doctors who might be doing a
particular procedure. For example, if you have a choice between surgery, external beam radiation, or seeds, you should
give strong consideration to meeting with each of the practitioners who will actually be doing the procedure prior to
making your decision. It's important that you have confidence in this doctor and that all your questions are answered
to your satisfaction. If the doctor is too busy to spend the
required time for you to feel confident that you're making
the right decision, I suggest you select another doctor.

The list of doctors in each specialty presented in this book
comes from a consensus of prostate cancer experts. In other
words, these are the "doctor's doctors," the ones they would
go to if they had prostate cancer. If you stick with the doctors
listed in this book, you can be assured of receiving the best
care available. Naturally, this doesn't necessarily mean that
you'll be cured or that you'll be free from side effects, but
your odds of successful treatment will improve.

Taking the Next Step

After consulting your family doctor, urologist, and medical oncologist, you'll know a lot about the available treat-

ment options. A little later we'll discuss appropriate treatment choices for differing stages of disease at the time of
diagnosis. First, though, let's take a general look at each type
of treatment. If you don't have a medical oncologist on your
team and you're depending solely on a urologist, I suggest
you read the following sections on available treatments particularly carefully.

6

WATCHFUL WAITING

"Watchful waiting" means closely monitoring prostate cancer under medical supervision, preferably by a medical oncologist specializing in prostate cancer.

I have a distinct dislike for this term. It has a fatalistic sound to me. Waiting for what? To be treated? To die? A survey of couples seeking advice on treatment choices conducted by Maureen O'Rourke, a registered nurse at the University of North Carolina, found that "watchful waiting" was consistently described by urologists as "doing nothing." This sounds a lot like "giving up," an unpalatable option for most men with prostate cancer. As one patient in this survey stated, paraphrasing his urologist: "He said you can do nothing, then die before long. I'm not a do-nothing guy." Nor should you be.

But what if we change the term "watchful waiting" to "attentive lifestyle therapy?" Doesn't this sound more positive? Although there's mounting evidence that lifestyle changes, such as nutrition, exercise, and stress reduction, may help slow the rise of PSA in men known to have prostate cancer, at this stage, there's no firm medical proof. Several studies are currently in progress evaluating the effects of lifestyle changes alone on cancer progression. These studies closely monitor PSA in relation to compliance with the new lifestyle program. However, it will be at least a few more

years before we find out how these men do on "active conservative" therapy programs.

To determine whether attentive lifestyle therapy is a possibility, it makes sense to look at the natural history of prostate cancer in men with escalating levels of tumor aggressivity,
as measured by the Gleason score. Just such a study was
done by none other than Dr. Gleason himself, with the help
of three associates. What they found was reported in *JAMA*
in 1998 and is summarized in the table below. This table
shows the risk of dying from prostate cancer within 15 years
of diagnosis with *no treatment* and no specific lifestyle adjustments.

Biopsy Gleason score	Risk of dying from prostate cancer within 15 years
2-4	4%-7%
5	6%-11%
6	18%-30%
7	42%-70%
8-10	60%-87%

From this table it's apparent that men with low Gleason
scores (2-5) have an excellent prognosis without aggressive
treatment. Obviously, they will also have no noxious side effects by choosing this course.

Men with Gleason scores of 7-10 have a better chance of
living 15 years or more with aggressive therapy.

The Gleason 6 group comprises the majority of men newly
diagnosed with prostate cancer. Whether to treat these men
aggressively or conservatively is not so clear-cut. They have
a 70%-82% chance of surviving 15 years without aggressive
treatment (unless they die of something other than prostate
cancer). Not bad odds. As mentioned previously, there is no
conclusive proof (yet) that surgery increases overall life expectancy in low-risk prostate cancer. Low-risk is defined as
a PSA of 10 or less, and a Gleason score of 6 or less, and
clinical stage T1c to T2a. Conducting studies that randomly

assign men to receive either surgery or no definitive treatment is difficult. Most men have a distinct preference for either aggressive or conservative treatment. To get a large group of men to agree to randomly receive either surgery or watchful waiting is no small to task.

The only clinical trial comparing surgery with watchful waiting that has been published so far comes from Scandinavia and was reported in the September 12, 2002, edition of the prestigious *New England Journal of Medicine*. Six hundred and ninety-five men with newly diagnosed prostate cancer were randomly assigned to surgery or were closely followed with no definitive treatment. The average age of the men was 65; they were clinically T1 to T2 and the median follow-up time was 6.2 years. Patients were followed until death from any cause. Of note is the fact that 75% of the men in this study had their tumor discovered by digital rectal examination; in the United States about 75% of prostate cancer cases are now discovered by routine PSA screening, rather than by DRE.

The results of this Scandinavian study are the subject of considerable controversy. During the study period, 31 out of 348 men assigned to watchful waiting died of prostate cancer, compared to 16 out of 347 men who received surgery. This is a statistically significant result and is the first conclusive evidence that surgery reduced the risk of dying from prostate cancer. Big news! But when all causes of death were considered, 62 men in the watchful-waiting group and 53 men who had surgery died. This is not a significant difference.

The thought that immediately leaps to mind is that some of the men in the surgery group may have died from complications of the surgery, such as anesthesia, blood loss, or infection. So, even though surgery seems to have reduced the chance of dying from prostate cancer in this study, it did not reduce the overall risk of dying when all causes of death were considered.

To further complicate the issue, men who had surgery had significantly fewer metastases than the men who received no treatment. Radical prostatectomy reduced the chance of distant metastases by 37%. Dr. Patrick Walsh of Johns Hopkins predicts that the advantages of surgery will become more pronounced over time, since these men with metastases are more likely to succumb to prostate cancer than those free from metastases because they had surgery. Sound logic, but it still remains to be proven.

As for side effects, 80% of the surgically treated men in this study were impotent after surgery and nearly half had at least some degree of incontinency. But as Dr. Walsh points out, in the younger American population (average age 60 versus 65), "experienced academic urologists" report impotency rates of 14% to 38% and incontinency rates of 5% to 8%. This is a strong argument for using great care in selecting a urologist, if you choose surgery. American surveys of individual private urologists (as opposed to those working in academic hospitals) show that the incidence of impotency and incontinence mirrors the greater side effects of the Scandinavian experience. Pick your surgeon carefully! (See pages 87-88 for a list of recommended surgeons.)

More time is needed for the Scandinavian study to yield more definitive conclusions. In the meantime the Department of Veteran Affairs in the United States is now studying 731 men similarly comparing surgery with watchful waiting. Half the men in this study were picked up by PSA screening. A study comparing surgery with radiation is also currently progressing.

So where does this leave us? Is making significant lifestyle adjustments really an option? What is the risk that the cancer might spread if you choose this route?

Studies evaluating the effect of changes in diet, exercise, and stress management on cancer progression are currently under way for men with low-risk cancer. A recent study by Dr. Carter and his group at Johns Hopkins indicates there is little added risk of the cancer spreading for men with low-volume low-risk prostate cancer. They studied 81 men with T1-c prostate cancer picked up by PSA screening with PSAs of 10 or less and Gleason scores of 6 or less. They followed them with PSAs every six months and annual repeat prostate biopsies. The median follow-up period was 23 months. They set strict criteria for surgery. Any man who had any Gleason grade 4 or 5 pockets of cancer in his repeat biopsy, or more than 2 positive cores, or if any biopsy core was 50% or more involved with cancer were promptly treated with surgery.

Sixty-nine percent of the men in this study had no observable progression of their prostate cancer during the study period. These men have avoided surgery at least so far. Of the 13 out of 81 men who did have their cancer advance, 12 were deemed to have cancer that was curable by surgery. The researchers concluded, "Expectant management may be suitable for men with small-volume low-risk cancers." Noteworthy is the fact that this study only covers 2 years. If this preliminary evidence continues to hold true, it will add strong support for the argument in favor of conservative management for this group of low-risk men.

Note that the men in this study apparently made no significant lifestyle adjustments. Although there is no conclusive evidence yet that these lifestyle changes reduce the risk of prostate cancer spreading, preliminary evidence and reports from doctors who encourage their patients to make these changes are encouraging. There is no question, however, that a low-fat diet with lots of vegetables and fruit, increased exercise, and stress reduction reduce the risk of heart disease (see "Nutrition"). Since the chance of dying from heart disease exceeds the chance of dying from low-risk prostate cancer, it seems logical that making these adjustments will increase your overall life expectancy, as well as your quality of life, whether or not you decide on definitive treatment of your prostate cancer.

So should you choose lifestyle changes with close medical supervision over surgery or radiation for low-volume low-risk prostate cancer? I can't answer that, but you can. For many men, perhaps most, having untreated cancer in their body is simply unacceptable. They want it out, or destroyed, and the sooner the better. If this is true for you, I'd recommend either surgery, radiation, or seeds. They are all about equally successful.

For those of you who can overcome the psychological effect of having a small slow-growing cancer, are under close medical supervision, and are prepared to take decisive action if the cancer progresses, conservative management may be an option. If your tumor is slow-growing, as many are, you may be able to avoid the potential side effects from more definitive treatments. With diligent monitoring, the chances of the tumor escaping the prostate appear to be present but small. How this limited risk compares with the risk of potential side effects from more definitive treatment is an individual decision to be made by a man and his partner. Adding significant lifestyle changes reduces your risk of heart disease, may reduce the risk of the cancer progressing, and will benefit your overall health and well being.

Some men have extremely slow-growing cancers. One way to determine how fast a cancer is growing is to follow the PSA and calculate the time required for the PSA to double. A recent study by Dr. Choo and his associates at the Toronto-Sunnybrook Regional Cancer Center found that in more than 200 men with low- to intermediate-risk prostate cancer who entered a study on the feasibility of watchful waiting, 42% of the men had a PSA doubling time of over 10 years. Twenty-eight percent of the men had a PSA doubling time of greater than 50 years! Obviously, it's exceedingly unlikely that these men will require treatment.

If you select conservative management with the fallback of definitive treatment, I suggest you select a medical oncologist familiar with this type of program to optimize your chances of success.

There's another reason why some men with slow-growing tumors might select attentive lifestyle therapy as a course of action. With the entire human genome now sequenced, it's possible that a cure for prostate cancer may be in hand before many men's disease becomes life-threatening, if at all.

A Quick Look at the Meaning of Medical Statistics

In the words of Dr. Chris Logothetis, a medical oncologist and prostate cancer expert at M.D. Anderson in Houston, Texas, "Statistics describe an average patient who never exists. Average statistical outcomes never apply to the individual patient. Treat medical statistics only as a rough guide. Then do everything possible to tip those numbers in your favor."

They may reason that they can avoid the side effects of definitive local treatment and still be cured of their cancer five or ten years or more down the line. Such thinking is not far-fetched, in my opinion, given the exponential growth of genetic medicine and the slow-growing nature of low-risk prostate cancer.

Ultimately, the choice you make depends a lot on your outlook, attitude, and tolerance for ambiguity. Attentive lifestyle therapy requires a high tolerance for ambiguity. Many men prefer the relative certainty of definitive treatment and are willing to risk the possible side effects. Let's have a look at those options.

Key References

O'Rourke M. Narrowing the options: The process of deciding on prostate cancer treatment. *Cancer Invest* 1999; 17: 349-359.

Albertsen P, Hanley J, Gleason D, and Barry M. Competing risk analysis of men aged 55 to 74 years at diagnosis managed conservatively for clinically localized prostate cancer. *JAMA* 1998; 280: 975-980.

Holmberg L et al. A randomized trial comparing radical prostatectomy with watchful waiting in early prostate cancer. *New Engl J Med* 2002; 347: 781-789.

Steinbeck G et al. Quality of life after radical prostatectomy or watchful waiting. *New Engl J Med* 2002; 347: 790-796.

Walsh P. Surgery and reduction of mortality from prostate cancer. *New Engl J Med* 2002; 347: 839-840.

Carter HB. Expectant management of non-palpable prostate cancer with curative intent: preliminary results. *J Urology* 2002; 167: 1231-1234.

Choo R et al. Feasibility study: watchful waiting for localized low to intermediate grade prostate carcinoma with selective delayed intervention based on prostate specific antigen, histological and/or clinical progression. *J Urology* 2002; 167: 1664-1669.

7

SURGERY

More than 40,000 radical prostatectomies (removal of the prostate and regional lymph nodes) are performed annually.

For many years surgery has been the "gold standard" for treating prostate cancer. We know more about the long-term results of surgery than we do about any other treatment. Although radiation has recently been accepted as a comparable alternative to surgery, data from surgery have been collected for a longer period of time.

Many men feel secure with this seasoned procedure. Perhaps the biggest benefit that can be derived from surgery is that you'll know where you stand. The surgeon and the pathologist can accurately stage the severity of your disease. If the tumor has spread beyond the prostate capsule, for example, or if the seminal vesicles or pelvic lymph nodes are involved, you'll be told. If the surgeon got all the cancer and the surgical margins are clear, you'll be so advised and reassured. As Dr. Paul Lange, Chairman of Urology at the University of Washington and a prostate cancer survivor succinctly put it, "I feel secure in knowing that my prostate cancer was found to be confined to the prostate gland at surgery. Knowing this is a great relief. The probability that I am cured is excellent."

Even if the news is not so good, information obtained

from surgery is useful in determining additional treatment that may be required. In some cases, radiation may be necessary to treat cancer that remains after surgery. In addition, if the disease is more extensive than expected, long-term remission is often achievable by immediately starting hormonal therapy (see page 102).

Lifestyle decisions might need to be made. You may choose to work less and devote more time to fighting your disease. Finances permitting, you may opt to retire to devote more time to quality of life, exercise, nutrition, and stress reduction. For many, perhaps most, knowing with certainty the extent of their disease is imperative to the decision-making process.

HELPFUL HINT

Although there are exceptions, surgery is recommended for otherwise healthy men under 70 with a life expectancy of at least 10 years, a high likelihood of organ-confined cancer, *and who prefer surgery.*

Besides knowing where you stand, a common motivator for men who select surgery is the desire "to get the damn thing out." Surgery seems definitive: Get rid of the tumor before it spreads. Surgery, for men who think this way, seems more certain than radiation. With radiation, they may wonder if all the cancer cells have been killed. What if a few survive the radiation and start to grow again? What then? Surgery puts an end to this kind of conjecture.

Another good reason for surgery is that in the event it's unsuccessful, additional treatment with radiation has up to a 50% cure rate. This is a nice fallback position given a worst-case scenario. If the chance of cure with surgery is 70%, the combined cure rate for surgery plus salvage radiation if surgery doesn't get all the cancer may be as high as 85%. Pretty good odds.

On the other hand, for men who have radiation therapy as their primary treatment, surgery as salvage for failed radiation is fraught with potential side effects, such as incontinence and impotency. It takes a skilled surgeon, indeed, to deal with the scar tissue caused by radiation, remove what's left of the prostate and any tumor, and preserve continence and potency. Certainly the risks from salvage, as a second procedure for remaining cancer is called, are considerably higher when radiation precedes surgery than when surgery comes first.

Some prostate cancer experts (and they're not all urologists, either) like to use surgery as a first-line treatment, because "the patients seem to do better." One such proponent is Celestia Higano, a medical oncologist specializing in prostate cancer at the University of Washington. "Getting the bulk of the cancer out, even if we can't get it all, significantly reduces the remaining tumor burden. Patients with reduced tumor burdens tend to respond better to subsequent treatments. I prefer surgery as a front-line treatment even in high-risk patients with aggressive cancers and high PSAs, as long as there's no evidence of bone metastases."

Although there's no hard evidence that "debulking" the tumor mass improves outcome, this belief is common in a number of astute clinicians. Since these professionals deal with prostate cancer on a daily basis, it seems imprudent to ignore their clinical impressions. They admit, however, that there's no hard data to support this belief. Additionally, as you'll read below, for low-risk patients other treatments have statistical cure rates equal to surgery. And it doesn't stop with low-risk disease. For more advanced cases, although some doctors have a preference for surgery, more are inclined to use radiation combined with hormones. Using hormones prior to radiation shrinks the tumor mass, effectively reducing tumor bulk. Hormones may also make tumors more susceptible to the effects of radiation.

Over the years surgery has improved. The "nerve-sparing" procedure pioneered by Dr. Patrick Walsh at Johns Hopkins is now widely practiced. This technique preserves the nerves responsible for erections on one, or both, sides of the prostate, depending on the extent of the cancer. Dr. William Catalona, a brilliant surgeon and Head of Urology at

Washington University in St. Louis, reported results in the August 1999 edition of the *Journal of Urology* on 1,870 of his patients. He used the nerve-sparing procedure whenever possible. For men under 70, sparing the nerves on both sides preserved potency for 71% of the men. If only one nerve was left, the chance of preserving potency was reduced to 48%. For men over 70, leaving one or both nerves was not dramatically different (48% versus 40%). In Dr. Walsh's own hands, in a much smaller study of only 70 men who had radical prostatectomies, only 14% reported impotency 18 months after surgery. These results compare with a 70% chance of erectile dysfunction before the nerve-sparing procedure was perfected.

Blood loss, a common complication a few years ago, has now been reduced. In top surgical hands, transfusions prompted by blood loss from surgery are uncommon.

Most importantly, incontinence, perhaps the most dreaded complication of radical prostatectomy, has been reduced to an acceptable risk for most men. The best surgeons are now reporting only a 2%-7% risk. And they define continence as requiring only a liner (a very thin pad that many women use daily), or nothing, within a year of the procedure. These results compare quite favorably with incontinence risks of 60% or more in earlier reports. Be aware that incontinence is much less common at big teaching hospitals than in private practice.

It's critical, therefore, that if you choose to have surgery, you find the most skillful and experienced surgeon available. The difference between a master, a surgical virtuoso if you will, and an average surgeon is huge. If a urologist tells you that in his or her hands, the chance of requiring a liner, or worse, for incontinence is greater than 7%, I suggest you find

---

HELPFUL HINT

If you decide on surgery, find the best urologist available. Surgery is an art. Finding a true artist is well worth the effort when the risks include impotence and incontinence.

another urologist, or choose a treatment other than surgery.

(Note that you might read the literature and discover that in a large series, the incontinence rate may appear to be higher than 7%. In Dr. Catalona's study, 8% reported incontinence. Keep in mind that this series was done over many years and surgical techniques are continually being refined and improved. A big series doesn't take these improvements into account.)

It's crucial to select a urologist who can get the job done while minimizing the risk of complications. But how do you know who is capable?

Selecting A Urologist

I have developed a list of top surgeons covering a wide geographic area. I got these names from the best urologists in the field. Again, these are the "surgeons' surgeons," the ones the top urologists would select if they needed prostate surgery. If you decide on surgery, you can depend on the competency of these surgeons. I can't guarantee that you won't get some undesirable complications from treatment, but by selecting one of these men, you'll significantly improve your chances of an excellent result. I'm sure there are competent surgeons who have not been included in this list. My goal is not the creation of an exhaustive list of great urologists, but rather to provide you with a list of men you can depend on to do a quality radical prostatectomy.

List of Qualified Surgeons
East Coast

William Dewolfe	Beth Israel Hospital	Boston, MA
David McLeod	Walter Reed Hospital	Bethesda, MD
Judd Moul	Walter Reed Hospital	Bethesda, MD

Carl Olsen	Columbia University	New York, NY
Jerry Richie	Peter Bent Brigham Hosp.	Boston, MA
Peter Scardino	Sloan Kettering Memorial Hospital	New York, NY
Patrick Walsh	Johns Hopkins University	Baltimore, MD

South

Ray Marshall	Emory University	Atlanta, GA
Dave Paulsen	Duke University	Durham, NC
Jay Smith	Vanderbilt University	Nashville, TN
Mark Soloway	Univ. of Miami Hospital	Miami, FL

Midwest

Herb Brenler	University of Chicago	Chicago, IL
William Catalona	Washington University	St. Louis, MO
Eric Klein	Cleveland Clinic	Cleveland, OH
Robert Myer	Mayo Clinic	Rochester, MN

West Coast

Peter Carroll	University of California	San Francisco, CA
Jean De Kernion	UCLA Hospital	Los Angeles, CA
Stuart Holden	Tower Urology Medical Group	Los Angeles, CA
Paul Lange	University of Washington	Seattle, WA

Reservations Regarding Surgery

Now that we've reviewed some of the advantages of the surgical approach, let's explore some of the possible downsides. Unquestionably, surgery is harder on bodies than radiation. Although the top surgeons will have you out of the operating room in three hours (perfectionists such as Dr. Catalona take longer) and out of the hospital in about three days, it will take four to six weeks for you to reasonably fully recover.

You'll leave the hospital with a catheter in your bladder.

Why? Because during surgery your urethra, the tube through which urine passes, must be severed and re-attached. It takes at least two weeks for this to heal well enough for the catheter to be removed. When the catheter is removed, most men will have urinary leakage to one degree or another. Pads will be required to make this a socially acceptable condition. Many will need these pads to lessening degrees for six months or more. For some, their use may become a permanent requirement. Other urinary complications, such as urinary retention, may require re-insertion of the catheter for varying periods of time. For most of the men I have talked with, dealing with urinary adjustments far eclipse any considerations of pain associated with surgery.

Incontinence is one of the two worst side effects of surgery. Impotence is the other (see later in this section). I've mentioned blood loss. Other side effects include rectal damage, infection, and swelling.

It's important to take a cold hard look before deciding whether surgery is the best procedure for you. Some patients have surgery pushed on them without having alternative treatment options fully explained. Just as surgery may be an obviously correct choice for some men with a particular outlook, it may represent unneeded risk, discomfort, and inconvenience for others. Remember, there's no universally correct procedure for treating prostate cancer.

Besides surgery, you have other choices that are reasonable. New studies show that for early prostate cancer, surgery, seeds, and 3-D conformal external beam radiation are all equally effective. This may make the decision process difficult. Since no treatment is clearly superior to another for early cancer, potential side effects from treatment may become significant factors in the treatment selection process.

This comment by Dr. Ken Russell, a top-notch radiation oncologist at the University of Washington, sums it up. It was made with specific reference to my case, "You have three choices: surgery, external beam radiation, or palladium seeds.

They're all about equally likely to be successful in your case. Therefore, you might want to review the side-effect profile of each treatment and make your decision based on which potential side effects are the most acceptable to you."

Sage advise and rarely given. Most doctors, by their own admission, have a therapeutic bias. The literature, however, does not support a bias. If you have a PSA of 10 or less, a Gleason score of 6 or less, and clinical stage T-2a or less, your chances of long-term cure are about the same whether you choose surgery, external beam radiation, or seeds. That's right. They're all about equal. And the majority of men with prostate cancer fit the above profile. Once you fully understand this dynamic, it makes treatment selection more pragmatic: Do what's best for your personal situation.

Besides side effects, convenience of treatment, work considerations, and local availability of a master treatment specialist are additional considerations. The quality and experience of the doctor treating you is paramount. I would much rather have seeds, or radiation, from a top man in the field than have surgery by an average urologist.

Conversely, I would choose surgery by an expert over a brachytherapist or radiation therapist of moderate experience. No matter what some urologists may tell you, there's nothing sacrosanct about surgery.

The consideration of lifestyle changes combined with close medical monitoring for men with low-risk low-volume prostate cancers has already been discussed.

When Is Surgery Inadvisable?

Generally speaking, surgery is not recommended for men over age 70. However, many men who are over 70 are as fit as a fiddle. If you're 72, in good shape, and prefer surgery, I see nothing wrong with this option. Men with heart conditions, diabetes, or other health problems may be well advised to seek other treatment options.

Most prostate cancer experts prefer external beam radiation combined with androgen ablation (hormones) for locally advanced disease. If there's a high probability that the cancer has penetrated the capsule of the prostate, surgery is unlikely to remove all the cancer. External beam radiation covers a wider area and can kill cancer cells beyond the reach of the surgeon's scalpel. Hormonal therapy has a good chance of killing cancer cells that may have migrated into the blood or lymph systems. The combination of treating a larger local area and going after aberrant cells that may have broken away makes sense when chances are high that the cancer has escaped the confines of the prostate.

Surgery and High-Risk Prostate Cancer

Due to the widespread use of PSA screening, prostate cancer is being picked up at an early stage. This early detection has made surgery a viable option for some men with high-risk Gleason grade 8-10 cancers. Eight percent of all prostatectomies at the Mayo Clinic are for Gleason 8-10 cancers. Recent data from Mayo shows that 31% of men in this high-risk group still had organ-confined cancers. Additionally, 80% were free from lymph-node metastases. Surgery alone, however, is generally considered to be insufficient. Hormonal therapy that reduces testosterone and other androgens has been shown to reduce the chances of these cancers progressing. How long to continue androgen-ablating hormonal therapy is debatable and will vary depending on the findings at surgery. If lymph

---

HELPFUL HINT

If you're considering surgery to treat Gleason 8-10 prostate cancer consider the following:
• The lower your PSA prior to surgery the better. Men with PSAs of 10 or under do better than men with PSAs over 10.
• It's best to have a negative DRE (no palpable tumor mass).
• Hormonal therapy reduces cancer progression.
• Men with Gleason 8-9 tumors do significantly better than men with Gleason 10 tumors.

nodes are found with cancer, hormones should be continued indefinitely.

Another study of men with high-grade cancers from M.D. Anderson Cancer Center in Houston, Texas, showed that 55% of men were free from cancer 7 years after surgery.

Key References
Lau WK et al. Radical prostatectomy for pathological Gleason 8 or greater prostate cancer: influence of concomitant pathological variables. *J Urology* 2002; 167: 117-122.
Mian B. Outcome of patients with Gleason 8 or higher prostate cancer following radical prostatectomy alone. *J Urology* 2002; 167: 1675-1680.

How Do I Know I've Been Cured?

Surgery removes the entire prostate gland. Since the prostate produces virtually all PSA in the body, your post-operative PSA blood tests should show undetectable levels of PSA. For the standard PSA test this means less than 0.1 ng/ml. If the PSA rises to 0.2 ng/ml, or more, and this is confirmed by repeating the test (eliminating the possibility of lab error), the PSA is coming from prostate cancer cells. These cells may be in the area of the prostate, or they may have spread to more distant places. Some studies use a PSA of 0.3 as an indicator of cancer relapse.

An ultra-sensitive PSA test is now available that may be able to detect a rising PSA level long before the standard assay. In one study, this ultra-sensitive test was able to diagnose a recurrence of cancer after surgery 2.5 years earlier than the more commonly used, but less sensitive, PSA assay. Knowing as early as possible that surgery has failed allows you to attack remaining cancer cells with radiation and/or hormones at the first signs of recurrence, although the timing on when to use these treatments is controversial (see "Advance Disease").

If you're cured by surgery, your PSA should stay at undetectable levels. According to some studies, like the one below by Dr. Catalona, after five years of undetectable PSA levels it's unusual to have a subsequent rise in PSA; after seven years it's rare. The result of other surgeons' work, notably Dr. Patrick Walsh's series of nearly 2,000 men, showed that 23% of patients had PSA recurrences within five years; 4% had recurrences after 10 years. But the only way to determine if you're cured is by monitoring your PSA. Overall, about 70% of men who have a radical prostatectomy are cured, and only 3% will die of prostate cancer within seven years.

Some men may have the cancer return, but it may grow so slowly that it literally takes years to see a measurable increase by standard PSA testing. Indeed, some investigators think these tortoise-like tumors may be the ones showing up 10 years, or more, after surgery, especially if a PSA cutoff for recurrence of 0.3ng/ml is used to determine recurrence. In these men the cancer may be growing so slowly that it takes more than 10 years for the PSA to reach 0.3ng/ml. These men may not need additional treatment even though some cancer cells survive. Lifestyle adjustments may slow cancer growth even more.

How do you know if you'll be one of those seven out of 10 men that are cured? Well, you don't. But there are some guidelines that can help evaluate your chances. A large study of nearly 1,800 men, all of whose surgery was performed by one man, Dr. William Catalona at Washington University in St. Louis, found that three factors independently predicted the chance of the cancer coming back: preoperative PSA, Gleason score (at time of surgery), and pathological stage of disease (stage at surgery).

Let's look at each of these parameters separately in Dr. Catalona's patients.

Preoperative PSA

With a PSA level of 0.0-2.5, your chance of being free of disease (PSA undetectable) at seven years after surgery is 93%.

With a PSA level of 2.6-4.0, your chance is 88%.

With a PSA of 4.1-9.9, it's 76%.
And at 10.0 or greater, it's 49%.

Gleason score

With a Gleason score of 2-4, your odds of being free of disease at seven years are 84%.

With a Gleason score of 5-7, your odds are 68%.

And with a Gleason score of 8-10, your odds are 48%.

Pathological Stage (Actual Extent of Tumor at the Time of Surgery)

If your pathological stage is T1 or T2 (organ confined), your odds are 81% of having an undetectable PSA seven years after surgery.

A T3a/T3b (tumor has escaped prostate, but is localized) and negative surgical margins will put you at 76%.

T3a/T3b and positive surgical margins will be 57%.

With T3c (seminal vesicle involvement), it's 26%.

And with lymph-node metastases, it's 19%.

Note: A negative surgical margin means there is no sign of cancer remaining outside of the removed tissue. See page 100 for an explanation of positive surgical margins.

As you can readily determine from this excellent summary of 14 years of work by a renowned surgeon, if your initial PSA is less than 10 at the time of surgery, you have an excellent chance of cure; if it's less than 4 your chance of cure is about 90%. In similar studies, the chance of cure is also consistently high (83%+).

Likewise, men with low Gleason scores have a higher rate of cure than men with higher Gleason scores. If your cancer is contained within the prostate at the time of surgery, the chance of being free from disease at seven years is high (81%). Similarly, if the cancer has spread into the tissues surrounding the prostate, but the surgeon apparently got it all (negative surgical margins), the probability of cure is almost as high (76%).

Men with a poor surgical profile should strongly consider immediate additional treatment. This group includes men who have positive surgical margins, or worse, men with high PSA levels before surgery (over 20) and men with Gleason scores that indicate aggressive tumors (Gleason 8-10).

Please note that some men with advanced disease, like lymph-node involvement, still have undetectable PSA levels seven years after surgery without the use of androgen-ablating hormones. By adding immediate continuous testosterone-suppressing hormones (or in some cases removing the testes), Dr. Messing and colleagues increased the number of men with undetectable PSA levels to 77%! So even if you're found to have more advanced disease at surgery than previously thought, a treatment plan now exists that promises excellent long-term results (see page 102).

On the other hand, if your disease is found to be organ-confined, although it augers well for cure, some men will still have recurrences. This is why it's important to have regular DREs and PSA blood tests after surgery. Most surgeons recommend checking these parameters every three months for the first year, every six months for the second year, and annually thereafter.

Important Factors to Consider With Surgery

Gleason score—Generally speaking, the higher your Gleason score, the greater the risk of surgery. Although surgery can be a successful treatment for aggressive cancers (Gleason 8-10), if the PSA is less than 10 ng/ml, it's not generally considered to be the treatment of choice for men with high Gleason scores and a PSA higher than 10 ng/ml.

PSA—Surgery works best for men with organ-confined tumors. When the pre-operative PSA is greater than 10 ng/ml, the chance of non-organ-confined disease increases. Surgery is not usually performed on men with PSAs over 20. PSAs between 10 and 20 are a gray area. Here, the decision depends on other test results. If tests like an endorectal MRI indicate the likelihood of organ-confined disease, surgery may be an excellent choice. If not, radiation, possibly with hormones, might increase the chances of cure. In Dr. Catalona's study of about 1,800 men, 51% of men with PSAs greater than 10 ng/ml prior to surgery ultimately had recurrence of their cancer.

Clinical Stage—Surgery is generally not indicated if the clinical stage is more advanced than T2. Men with T2c disease (both sides of prostate have tumor) have significantly higher cancer recurrence rates after surgery than men with T2a disease (less than 50% of one side of the prostate has tumor).

General health—Men selecting surgery should be in good general health. Heart disease, diabetes, and other significant medical conditions must be carefully evaluated prior to selecting surgery. Many men with these conditions opt for radiation instead.

Some Surgical Results

I thought it might be useful to review the results of surgery alone, by an excellent surgeon, on a series of 1,000 consecutive men that he treated. The surgeon, Dr. Peter Scardino, is at Sloan Kettering Memorial Hospital in New York (see list of recommended urologists). If men received any additional treatment, they were considered a surgical failure.

• Only 11 out of 1,000 died of prostate cancer during the study, while 40 out of 1,000 died of other causes during the study period (median time 46.9 months). Deaths from prostate cancer were only 22% of all deaths.

• At 10 years, the actuarially derived probability of dying from prostate cancer was 2.4%!

• The chance of having metastases at 10 years was 15.3%.

• The odds of being free from cancer at 5 and 10 years respectively were 78% and 75%.

• Men with low-risk cancer had an 88% chance of being cancer-free after 10 years; intermediate risk (Gleason 7, or PSA 10.1-20, or clinical stage 2b) men had a 77% chance of being cancer-free at 10 years; high-risk men's (PSA greater than 20, or clinical stage T2c, or Gleason 8-10) probability of cancer-free survival at 10 years was 57%.

• In this study men with positive surgical margins were 4 times more likely to have their cancer recur than men with negative margins. The skill of the surgeon has substantial influence on margin status.

• Surgery was effective even for high-risk patients.

Bottom line (mine): For an excellent surgical result and to maximize your chances of cure, pick the best surgeon you can find. The list provided in this book is reliable.

Key Reference

Hull G, Scardino P et al. Cancer control with radical prostatectomy alone in 1,000 consecutive patients. *J Urology* 2002; 167: 528-534.

A Rising PSA After Radical Prostatectomy

The greatest fear for men who undergo surgery for prostate cancer is that their PSA will start rising after the operation. Most men have an undetectable PSA shortly after surgery. With the exception of rare lab errors, a rising PSA means that cancer cells remain.

Before discussing how to approach a rising PSA, it may be helpful to look at what happens to men with a rising PSA who have no other forms of therapy. How do they fare? Data on this are provided in an excellent study from Dr. Patrick Walsh and his group at Johns Hopkins Hospital. As you'll recall, Dr. Walsh is the inventor of the nerve-sparing procedure to help preserve potency after prostatectomy.

In this report, published in the May 5, 1999 issue of *JAMA*, Dr. Walsh, Dr. Partin, and Dr. Pound studied a group of nearly 2,000 patients on whom Dr. Walsh had performed radical prostatectomies. Of this group, 315 men, about 15%, developed rising PSA levels at various times after surgery. Eleven of the 315 had immediate hormone treatment. The remaining 304 men had no treatment unless clinical metastatic disease was confirmed. In the 15 years between 1982 and 1997, 103 (34%) of the 304 men with rising PSAs developed metastases. The median time from elevated PSA to metastases was eight years! So even with no treatment for a rising PSA, it took an average of eight years for the cancer to spread to the point where it could be picked up by tests.

Additionally, this study showed that the median time to death, after the cancer had spread, was five years. Adding these two numbers together, the median survival time from a rising PSA after surgery to death in this group was 13 years. To be sure, not all men live this long. "Median survival" means that half the men live longer than 13 years and half the men live less. Early use of hormones may extend survival time still further.

Is there any way to determine the likelihood of being free from metastases for a long time? Dr. Walsh believes there is. He points to three factors: Gleason score, time from surgery to elevated PSA, and PSA doubling time.

If a man has PSA failure (elevated PSA) and a Gleason score of 8-10 (most aggressive), his chance of being free from metastases five years from the time of his first elevated PSA test, right after surgery, is 40%. Men with Gleason scores of 5-7 have a 73% chance of being free from metastases five years later.

At seven years, a man with a Gleason score of 8-10 has only a 29% chance of freedom from metastases; for a Gleason score of 5-7 the chance is 62%.

But if a man has a Gleason score of 8-10 and his elevated PSA is not detected until more than two years from the time of surgery, the probability of his being free from metastases at five years increases from 40% to 60%. At seven years his chance increases from 29% to 47%. This compares with 31% and 21% freedom from metastases for five and seven years, if the PSA failed in less than two years. For men with Gleason scores of 5-7 and the PSA doesn't rise for two or more years, the chance of being free from metastases in five years is 82%, after seven years 77%. If the PSA rises in less than two years, these figures drop to 62% and 47%.

Additionally, if it took more than 10 months for the PSA value to double and more than two years from surgery to PSA recurrence, men with Gleason scores of 5-7 had an 82% chance of being metastasis-free at seven years. If the PSA doubled in 10 months or less, there was only a 60% chance of being free from cancer seven years later.

The reason I've gone into detail on this important study is to demonstrate that, even if you're unlucky enough to be in the minority group that has an elevated PSA at some point after surgery (remember, it was only 15% of Dr. Walsh's 2,000 patients), there's a very real chance that you'll be able to live a long time. With gene therapy, vaccines, and sophisticated methods of delivering cancer-killing chemicals directly to the cancer cells (see "New and Future Developments"), you may have an excellent chance of surviving until a cure is in hand. Proper nutrition, exercise, and the early use of hormones may further extend life expectancy.

Summary of the Johns Hopkins Analysis for Men With a Rising PSA After Surgery

- Only 34% developed metastases within 15 years.
- The chance of dying was 6% at 10 years, 9% at 15 years.
- At eight years, 50% had no measurable metastases.
- Median survival was five years from the time of measurable metastases.
- Favorable indications:
  - Gleason score of 6 or less;
  - two years or more from the time of surgery for PSA to start rising;
  - greater than 10 months for the PSA to double.
- Unfavorable indications:
  - Gleason score of 8 to 10;
  - PSA rising less than two years from the time of surgery;
  - less than 10 months for the PSA to double.
- Men with a Gleason score of 8-10 had a 29%-47% chance of being free from metastases after seven years, depending on when their PSA started rising after surgery and how fast it doubled.

Before leaving Dr. Walsh's work, I want to make an important point that is often misunderstood by men with prostate cancer. In Dr. Walsh's series of nearly 2,000 patients, at the time of surgery only 911 (45.6%) had organ-confined cancer. Eight hundred sixty-one men (43%) had cancer that had penetrated the capsule of the prostate gland; 105 men (5%) had seminal vesicle involvement and 120 men (6%) had cancer in their pelvic lymph nodes. So 55%, nearly 1,100 men in this series, had cancer that had escaped the confines of the prostate. But only 315 men had a subsequent rise in PSA during the study period.

It's clear from these statistics that for the wide majority of men who had cancerous prostates surgically removed, penetration of the prostate capsule by cancer did not lead to disease recurrence. I think there's a common misconception that if the cancer has escaped the prostate by any amount, it's tantamount to a death sentence. This just isn't true.

What To Do About Positive Margins

A "positive margin" means that the pathologist who examines the prostate gland after its removal by surgery sees cancer cells right up to the edge (margin) of the specimen. Although this is not a good prognostic sign, only half of these men will have their cancer recur. These odds can be shortened by an additional 10% to 20%, according to Dr. Catalona's work, by using external beam radiation on this high-risk group. The dose of radiation varies from 48 Gy to 68 Gy; 64.8 Gy is probably most common at present. The idea is to kill any cancer cells left in the prostate bed. Obviously, follow-up radiation cannot reach cancer cells that may have migrated to distant locations. Patients who are found to have cancer in their lymph nodes are, therefore, generally treated with hormones in an attempt to control cancer cells throughout the body.

It is not clear that Dr. Catalona's work will be the final word on what to do about positive margins. There are many variables to consider. The issue is highly controversial and rapidly evolving. Experts disagree and there are ongoing studies. Although radiation after surgery is likely to play a role in the treatment of some men with positive margins, that role hasn't yet been clearly established.

High-risk prostate cancer has a greater chance of resulting in positive margins than low-risk disease. Reported studies show positive margins for low-risk cancer of between 7.7% and 39%, for high-risk tumors 18% to 59%. As discussed, surgical technique definitely makes a difference in the probability of having undesirable positive surgical margins.

The number of positive margins is also significant. Men with only one positive margin have half the risk of the cancer returning as men with more than one positive margin in the removed prostate. About 75% of men with positive margins can expect to have only one.

In one study of 210 patients, 25% of men with positive margins had their cancer recur with a median follow-up time of 22 months from the time of surgery. Longer follow-up is needed to evaluate the full influence of positive margins.

Key References

Hull G et al. Cancer control with radical prostatectomy alone in 1,000 consecutive patients. *J Urology* 2002; 167: 528-534

Sofer M et al. Positive surgical margins after radical retropubic prostatectomy: the influence of site and number on progression. *J Urology* 2002; 167: 2453-2456

Kupelian P et al. External beam radio-therapy versus radical prostatectomy for clinical stage T1-2 prostate cancer: therapeutic implications of stratification by pre-treatment PSA levels and biopsy Gleason scores. *Cancer J Sci Am* 1997; 3: 78

Using Hormones for Lymph-Node Metastases Found at Surgery: Immediate Versus Delayed

A recent article in the *New England Journal of Medicine* by Dr. Ed Messing (mentioned earlier) strengthens the case for surgery for locally advanced disease. This landmark study combines data from several major hospitals. As in all of the best studies, it was prospective and randomized.

The objective of this investigation was to determine, in

men who were discovered to have lymph-node metastases at the time of surgery, whether immediate hormone therapy was better than delayed hormone therapy. Ninety-eight men were found to have involved lymph nodes; 47 received immediate hormones, while 51 were observed and treated with hormones only if their disease progressed. After an average (median) time of more than seven years, only three out of 47 men in the treated group (6%) had died from prostate cancer. Over this same time period, 16 of 51 men (31%) who had not received hormones died. These results are statistically significant. They show that for men with lymph-node involvement at the time of surgery, the use of hormones immediately after surgery significantly increased life expectancy. This is big news!

Even more striking is the fact that in the treated group of 47 men, 34 (77%) of those still living had no evidence of prostate cancer; their PSA level was also undetectable. However, only 18% of those still alive in the untreated group (six of the 35) had no sign of recurrent disease and undetectable serum PSA. When treated with immediate hormone therapy, Dr. Messing and his colleagues found that their surgical patients with documented lymph-node metastases did about as well as men with low-risk disease!

Now that it appears as though immediate complete androgen blockade often leads to long-term remissions, knowing that the disease has spread to the lymph nodes is particularly valuable information. While Messing's well-done and rigidly controlled study needs to be confirmed by other investigators, it has made surgery a more viable option for men whose cancer may have already spread beyond the prostate. In my own case I would have given sur-

> **HELPFUL HINTS**
>
> Men with lymph nodes involved with cancer at the time of surgery should start hormone therapy immediately and stay on hormones indefinitely.
>
> Men who follow this course of action appear to do about as well as men with low-risk disease.

gery more consideration. Since the chance that my cancer had at least penetrated the prostate capsule was high, I opted for hormones for more than 2 years combined with 3-D conformal external beam radiation. If the diagnosis of prostate cancer were made today, I'd be hard-pressed in choosing between this treatment and surgery combined with hormonal therapy.

Prospective and Randomized

Prospective randomized studies are the most high-powered medical studies. They take people with similar degrees of disease and randomly (like drawing a name out of a hat) assign them to one form of treatment or another. Then they monitor each group as time progresses (prospective) and compare the results. When a medication is being tested, it is compared with an identical-looking but inactive placebo (sugar pill). The best studies are "double-blind"; neither the patient nor the doctor knows whether the drug or the sugar pill is being administered.

Using Hormones Prior to Surgery (Neoadjuvant Hormonal Therapy)

Speaking of hormones, one of the more controversial areas in the initial treatment of prostate cancer is whether, and for how long, to use hormones prior to surgery. Part of the reason for the lack of consensus on this issue is that the clinical data is perplexing. Most of the studies have evaluated the effects of three months of hormones (complete androgen blockade) prior to surgery. Nearly all prospective randomized studies, comparing three months of neoadjuvant hormones to surgery alone, report a significant increase in cancer confined to the prostate, compared to cancer that has penetrated the capsule, in the group receiving hormones. The hormone-treated group also had substantially fewer positive margins.

One such trial was done at Sloan Kettering Memorial Hospital in New York City. Of the first group of patients who had three months of hormones followed by surgery, 74% of the men had organ-confined disease and only 13% had positive margins. The second group of men had surgery alone. Only 49% had cancer contained within the prostate and 36% had positive margins.

While these results seem impressive, the benefits began to blur when these patients were followed up in the clinic. One would expect the hormone-treated group to do a lot better. The standard used for freedom from prostate cancer is the PSA response. If the cancer is gone, the PSA should remain basically undetectable. Yet the Sloan Kettering researchers found that at both 35 months and 57 months, there was no significant difference in the PSA recurrence rate in the two groups. So, even though at the time of surgery it seemed as though the hormone-treated group had benefited substantially, this was not borne out on long-term follow-up. Because there appeared to be no increase in the time free from cancer and no survival advantage with neoadjuvant hormone use, urologists have shied away from them. Why subject patients to the side effects of hormones if they're no better off in the long run than with surgery alone? Why indeed?

Still, perhaps the reason hormones didn't have a lasting effect had to do with the length of time they were used. To test this hypothesis, a Canadian group led by Dr. Gleave used an eight-month course of androgen deprivation therapy instead of the standard three-month course prior to surgery. After eight months of hormones, nearly 90% of patients had reached a low point in their PSAs. Interestingly, after five months only 46% of men had reached a PSA nadir. At three months, only 28% had PSAs that had bottomed out. It appears that a wide majority of patients require more than three months to reach a PSA nadir. In Gleave's group of men, 74% had no sign of cancer outside their prostate and only 6% had positive margins when they finally did have surgery. More impressively, after a two-year follow-up, only 9% of the hormone-treated men had a PSA relapse. This might be due to long-term lingering effects of the hormones. More time is needed for evaluation. The medical community will closely follow the progress of these men over the next few years.

More studies need to be done to confirm Gleave's findings. Even so, his results, combined with the results of other investigators, indicate that longer use of hormones prior to surgery may be advantageous. Studies done combining hormones with radiation, as an alternative to surgery, strongly indicate that at least eight months of hormone therapy may be necessary for optimal results for all but low-risk cancers, and perhaps as long as three years. For T-3 disease, at least two years of hormones combined with external beam radiation is becoming the standard. Since many men have their cancer understaged (the extent of the disease is worse than previously assessed), it seems reasonable that men who are found to have T-3 disease at the time of surgery might also benefit from a longer course of hormones. Just how long is enough is a key issue. In both surgery and radiology, studies are currently underway to determine the optimal time for using hormones. What seems clear, however, is that more than three months is required.

Another open issue is whether hormones have any role after surgery, as they do after radiation. I think that over the next few years you'll see hormones play an increasingly important role in combination with both surgery and radiation in the treatment of prostate cancer.

Key References

Messing E et al. Immediate hormonal therapy compared with observation after radical prostatectomy and pelvic lymphadenectomy in men with node-positive prostate cancer. *New England Journal of Medicine* 1999; 341: 1781-1788.

Catalona WJ and Smith DS. Cancer recurrence and survival rates after anatomic radical retropubic prostatectomy for prostate cancer: intermediate term results. *J Urology* 1998; 160: 2428-2434.

Pound C, Partin A, Walsh P et al. Natural history of progression after PSA elevation following radical prostatectomy. *JAMA* 1999; 281: 1591-1597.

Valicenti et al. Durable efficacy of early postoperative radiation therapy for high-risk pT3 N0 prostate cancer: the importance of radiation dose. *Urology* 1998; 52: 1034-1040.

Klotz L et al. CUOG randomized trial of neoadjuvant androgen ablation before radical prostatectomy: 36 months post-treatment PSA results. *Urology* 1999; 53: 757-763.

Klein E et al. Initial dissection of the lateral fascia reduces the positive margin rate in radical prostatectomy. *Urology* 1998; 51: 766-773.

Walsh P. Anatomic radical prostatectomy: evolution of the surgical technique. *J Urology* 1998; 160: 2418-2424.

Seminal-Vesicle Involvement Found At Surgery

If cancer is found in the seminal vesicles (small sacks) at surgery, this is a poor sign. But it's not as serious as lymph-node metastases. We know from Dr. Messing's work that the immediate use of hormones often results in long-term remission in men with lymph-node involvement. But what if the seminal vesicles are involved? Should hormones be started immediately?

First, it's important to note that seminal vesicle involvement (SVI) can be broken down to evaluate the risk of the cancer progressing. According to a study led by senior author Dr. David Wood, Professor of Urology at Wayne State University in Detroit, not all SVI cases have the same risk. Dr. Wood's group evaluated 93 men who had SVI without lymph-node metastases. He reported his results in the *Journal of Urology*. The following charts summarize this group's findings:

Lowest Risk Profile for Progression of Cancer with SVI
> Negative surgical margins
> Pre-surgery PSA of 10 or less
> Gleason score of 6 or less

Highest Risk Profile for Progression of Cancer with SVI
> Positive surgical margins
> PSA greater than 10
> Gleason score 7 or more

Dr. Wood found that each of these factors independently predicted risk, but that the status of the surgical margins was a highly significant factor. Put another way, men with negative surgical margins have a much better chance of being free from metastases seven years or more after surgery than men with positive surgical margins.

There's no question that men with SVI and positive margins need to be treated aggressively. Local external beam radiation and hormonal therapy are probably indicated for this high-risk group. But if the surgical margins are clear, the appropriate treatment is not as clear. Some doctors will closely monitor the PSA and add hormones if the PSA rises. Others will recommend starting hormones immediately for two years. If it were my decision, I'd want two years of hormones, even if the surgical margins were negative. If the cancer has reached the seminal vesicles, in my view, there's a good chance that cancer cells have escaped into the blood or lymph systems. Hormones can help kill these cells. I wouldn't want to risk letting them get established. So I'd go for the hormones and deal with the side effects.

Having used hormones for 27 months, I believe the side effects are manageable for most men, especially if they're willing to modify their lifestyles (see "Hormones"). This decision must be made in close consultation with your doctors. As previously stated, having a medical oncologist on your team who specializes in prostate cancer will be a big help in the on-going decision-making process. The risk of the cancer advancing must constantly be weighed against the side effects from treatment. In each case, the ultimate decision is a personal one between a man and his partner.

Key References
Tefilli M et al. Prognostic indicators in patients with seminal vesicle involvement following radical prostatectomy for clinically localized prostate cancer. *J Urology* 1998; 160: 802-806.

How to Estimate Your Risk of Future Distant Metastases After Surgery

What every man wants to know after surgery is, "Am I cured?" No doctor can tell you with certainty that you're cured. Even men with the lowest Gleason scores (2-4) and pre-surgical PSAs (0-4), and organ-confined disease, have a 5%-10% chance of having a rising PSA at some point. Although this is not certainty, the chance of cure is excellent. At the other end of the spectrum, men with a Gleason score of 8-10 with an initial PSA of 35, SVI, and positive surgical margins have virtually a 100% chance of having a rising PSA within two years without additional treatment.

Studies have shown that if PSA starts rising within the first year after radical prostatectomy, there's a high probability that the cause of this increase is distant (away from the prostate) microscopic areas of cancer. Dr. Cadeddu and his colleagues at Johns Hopkins found that when radiation was used to try to control rising PSAs within a year of surgery, only 6% of the men treated responded. This strongly indicates that the cancer cells are outside the reach of the radiation beam (e.g., in distant locations). Men with rising PSAs in the first year after surgery (10 months in the Johns Hopkins study) should give serious consideration, in consultation with their doctors, to starting hormones immediately. Most medical oncologists now believe it's best to attack remaining cancer cells before they increase in number and be-

---

• A rising PSA in the first year after surgery is associated with micro-metastases in places distant from where the prostate was removed. Hormonal therapy is often needed to treat this, especially if tests fail to show local recurrence.

• A rising PSA two of more years after surgery is more likely to be associated with cancer recurring in the area of the removed prostate. Radiation therapy is often more suitable for these men.

• A rising PSA more than 1 year but less than 2 years after surgery is more favorable than one that rises in the first year, but not as favorable as a rising PSA 2 or more years from the time of surgery.

• All men with a rising PSA after surgery should have tests, like an endorectal MRI and a ProstaScint scan, to try to establish where the cancer has recurred.

come well-established.

If the PSA rises after two years, there's a greater chance that the recurrence is in the area where the prostate was removed. You have a decent chance of this being cured by radiation (see page 133). As you can see, *when* the PSA starts rising, if it does at all, makes a difference. The further away from the time of surgery the better.

So is there a way to determine your chances of having a rising PSA within the first two years after surgery? There is. Once again, credit for this work goes to Dr. Anthony D'Amico and his group at Harvard. They combined the preoperative PSA with several parameters determined at surgery—Gleason score in the removed cancer, margin status (positive or negative), and pathological stage (organ-confined, extra-capsular extension, SVI, etc.). Then they determined the chances of a rising PSA within two years of surgery using these parameters in combination. Their results are presented below courtesy of Dr. D'Amico and the *Journal of Urology*.

From these graphs you can determine your risk of PSA failure. Then you can decide if this risk is great enough to consider additional treatment.

How much risk is enough to get treatment? This question must be answered individually. Dr. D'Amico considers a more then 50% chance of PSA failure to be "high-risk." But he's quick to caution that this assessment will vary amongst doctors and patients. By starting with knowledge of the probabilities of PSA failure, it's easier to make a cogent decision on additional treatment.

Key Reference

D'Amico A et al. The combination of preoperative prostate specific antigen and postoperative pathological findings to predict specific antigen outcome in clinically localized prostate cancer. *J Urology* 1998; 160: 2096-2101.

Predicting Postoperative Prostate
Specific Antigen (PSA) Outcome

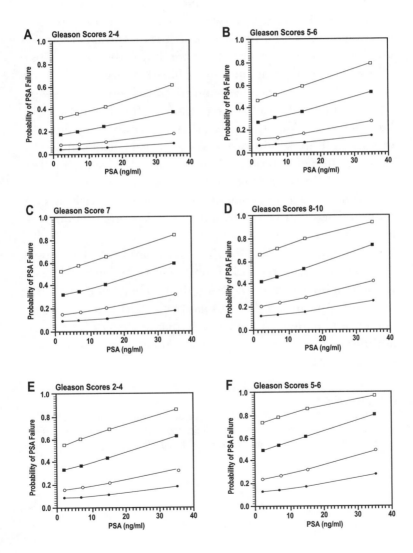

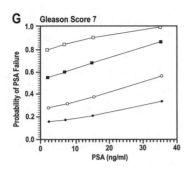
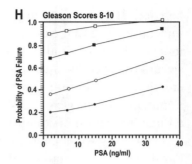

Reprinted by permission from Anthony D'Amico, M.D., and the *Journal of Urology*.

The Effects of Surgery or Radiation on Sexuality

One of the most common problems, but least discussed by both doctor and patient, is the impact of treatment on sexual function. The most common sexual side effect from treatment with surgery, radiation, or seeds is the inability to attain and maintain erections. Medically known as "erectile dysfunction" or "impotency," this problem is estimated to affect 20-30 million American men in the population at large, yet according to Dr. Hellstrom at the 2002 annual AUA meeting, "Surprisingly only 1 in 10 of these men has conferred with his physician about his 'problem.'"

Given this situation in the general male population, it's small wonder that many men being treated for prostate cancer don't discuss sexual implications with their doctors. Even when the subject of sex is broached, discussions are often brief.

Here are some facts that I believe are important for men to know.

• Doctors define potency as the ability to have an erection sufficiently durable for sexual penetration. Treatment often results in a semi-hard erection capable of penetration, but less than fully satisfactory to its wielder. Oral agents, like Viagra or Cialis, may help sustain hardness and should be tried. If they fail to improve the situation, Caverject, an injectable drug that can be self-administered, often provides long-lasting sustainable erections. A close friend of mine swears by Caverject, claiming that he is able to maintain an erection for 2 hours! Considering that he was completely impotent after surgery and Viagra was no help, this has made a huge impact on his quality of life.

• Surgery (by a good surgeon) and radiation have comparable rates of erectile dysfunction.

• Treatment for prostate cancer usually causes "dry" orgasms. Although there is often no decrease in sensation or contractions, you may well be shooting blanks. So long as you're aware of this possibility, it's usually no big deal.

• Some men may wind up with a curved penis when erect. This condition, known as Peyronie's Disease, may be the result of scarring from treatment. A new treatment for this difficult-to-treat condition is being developed in Switzerland. Using a machine called the Minilith that delivers small electrical shocks to the penis, a new study shows that 79% of men experienced significant improvement in the penile curvature and there was also a significant improvement in the ability to have erections. This machine is being developed by Storz Medical in Kreuzlingen, Switzerland. If you suffer from Peyronie's Disease, you might want to contact this company for an update on availability.

• Viagra should be used early in men who have had nerve-sparing radical prostatectomies, according to a new study. One hundred milligrams of Viagra taken every other night for 6 months after surgery increased the smooth muscle content of the penis. Theoretically, this should improve potency, although this has yet to be proven. (For more on the use of Viagra and other new impotency drugs see page 124.)

Key Reference
Hellstrom W. Update: Managing Sexual Dysfunction. Disclosures from the American Urological Association 97th Annual Meeting, May 25-30. 2002.

As you can see, there are a number of significant sexual issues that arise from treatment of prostate cancer. For men who are still sexually active, an in-depth discussion of these issues with your doctors is advisable.

Risk of Impotency After Surgery

For most men, one of the scariest things about prostate surgery is the risk of impotency. We discussed this briefly earlier in the section, but it's important to explore this area more extensively.

First of all, all men are infertile (they can't make babies) after radical prostatectomy due to removal of the seminal vesicles. This doesn't mean that you can't achieve an erection and climax. However, ejaculations are "dry." The contraction (feeling) is there, but no fluid comes out. Don't be alarmed about this. It's normal.

The question is whether or not you'll retain sexual potency. Sexual potency, in medical terms, refers to the ability to achieve an erection sufficient to have intercourse without medical assistance. Medical assistance includes penile injections and the use of prosthetic devices. Viagra is a special case. Since it's so easy to use and its use is becoming so widespread, some investigators lump it in with their general results of success in restoring sexual function.

I've covered it before, but it can't be overemphasized: The single most important factor in regaining sexual potency after a radical prostatectomy is the skill of the surgeon. No guarantess, but you'll significantly improve your chance of remaining sexually competent.

The standard of comparison for urologists when it comes to the ability to have erections after surgery is the work of Dr. Patrick Walsh at Johns Hopkins. As you'll recall, Dr. Walsh invented the nerve-sparing operative procedure. This resulted in many men retaining their erectile function after surgery. In Dr. Walsh's hands, including the use of Viagra, sexual function returned gradually to most men post-surgery. By 18 months, 86% of the men who were potent prior to surgery had regained their potency.

It should be noted that this data, reported in the June 2000 edition of the *Journal of Urology*, referred to only a small sample of 62 men.

Earlier in this chapter we discussed Dr. Catalona's experience with potency. In this study (presumably without Viagra), 68% of men (543 out of 798) whose erectile nerves were saved bilaterally (on both sides) regained potency; 47% (28 out of 60) regained potency with unilateral (one-side) nerve-sparing surgery. Viagra is particularly helpful for this group of men with only one nerve bundle left. Sometimes it's necessary to remove the nerve bundle on one or both sides due to cancer involvement. If both nerve bundles are cut, there's no chance of a spontaneous return of erectile function—unless a sural nerve graft is done at the time of surgery (see next section).

Key References

Walsh P. Radical prostatectomy for localized prostate cancer provides durable cancer control with excellent quality of life: a structured debate. *J Urology* 2000; 163: 1802-1807.

Catalona W et al. Potency, continence and complication rates in 1,870 consecutive radical retropubic prostatectomies. *J Urology* 1999; 162: 433.

A New Procedure During Surgery To Help Reduce Impotency

When men go to sleep prior to prostate surgery, one of their last memories often includes worries about impotency. The surgeon has told him that, although he will try to save the cavernous nerves responsible for erections, he can make no guarantees. If the cancer involves one or both nerve bundles, he will have to remove the involved nerves to give the man the greatest chance of cure.

And when men wake up, their first question is usually about their erectile nerve bundles.

A new procedure has been developed by urologists at Baylor and M.D. Anderson in Texas. They remove a small nerve, called the sural nerve, from behind a man's ankle and attach it to the severed stump of the nerve that has had to be removed due to cancer. This procedure must be done at the time of the radical prostatectomy. It can't be done later. Although by late 1999 they had performed this transplant on only 14 men, four (28%) had complete return of sexual function and seven others (50%) had partial erections. Since nerves grow very slowly, it remains to be seen whether the seven men with partial erections can continue to improve.

If this procedure continues to look as good as is indicated by these preliminary cases, it will unquestionably become part of standard surgical practice. A great number of cases of impotency from surgery will then be a thing of the past.

8

RADIATION

What Is Radiation Therapy?

Radiation therapy uses high-intensity beams to destroy cancer cells. Because prostate cancer is often growing in multiple locations in the prostate, radiation attempts to destroy the entire prostate—both cancer and normal prostate cells.

There are two classes of radiation treatments. The first, called external beam radiation therapy (EBRT), uses a device that looks like an extra-large version of the X-ray machine you see in almost all dental offices. But instead of employing the low-energy particles used for dental diagnoses, this machine uses a linear accelerator that creates a high-energy beam of radiation that kills cells by disrupting their DNA. Since the beam comes from outside the body, it's called external beam radiation.

The beams are formed by tiny sub-microscopic particles, such as photons, protons, neutrons, or combinations thereof. Photons are by far the most common. But in qualified hands, a combination of proton and photon radiation also appears to produce excellent results. Neutrons are not used clinically, because studies have shown no increased long-term response to these particles. Also, they have more side effects and are more expensive. Neutrons are being tried experimentally as a follow-up treatment, when surgery fails to provide cure.

The second category of radiation therapy uses internal emissions of radiation directly into the prostate from small radioactive "seeds," each about the size of the point of a pencil. These seeds can be placed permanently, using radioactive Iodine-131 or Palladium-103, or temporarily using Iridium-192 placed in removable tubes. This temporary set-up is known as "high-density radiation therapy." This technique was in the public spotlight a few years back when Andy Grove, Chief Executive Officer of Intel Inc., chose it as part of his therapeutic regime. Internally generated radiation is called brachytherapy. More commonly, it's referred to simply as "seeds."

Modern computer technology and improvements in imaging techniques, like the endorectal MRI, have allowed for significant improvements in both EBRT and brachytherapy. Let's examine the current state of the art.

External Beam Radiation Therapy (EBRT)

With all radiation, generally speaking, the higher the radioactive dose to the cancer cells, the greater the chances of cure. The problem is that radiation also kills normal cells in the organs surrounding the prostate—specifically, the bladder and rectum. The trick is to provide a maximal dose to the cancer, while minimizing the amount of radiation exposure to the bladder and rectum.

3-D Conformal Radiation Therapy (3-D CRT)

Conventional radiation for prostate cancer treats a square-shaped area. Everything in this area gets blasted. Therefore, this technique is limited in the amount of radiation that can be administered without serious bowel or bladder complications.

3-D conformal radiation therapy uses modern science and computer technology to create a radiation beam that closely conforms to the shape of a man's prostate. The radiologist usually factors in about a one-centimeter margin to account for daily movement of the prostate, as well as any tumor that may have penetrated the capsule. With the help of biophysicists, the exact angle and shape of the radiation beam from six to eight different positions is carefully calculated. The beam is shaped exactly to the prostate. This way the prostate gets far more radiation than the surrounding tissues. In addition, sophisticated blocking techniques are used to shield the bladder and rectum from receiving too much radiation. With 3-D CRT, substantially higher radiation doses can be delivered to the prostate than with conventional radiation. This dose escalation delivers more cancer-killing radiation to the tumor. There are also fewer serious side effects with 3-D CRT.

3-D CRT isn't available everywhere, but it is available in enough places in the U.S. that conventional radiation should not be considered. Outside the U.S. is a different story. In New Zealand, for example, 3-D CRT generally uses only four positions and delivers just 66 Gy of radiation, compared to 73.8 Gy, or more, in the United States (see "Treatment Down Under").

Besides precise planning of the contours of the radiation beam, 3-D CRT also depends on exact positioning of the patient each day. To accomplish this, the patient must be immobilized. The feet can be kept from moving using what's called a "cradle," a foam-like plastic mold that is contoured to the back of a man's legs up to just past his knees. By fixing the cradle in the same place on the radiation table every day and placing the patient in the same position in the cradle, his position is fixed. With 3-D CRT precision is the name of the game. As techniques continue to improve, higher and higher doses can be safely delivered.

Within the prostate itself, particularly high doses can be focused specifically on the main tumor areas. This technique is termed "intensity modulated radiation therapy (IMRT)." We'll discuss this exciting new technique in detail later. Top radiologists believe this will become the new standard for radiation treatment in the near future. It's currently available only at selected institutions in the United States.

3-D CRT Dose Escalation

The dose of radiation is measured in units called "rads." A hundred rads equals one Gray (Gy). Conventional prostate radiation delivers 6,400-6,600 rads, or 64 to 66 Gy. 3D-CRT delivers much more. I had 73.8 Gy. At the time of my radiation therapy in April 1999, the highest doses in the United State were 81 Gy. This was available only at one hospital—Sloan Kettering Memorial in New York City. At the time of this writing, some 15 months later, Sloan Kettering is still the leader in dose escalation. Now they can safely deliver 90 Gy to the tumor by combining IMRT with 3D-CRT. Other hospitals have also increased their doses. The hospital where I was treated, the University of Washington in Seattle, now goes up to 81 Gy using IMRT.

Radiation is given daily for eight to nine weeks. The actual time under the machine is just a few minutes, but with waiting time, dressing, and undressing, it takes an hour at the hospital. The usual dose is 1.8 Gy per day. There is no treatment on weekends or holidays. There is no pain whatsoever from the radiation itself.

The radiologists at Sloan Kettering have found that increasing the radiation dose is especially important in men with intermediate and unfavorable outlooks. They define the intermediate group as men with one of the following:
- PSA greater than 10;
- Gleason score greater than 6;
- clinical stage greater than T2;
- men with an unfavorable prognosis have at least two of the above signs.

Another leading radiation group is based at the Fox Chase Cancer Center in Philadelphia, Pennsylvania. Here, prolific researcher, Dr. Gerald Hanks, an artist in radiation therapy, has also studied the impact of dose escalation. He and his staff discovered that dose increases made a significant difference for most men, but not for men in either the lowest or highest risk groups. Favorable characteristics in this study included a PSA of less than 10 Gleason score of 6 of less, a T1 or T2a clinical stage, and no perineural invasion. Unfavorable characteristics included a PSA of 20 or more, Gleason score of 7-10, T2b-T3 clinical stage, and perineural invasion. PSAs of 10.0-19.9 were intermediate in outcome.

The group that seemed to benefit most from dose escalation consisted of men with PSAs over 20ng/ml and Gleason scores of 2 to 6. Here, dose increases to 76-77 Gy improved outcome, as determined by five-year PSA data, by 40%! Most other groups responded positively to dose escalation, though not so dramatically. But men with PSAs over 20 and a Gleason score of 7 to 10 did not benefit from this dose escalation. Most medical oncologists would combine hormones with radiation in this high-risk group. Dr. Hanks' work reaffirms the appropriateness of this approach, while also showing the improvement that most men will reap from higher doses of 3D-CRT. He concludes, "The national practice must be upgraded to allow the safe administration of 75-80 Gy 3-D CRT."

In a report given at the 40th Annual ASTRO Meeting in 1999, Dr. Hanks also presented data showing that radiation doses of less than 74 Gy (median 72 Gy) were associated with a significantly higher rate of metastases than higher doses (median 76 Gy).

This is the first report to strongly indicate that lower doses have more risk of metastases. Ultimately, this conclusion should translate into a diminished life expectancy for low-dose radiation as compared with higher doses, but this has yet to be conclusively proven—due, primarily, to the slow progression of many prostate cancers, which makes mortality comparisons difficult. Of course, none of us prostate cancer survivors finds this slow cancer progression to be objectionable, despite the difficulties this presents to investigators.

The clear direction being taken by radiology departments

across the nation is to continue to perfect dose-escalating procedures. If your PSA is over 10 or your Gleason score is 7 or higher, or if you have perineural invasion on biopsy, shoot for at least 75-80 Gy if you choose radiation. Look for a center that offers IMRT. Also, give strong consideration to adding androgen-blocking hormones to your treatment plan. I chose to add 27 months of androgen-ablating hormones to my 73.8 Gy of radiation for my Gleason 7, PSA 11.2 cancer, and I'm glad I did. My PSA is now 0.3 and stable four years after radiation.

Key References

Zelefsky M et al. Dose escalation with three-dimensional conformal radiation therapy affects the outcome in prostate cancer. *Int J Radiat Oncol Biol Phys* 1998; 41: 491-500.

Hanks G et al. Dose selection for prostate cancer patients based on dose comparison and dose response studies. *Int J Radiat Oncol Biol Phys* 2000; 46: 823-832.

Side Effects From 3-D CRT

Although 3-D CRT has fewer side effects than conventional radiation therapy, a number of men will develop bowel and/or bladder symptoms. Fortunately, these are usually minor and controllable with medication. Bowel symptoms can include diarrhea, bloating, cramping, and mucus and/or blood in the stools. Although no medical studies prove it, a man's attitude, activity level, and general state of health seem to reduce symptoms.

Diarrhea is the most common bowel symptom. It can generally be controlled with Lomotil. Occasionally, it's sufficiently severe that radiation therapy must be suspended for up to a week. For most men, however, if they get diarrhea, it's a controllable nuisance during therapy. Some men have little or no diarrhea. I was fortunate enough to be one of them.

Mucus or blood in the stools can sometimes alarm men

having radiation. These are usually painless discharges that come from irritation and inflammation of the cells lining the rectum. Blood can appear in the form of thin strands, often mixed with mucus, in bowel movements, or it may be visible on the toilet tissue. Occasionally, greater quantities of bright red blood are excreted. It's rare, however, for medical intervention to be required to stop the bleeding.

Note that there's an increased risk of bowel problems in diabetics and in men receiving radiation doses higher than 75.6 Gy without IMRT.

Bladder symptoms include frequent urination (both day and night), urgency (need to quickly find a toilet), start-and-stop urination, and more rarely, burning (usually mild) on urination. As with the bowel symptoms, these are generally manageable with medication.

Both bowel and bladder symptoms, if any, usually disappear gradually within a few weeks of the end of treatment.

How Common Are Bowel and Bladder Side Effects?

In a report from the Joint Center for Radiation Therapy at Harvard Medical School, researchers observed that 39% of men undergoing EBRT had some rectal complications after treatment. However, only 14% of the men receiving EBRT had symptoms severe enough to require treatment. Similarly, 33% had bladder-related symptoms, but only 9% required treatment.

Men with diabetes, however, have a significantly higher chance of developing lingering bowel and bladder problems after EBRT. These men are more prone to rectal bleeding requiring medical attention. They're also at significantly greater risk of rectal blockage, according to a study by Dr. Hanks at Fox Chase in Philadelphia. Dr. Hanks recommends more shielding of the rectum of diabetic men during radiation and careful consideration in selecting the radiation dose in these men.

Key References

Beard C et al. Radiation-associated morbidity in patients undergoing small-field external beam irradiation for prostate cancer. *Int J Radiat Oncol Biol Phys* 1998; 41: 257-262.

Herold D, Hanlon A, and Hanks G. Diabetes mellitus: An independent predictor of significant late complications after external beam radiotherapy. Proceedings of the 40th Annual ASTRO meeting. 1999; *Abstract 2167*.

Impotency and Radiation Therapy

As with all treatments for prostate cancer with the exception of lifestyle changes, external beam radiation therapy (EBRT) increases the risk of impotency. About 60% of men capable of erections sufficient for intercourse before EBRT will still be capable of having intercourse after EBRT. With Viagra this percentage increases. The risk of impotency with EBRT is comparable to nerve-sparing surgery.

A small study led by Dr. Sumita Kedia from the Cleveland Clinic was done on 21 men who had lost the ability to have erections after radiation. Seventy-one percent of these men regained the ability to achieve firm erections immediately after the use of Viagra. This is great news. Similar results have been reported with Viagra for impotency secondary to seed implants (see "Brachytherapy"). For many men it now appears that, if radiation therapy results in impotency, there's now an answer: Viagra. Two new drugs for impotency with fewer side effects than Viagra, according to studies, should be out by the end of 2003. One of these, Cialis, is currently available in New Zealand. Not only does it seem to have fewer side effects than Viagra, its effects last up to 36 hours, providing more flexibility as well as more rigidity.

Key Reference

Kedia S et al. Treatment of erectile dysfunction with sildenafil citrate (Viagra) after radiation therapy for prostate cancer. *Urology* 1999; 54: 308-312.

Intensity-Modulated Radiation Therapy (IMRT)

IMRT is a new innovation that improves the effectiveness of conformal radiotherapy. IMRT uses computer-control to "paint" the prostate with different doses of radiation. This technique, pioneered at Sloan Kettering Memorial Hospital in New York City, selectively and precisely increases radiation doses to areas of the prostate involved with cancer. The results are impressive. Here are the 3-year results of treatment with IMRT on 772 men at Sloan Kettering (698 received 81 Gy and 74 received 86.4 Gy):

Non-Rising 3-year Actuarial PSA Stratified by Risk (no PSA rise)

low-risk—92%

intermediate-risk—86%

high-risk—81%

Because IMRT zeros in on the prostate, it creates fewer urinary and rectal side effects. Twenty-eight percent of men in this study had manageable urinary symptoms shortly after radiation. Only 4.5% had moderate, manageable, rectal symptoms during radiation therapy.

As for late side effects from radiation that occur about 2

• IMRT increases the effectiveness and decreases the toxicity of radiation therapy.

• IMRT delivers increased radiation to areas involved with cancer with high precision.

• IMRT is becoming the standard for external beam radiation therapy. New methods are currently being developed to determine tumor sensitivity to radiation and to increase the dose of radiation to tumor areas that may be more resistant to the effects of radiation.

years or more after radiation, 9% had urinary symptoms and 1.5% had rectal bleeding. Only 4 men out of the 772 treated required laser treatment or transfusions (0.1% of the men) to stop this bleeding.

IMRT is now the standard mode of external beam radiation therapy at Sloan Kettering and will soon become the national standard. It is currently also available on the West Coast at the University of California Hospital in San Francisco. Contact Dr. Mack Roach. In the Philadelphia area, contact Dr. Gerald Hanks at Fox Chase. At the University of Washington in Seattle, contact Dr. Ken Russell.

Key References
   Zelefsky MJ et al. High-dose intensity-modulated radiation therapy for prostate cancer: early toxicity and biochemical outcome in 772 patients. *Int J Radiat Oncol Biol Phys* 2002; 53: 1111-1116.
   Zelefsky MJ et al. Intensity-modulated radiation therapy for prostate cancer. *Semin Radiat Oncol* 2002; 12: 229-237.
   Leibel SA et al. Intensity-modulated radiotherapy. *Cancer Journal* 2002; 8: 164-176.

Radiation Side Effects Compared to General Population

One study that particularly caught my eye came from biostatistician Alexandra Hanlon, in conjunction with Dr. Hanks at Fox Chase. They astutely observed that the effects of radiotherapy had never been compared with same-aged normal men. They reasoned that some older men had problems with urinary control and diarrhea and they compared the symptoms reported by men after EBRT with those normal men. What they found was remarkable. The number of "normal" men with these symptoms was about the same as men who had EBRT! Thirty-seven percent of men after EBRT had a minor problem with urinary control (dribbling); 38% of normal men had the same problem. Similarly, 33% had frequent urination after EBRT, but 31% of comparable aged men without prostate cancer also complained of this symptom.

With diarrhea, 37% of men who had 3-D CRT reported some problems, and 28% of men in the general population complained of similar problems.

This study indicates that the side effects of 3-D conformal EBRT may be over-reported in medical studies, since the incidence of these problems in elderly men in general has not been taken into account.

Proton Beam Radiation Therapy

As we've seen, the effectiveness of radiation therapy depends on two factors: the dose of radiation delivered to the cancer and its accuracy. The theory behind proton radiation therapy is that it's easier to control than standard photon radiation. Because protons are heavy particles, they don't scatter as much as photons. They can be directed to a precise shape and depth, which allows exact targeting of the cancer. This precision permits a high dose of radiation to the cancer, while minimizing the impact on healthy surrounding tissues.

Proton therapy was pioneered at Massachusetts General Hospital in the mid-1970s. It's currently only available at two hospitals in the United States: Massachusetts General in Boston and Loma Linda University Medical Center in San Bernardino, California. The equipment is very expensive, as is the treatment. Some medical insurers however, will pay for proton therapy.

Up until recently, no studies had been done that evaluated the five-year outcome of proton therapy. Now there are. And the results are impressive. The group at Loma Linda, under the direction of Dr. Carl Rossi, Jr., reported their five-year results in 1998. A group of 643 patients were treated with either protons alone, or protons combined with photons. Patients received a total of 74-75 Gy, comparable to current doses of 3-D conformal EBRT. Five years later, 89% of the treated men were clinically free from disease (no physical signs of cancer). With the more sensitive PSA testing, 79% had no elevation of PSA after five years. This compares very favorably with surgery and is better than most other radiation studies with the possible exception of IMRT. Five-year data for IMRT is currently unavailable, so a direct comparison is not possible yet.

The chart below shows the percentage of men that did not have a rising PSA after five years, categorized based on their initial PSA prior to proton therapy.

PSA prior to proton therapy	% of men free from rising PSA at five years
0.0-4.0	100%
4.1-10.0	89%
10.1-20.0	72%
Over 20.0	53%

A more recent report, this one in 1999 in the journal *Urology*, was even more impressive. Three hundred and nineteen men with early-stage prostate cancer were treated with a combination of protons and photons, or protons alone. Early-stage disease was defined as clinical stage T1-T2a or T2b and a pre-treatment PSA of 15 ng/ml, or less. In this group, 97% had no clinical signs of cancer, and 88% had no PSA rise, at five years. As before, 100% of men with pre-treatment PSAs of 0.0-4.0 were biochemically (as measured by PSA) free from cancer; 92% with initial PSA of 4.1-10.0, and 73% with pre-treatment PSAs of 10.1-15.0, were also biochemically disease-free. These results compare favorably with the best surgery and radiation reports.

I visited Loma Linda before deciding whether to have 3-D conformal EBRT (photons) or proton therapy. I was most impressed with the facility, the staff, and the technique. I met with Dr. Rossi and Dr. Nancy Reyes-Molyneux. They were as well-informed as any doctors I had spoken with, and better informed than most. They presented their results in a frank open fashion. The results spoke for themselves. I talked with a number of men undergoing the treatment. They were all delighted. Side effects appeared to be minimal.

The biggest complaint the men had related to the minor discomfort of having a balloon containing 120 cc of water inflated in their rectum each day prior to radiation. The purpose of this balloon is to immobilize the prostate so it doesn't move during proton therapy. The rest of the patient is immobilized in a full-body plastic cast so that they can't move during treatment. When body immobility is combined with the water balloon that fixes the prostate, pinpoint accuracy can be achieved.

I was nearly convinced while at Loma Linda that this technique was better than 3-D conformal radiation therapy, especially for men like me with a PSA between 10 and 15 and a moderately aggressive Gleason score of 7. The results available at the time were about the same as 3-D conformal EBRT, and the cost for protons (about $50,000) was more than twice that of EBRT. With the release of data in the 1999 study, were I to make the decision today on radiation therapy, I believe I would select protons or IMRT—if I could afford them or convince my insurance company to pay for the treatment.

Key References

Slater J et al. Conformal proton therapy for prostate carcinoma. *Int J Radiat Oncol Biol Phys* 1998; 42: 299-304.

Slater J et al. Conformal proton therapy for early-stage prostate cancer. *Urology* 1999; 53: 978-984.

Can The Effectiveness
of Radiation Be Predicted?

Regardless of whether you chose photons or protons, after you finish radiation you'll want to know if it worked.
Tracking your PSA will give you the best indication. Radiation works gradually, killing cancer cells as they attempt to
multiply. Radiation damages DNA and kills cells as they divide. Prostate cancer is slow growing, hence slow dividing as
well. Radiation takes two years of more to kill all the cancer
cells in the prostate and surrounds. So your PSA should slowly
decline. Although it may seem counterintuitive, the longer
your PSA takes to reach a low point the better, so long as it
keeps steadily declining. The lowest point your PSA reaches
is called the "PSA nadir."

Men with a PSA nadir of 0.5 ng/ml or less have the best
prognosis. When this nadir is reached two or more years after radiation, the chances of cure are superb. A 1998 study
by Dr. Mark Ritter and his colleagues at the University of
Wisconsin Medical School showed that 92% of men who
reached a PSA nadir of 0.5 ng/ml or less within one to two
years of treatment maintained PSAs at this level five years
later. When the PSA nadir was reached in two to three years,
100% remained biochemically free from cancer as measured
by their PSAs.

With proton therapy and PSA nadirs of 0.5 ng/ml or less,
similar outcomes are found. In men with T1, T2a, or T2b
disease, 98% who reached this nadir level were biochemically
free from cancer five years later. Note that this report included
all men who received proton therapy, including those who
reached a PSA nadir in less than two years. Sixty-five percent
of the men with early-stage cancer achieved a PSA nadir of
0.5 ng/ml, or less; 23% reached a nadir between 0.51 and
1.0; 12% had a PSA nadir of greater than 1.0 ng/ml. Remember, even if you don't reach a PSA nadir of 0.5 ng./ml, you still
have an excellent chance of cure. In the proton therapy study,

88% of men with nadirs of 0.51-1.00 did not have a rising PSA five years after radiation, nor did 41% of those with nadirs greater than 1.0 ng/ml.

Is there a way to get a handle on the likelihood that your PSA nadir will be 0.5 ng/ml, or less? There is. The best indicator of PSA nadir is pre-treatment PSA level. With proton therapy, 83% of men with T1-T2b prostate cancer and a pretreatment PSA of 0.0-4.0 ng/ml had PSAs that dropped below 0.5 ng/ml at some point after treatment. This compares with 66% of men with PSAs of 4.1 to 10.0 ng/ml and 48% for men whose starting PSA was 10.1-15.0 ng/ml. Here again, early detection through PSA screening can detect cancers while PSA levels are still low (under 10). As you can see, most of these cancers are curable.

Pretreatment PSA levels also predict the outcome with photon EBRT. In a multi-institution study of more than 1,500 men coordinated by Dr. William Shipley at Massachusetts General Hospital, men with starting PSAs of 9.2 ng/ml or less had an 81% chance of having a low stable PSA five years out. This dropped to 69% if the PSA was between 9.2 and 19.7 ng/ml. Out of the 302 men in this study who were biochemically free of disease by PSA testing and were followed for more than five years, only 5% (16/302) started having a rising PSA between five and eight years out. This is comparable to late PSA rises after radical prostatectomy.

Key Reference
Shipley W et al. Radiation therapy for clinically localized prostate cancer: a multi-institutional pooled analysis. *JAMA* 1999; 281: 1598-1604.

Selecting A Radiation Oncologist

As with surgeons, there are vast differences between radiation oncologists. Precision is the key. If the radiation misses the mark, and this happens more often than you might think, there will be two unpleasant consequences. First, obviously, not all the cancer will be killed. And second, the radiation is more likely to damage healthy tissues. Although I'm sure there are excellent radiotherapists who are not on the ensuing list, I'm confident you can rely on the doctors that are recommended here. Some of the top hospitals have more than one recommended therapist.

Recommended Radiation Oncologists

East

Anthony D'Amico	Harvard Univ. Med. School	Boston, MA
Zvi Fuks	Sloan Kettering Memorial Hospital	New York, NY
Gerald Hanks	Fox Chase Cancer Center	Phila., PA
Steven Leibel	Sloan Kettering Memorial Hospital	New York, NY
William Shipley	Mass. General Hospital	Boston, MA
Anthony Zietman	Mass. General Hospital	Boston, MA
Kent Wallner	Sloan Kettering Memorial Hospital	New York, NY
Michael Zelefsky	Sloan Kettering Memorial Hospital	New York, NY

South

Mitchell Anscher	Duke Univ. Medical School	Durham, NC
Brian Butler	Baylor Univ. Med. School	Houston, TX
Michael Dattoli	Tampa University	Tampa, FL
Deborah Kuban	East VA Medical School	Norfolk, VA
Alan Pollack	M.D. Anderson Hospital	Houston, TX
Scott Sailar	U. of North Carolina	Chapel Hill, NC
Gunnar Zagars	M.D. Anderson Hospital	Houston, TX

Midwest

Jeff Forman	Wayne State University	Detroit, MI
Coleen Lawton	Med. College of Wisconsin	Milwaukee, WI

Carlos Perez	Washington University	
	School of Medicine	St. Louis, MO
Howard Sandler	University of Michigan	Ann Arbor, MI
Srinivasan Vijayakumar		
	U. of Chicago Med. School	Chicago, IL

West

John Blasko	Private practice	Seattle, WA
Mack Roach III	U. of CA Medical School	San Francisco, CA
Ken Russell	Univ. of WA Hospital	Seattle, WA
Carl Rossi, Jr.	Loma Linda U. Hospital	San Bernardino, CA
Nancy Reyes-Molyneux		
	Loma Linda U. Hospital	San Bernardino, CA
Steven Hancock	Stanford U. Medical School	Palo Alto, CA
Zbigniew Petrovich	U. of S. California	Los Angeles, CA

Radiation After Unsuccessful Surgery (Salvage Radiation)

As previously discussed, one of the arguments favoring surgery is this: If it leaves any cancer cells behind, radiation is often successful in killing off the remnants. How successful is radiation after surgery? Dr. Thomas Pisansky at the Mayo Clinic in Minnesota reports that nearly half of the men who undergo both treatments can expect to be free from prostate cancer five years later, with undetectable PSA levels. In this study, Dr. Pisansky followed more than 100 men who had a rising PSA sometime after a radical prostatectomy. The average time after surgery was 17.5 months. The average PSA at the time of radiation was 1.3 ng/ml. Eighty-two percent of these men had reductions in their PSA levels immediately after radiation therapy. Note that these men received radiation while their PSA levels were still low (average 1.3 ng/ml).

A more recent study confirmed that men treated when

their PSA was 1.2 ng/ml or less were nearly twice as likely to be free of cancer five years later as those with higher PSAs.

Other investigators have confirmed the importance of early radiation treatment when surgery fails. So what's the best approach if there are positive surgical margins? Should men start radiation shortly after surgery or should they wait till the PSA starts rising? Since we know that in some studies about 50% of men with positive margins will have undetectable PSAs five years later without any treatment, it may seem tempting to wait and see what happens. Recent studies indicate, however, that waiting increases the risk of the cancer coming back.

Dr. Richard Valicenti and co-workers at Jefferson Medical College in Philadelphia studied men who were found to have T3 cancer at the time of surgery, but had undetectable PSA levels immediately after surgery. Some of these men received radiotherapy within three to six months of surgery, regardless of their PSA level. Others received treatment only if their PSAs started to rise. Dr. Valicenti's team matched these men in pairs, according to pre-operative PSA level (less than 10 vs. more than 10), Gleason score (less than 7 vs. 7 or more), seminal vesicle involvement, and positive surgical margins. Eighty-eight percent of the men who received early radiation regardless of their PSA levels had negligible stable PSAs 5 years later, compared to 53% of those who received only surgery. When the men with positive surgical margins were compared, 87% of those that got early radiation were biochemically disease-free by PSA measurements, compared to only 31% who got no immediate treatment.

Dr. Vicini and his colleagues at the Department of Radiation Oncology at William Beaumont Hospital in Michigan also found that treating with radiotherapy within six months of surgery due to unfavorable findings at surgery made a significant difference in five-year outcome. In this study, 67% of the men treated with radiation shortly after surgery could expect to have negligible PSA levels five years later.

In light of these two studies, and others, it's clear that

post-operative early radiation therapy is clearly warranted in men who have positive surgical margins after surgery, even if PSA levels are undetectable. I would certainly choose this route, and most radiation oncologists would concur. Side effects from post-operative radiation are usually minor, because the dose administered is less than that used when radiation is the primary treatment. In my opinion the rewards generally outweigh the risks. Exception would be men with long PSA doubling times where the PSA stays below 1.0 ng/ml for prolonged periods. Salvage radiation is always an option for these men, but some will never need it. Their cancers are so slow-growing that they're likely to die of other causes. Constructive lifestyle changes may slow these cancers down even more, while helping to protect against heart disease.

What to do about positive surgical margins if the PSA doesn't decline to undetectable levels after surgery? Since there's now an increased chance that some cancer cells have escaped beyond the target area, I would add hormonal therapy to the radiation. For how long? Probably two to three years. Hormonal therapy can reach cancer cells that have escaped into the blood or lymph systems.

Key References

Pisansky T et al. Radiatherapy for isolated serum prostate specific antigen elevation after prostatectomy for prostate cancer. *J Urology* 2000; 163: 845-850.

Vicini F et al. Treatment outcome with adjuvant and salvage irradiation after radical prostatectomy for prostate cancer. *Urology* 1999; 54: 111-117.

Valicenti R. The long-term efficacy of early adjuvant radiation therapy for pT3N0 prostate cancer: a matched-pair analysis. *Int J Radiat Oncol Biol Phys* 1998; 42 (supp): 178 (abstract 108).

Chawla A et al. Salvage radiotherapy after radical prostatectomy for prostate adenocarcinoma: analysis of efficacy and prognostic factors. *Urology* 2002; 59: 726-731.

Importance of PSA Level After Surgery for Successful Salvage Radiation

What happens to PSA after surgery is important in determining what to do next. If the PSA drops to undetectable levels initially, this is a good sign. Even if there are unfavorable findings at surgery, such as positive margins or seminal vesicle involvement, men with undetectable PSA levels after surgery do substantially better than men with continued elevation of PSA.

Dr. Ken Russell and his team at the University of Washington in Seattle found that men with undetectable PSAs after surgery did better with salvage radiotherapy, especially if their PSA was less than 1.0 ng/ml prior to radiation. He conducted a trial with neutron radiation in a small group of men with adverse findings at the time of surgery. Neutron radiation is experimental. It uses a heavy particle that has no charge. These characteristics theoretically allow for better targeting of the radiation beam and less scatter, similar to protons.

Dr. Russell studied 21 men, 16 of whom had seminal vesicle involvement or lymph-node metastases found at surgery. All of them had locally invasive cancers or worse. Dr. Russell found that if a man had an undetectable PSA after surgery and had a PSA of 1.0 ng/ml or less at the time of neutron radiation, he had a 76% chance of having an undetectable PSA level three years later. If the PSA either did not reach undetectable levels after surgery, or the PSA level exceeded 1.0 ng/ml at the time of radiation, only 14% had undetectable PSA three years later.

Other studies have confirmed the importance of PSA dropping to undetectable levels after surgery. If this does not occur, men should consider more aggressive treatment with immediate hormonal therapy, either by itself or combined with radiation.

New Ways to Rate the Chance of Radiation Therapy Failure

We've previously discussed the negative impact of the bcl-2 oncogene and mutations in the p53 tumor suppressor gene. A 1999 study out of Johns Hopkins shows that these two genetic events can significantly impact the outcome of radiotherapy. Eighty-five percent of men with positive bcl-2 tests (too much bcl-2) ultimately failed radiotherapy. Similarly, 88% of men with p53 mutations had unsuccessful radiation therapy. When both bcl-2 over-expression and p53 mutations tested positive, 100% of the men ultimately had cancer recurrence. In my mind, testing positive for either of these genetic abnormalities is an indication for sustained hormonal therapy. Drugs specifically designed to reduce bcl-2 levels are being developed. In the not-too-distant future, genetic modifications of bcl-2 and p53 will be possible.

Key Reference

Scherr D et al. Bcl 2 and p53 expression in clinically localized prostate cancer predicts response to external beam radiotherapy. *J Urology* 1999; 162: 12-16.

PSA Rising After Radiation

Once the PSA hits a low-point, if a man is cured, it should stay down. The longer it stays down, the better the chance of cure. Studies show that if the PSA nadir reaches 0.5 ng/ml or less and stays at this level for a year, the chance of a low, stable PSA 5 years out is 92%. If the PSA nadir is 0.5-1.0 ng/ml and stays there for a year, the chance of a low stable PSA five years later is reduced to 69%.

A recent study at the University of California-San Francisco showed that 70% of men with PSA nadirs of less than 1.2 ng/ml were biochemically (by PSA) free from cancer 4 years after radiation, compared with 40% of men with PSA nadirs of 1.2 ng/ml or more.

As you can see from the above statistics, some men will have a rising PSA at some point after radiation. An isolated increase in PSA doesn't necessarily mean that cancer cells still exist. The standard used for failure as measured by PSA is 3 *consecutive* increases in PSA. This standard was set by the American Society for Therapeutic Radiation Oncology

(ASTRO). This consistent rising PSA is usually accompanied by considerable anxiety. It means that radiation did not kill all the cancer cells. Additional radiation is not an option at this point, because the risk of irreparable damage to vital tissues is too high.

• The ASTRO standard to determine radiation failure for prostate cancer is 3 consecutive increases (of any amount) in PSA level.

• Men with a rising PSA within the first year of completed radiation therapy are considerably more likely to develop early metastases than men whose PSA starts rising later.

• The PSA nadir (lowest point after radiation) is important. Men with PSA nadirs of 1.2 ng/ml or more have nearly twice the risk of cancer recurrence as men with PSA nadirs of less than 1.2 ng/ml.

The first thing to do is to try to locate the remaining cancer cells. A ProstaScint scan and endorectal MRI may reveal the location of the recurrence. If it's found to be localized to the prostate, surgery, cryotherapy (freezing), or brachytherapy (seeds) are all viable options. Of course, at the risk of hammering this point home ad nauseum, the skill and artistry of accessible practitioners, in my opinion, should be the determining factor in treatment selection. It's especially critical after radiation, which leaves scar tissue in the prostate and surrounds. This makes any additional procedure more difficult than it would have been before radiation and, in turn, increases the risk of significant side effects.

So you've got to select whom to use carefully. This is a salvage procedure. Ask the prospective doctors about their experience with this procedure, their results, and side effects. Try to get as much information as to which side effects you might expect and how often other men undergoing the same procedure by the same doctor experienced these effects. If you're not satisfied that the rewards justify the risks, I suggest you not rush into anything. Explore other options. Choices other than an invasive procedure are available. Hormonal therapy is a viable option. Aggressive lifestyle adjustments may also help slow the growth of remaining cancer cells.

As always, each man must measure the potential benefits of any treatment against his individual tolerance to possible side effects. Each man views this equation a little differently. It comes down to a personal decision between a man, his partner, and his doctors.

Often, no cancer can be found despite extensive testing. When to receive treatment (usually hormone therapy) is the subject of much debate in the medical community. This is extensively reviewed in the chapter "Advanced Disease."

Key References

Boyd T et al. The prognostic significance of stable PSA intervals at varying follow-up times after definitive radiation therapy. *Int J Radiat Oncol Biol Phys* 1998; 42(supp): 298 (abstract 2141).

Raymond J, Vuong M, and Russell K. Neutron beam radiotherapy of recurrent prostate cancer following radical prostatectomy. *Int J Radiat Oncol Biol Phys* 1998; 41: 93-99.

Small E and Roach M. Prostate-specific antigen in prostate cancer: a case study in the development of a tumor marker to monitor recurrence and assess response. *Seminars in Oncology* 2002; 29: 264-273.

The Radiation Diet

At most radiation centers, a dietician will review your diet prior to radiation. Typically, he or she will recommend a low-fiber bland diet during therapy. Radiation can cause inflammation of the rectum, which can result in diarrhea. A low-fiber diet that includes ripe bananas helps to reduce diarrhea.

On the other hand, if you're eating a prostate cancer and heart-friendly diet as recommended in this book, you're consuming a lot of high-fiber foods. Abruptly reducing fiber intake can cause constipation in men eating a high-fiber diet at the time of radiation. Constipation is also undesirable because it can lead to straining and additional discomfort to an already irritated rectum. For this reason, dietary changes should be made gradually and proportionally to symptoms from the radiation.

If you're used to a high-fiber diet, as I was, it may be best to stay on your current diet with some modifications. Avoid uncooked vegetables and fruits, with the exception of ripe bananas. Using a blender to puree cooked fruits and vegetables will make them more digestible. Chewing food extra-thoroughly is also helpful.

Avoid foods that stimulate intestinal motility: coffee, alcohol, chilis, and raw fruits and vegetables.

Avoid foods that may be irritating to the intestines: chilis, horseradish, *wasabi* (Japanese horseradish used in sushi), corn, citrus fruit, fatty food, fried food, dairy products, raw onions and garlic (OK to eat cooked, especially if ground first).

> **HELPFUL HINTS**
>
> • Chew food extra thoroughly before swallowing. The better you chew, the easier to digest.
> • Puree vegetables in a blender after cooking. Mix with cooked fruits for great flavor combinations. Avoid raw fruits and vegetables.
> • Rice, pasta, potatoes, squash, spinach, carrots, tomatoes, beets, peas, zucchini, mushrooms, and fish (if you eat it) are easily handled. I continued to eat tofu with rice to get complete protein.
> • The better your starting health, the fewer dietary modifications will be required. Men in excellent health (except for the prostate cancer) should stick to their normal healthy diet with a few precautions as mentioned above until/unless symptoms develop. Avoiding stress may help reduce symptoms.
> • If you eat beets, it may turn your urine and/or feces red. Don't mistake this for blood.

Avoid gas-producing foods (unless you tolerate them well, they're well-cooked, and you use a blender): cruciferous vegetables (broccoli, cabbage, cauliflower, Brussels sprouts, bok choy, arugula, radishes), beans and lentils, and high-fiber cereals, like All Bran and Grape Nuts.

Unfortunately, most of the yummy things on a heart- and prostate cancer-friendly diet are high in fiber and could potentially be a problem. Pureeing helps. I was able to eat cooked pureed vegetables and fruits of all kinds, including crucifers, during radiation therapy. Some of my favorites: cooked spinach pureed with baked pears, cooked cauliflower pureed with baked apples, well-cooked potatoes pureed with soy milk to make mashed potatoes, baked spaghetti squash with pureed cooked tomatoes and pureed baked garlic, cooked rhubarb pureed with baked strawberries and baked apples, pureed baked apples and pears and berries served over sliced bananas, well-boiled summer squash soup, soy protein isolate drink with banana and baked pureed berries (I drank one each day). Although contemplating eating pureed foods may precipitate thoughts of regression to childhood, I can assure you based on personal experience, that this association can be overcome, and that this way of eating is highly effective during radiation.

9

BRACHYTHERAPY (SEEDS)

Brachytherapy (pronounced "brake-ee-therapy"), also known as seeds, uses internally placed rice-sized capsules of radioactive material. Seeds are made either of Iodine-125 or Palladium-103. The radioactive iodine seeds emit radiation of lower intensity, but longer duration, than palladium seeds. The seeds are implanted directly into the prostate. The brachytherapist uses an ultrasound monitor to guide the placement of the radioactive seeds into precise positions within the prostate. Proper seed placement insures accurate distribution of the radiation. This also can help reduce side effects by sparing the urethra from unneeded radiation. As you probably recall, the urethra passes through the middle of the prostate. Too much radiation to the urethra can produce significant urinary complications.

Seeds are an attractive option for many men. The procedure requires little or no hospitalization. There's no scar. Computers work out the correct number of seeds and their placement. The pellets are introduced into the prostate through thin tubes inserted just beneath the scrotum. The patient is either temporarily numbed from the waist down or put to sleep. The procedure is quick and it doesn't have some of the potential complications of surgery, such as bleeding.

The seeds remain in place permanently, but lose their radioactivity over time. Because the source of radiation is directly within the prostate, high doses of radiation can be delivered without harming surrounding tissues. The radioactivity of each seed only penetrates the area immediately surrounding it (about five millimeters).

It's perfectly safe for men to have children sit on their laps after seed implantation. There's also no danger to a man's sexual partner. Many men have sex within a few days of implantation. Don't be alarmed if your semen is dark red or black. This is normal after the procedure and may last for a month or so.

When Should Seeds Be Considered?

Although no randomized studies comparing seeds with other treatments for prostate cancer have been reported, substantial work has been done recently to determine which men with prostate cancer are most likely to benefit from seeds. It turns out that for low-risk cancer, seeds seem equally as effective as either surgery or EBRT. Low-risk is defined here and elsewhere in this book as a PSA of 10 or less, a Gleason score of 6 or less, and a clinical stage of T2a or less.

In a presentation made at the 40th Annual ASTRO meeting in 1999, Dr. D'Amico and his team at Harvard compared 1,800 men who had been treated with either surgery, EBRT, or seeds. For men in this low-risk group, roughly 85% had low and stable PSAs five years after treatment regardless of which of these three treatments they selected.

For intermediate cancers, seeds were less effective than either of the other two treatments. Intermediate disease was defined as a PSA of more than 10 but less than 20, and/or a Gleason score of 7 and/or clinical stage T2b. About 60% of men in this category were biochemically free from cancer as measured by PSA five years after either radical prostatectomy or EBRT. However, only 28% of men with this category of disease had comparable results using seeds. Interestingly, if hormonal therapy was administered for three months prior to seed implants, this group's five-year freedom from disease was again comparable to surgery and

EBRT! Adding three months of hormones significantly improved outcome in intermediate-risk patients who got brachytherapy.

In high-risk patients (PSA greater than 20, and/or Gleason score of 8 or more, and/or clinical stage T2c or more), seeds performed much more poorly than either surgery or EBRT. Even adding three months of hormones didn't help this group. While about 30% of high-risk patients who had surgery or EBRT were biochemically free from disease at the five-year mark, none of the high-risk patients treated with seeds, either with or without three months of hormones, had low and stable PSAs. They all had either rising PSAs or clinical signs of cancer.

These results were confirmed and amplified for low- and intermediate-risk patients by Dr. Nelson Stone and Dr. Richard Stock at Mt. Sinai Medical Center in New York City. Drs. Stone and Stock found that 91% of low-risk men treated with seeds alone were disease-free by PSA after four years. This will likely fall closer to the 85% of the D'Amico study when five-year data are available. The intermediate group in this study was treated with five months of hormones instead of three months, then seeds. Four-year results showed 85% percent were free from cancer (by PSA). These results look more promising than the D'Amico figures, quite possibly because the men in the Mt. Sinai study received an extra two months of hormones. Note that both of the above studies compared seeds with 3D-conformal EBRT without IMRT. Recent IMRT data indicate greater effectiveness and fewer side effects than standard 3D-conformal EBRT. IMRT may therefore be preferable to seeds plus hormones for intermediate-risk disease. Hormonal therapy can also be combined with IMRT to kill cancer cells that may have escaped into the system.

The high-risk group in this study was treated aggressively with seeds, plus EBRT and nine months of hormonal therapy. This group included men with PSAs greater than 15ng/ml, Gleason scores of 8 or higher, and/or clinical stage

T2c to T3. There were 40 men in this group. Half of them had biopsy-proven seminal vesicle involvement.

Whereas none of the high-risk men in Dr. D'Amico's study were free from disease after five years, even if they had three months of hormones before seeds, 71% of the high-risk men in Dr. Stone's study were disease-free by PSA after three years. These results must be viewed with caution until five-year results are available. Remember, these men received EBRT and hormones in addition to seeds, so they could reasonably be expected to do better than the men that received EBRT alone in Dr. Amico's high-risk group (30% disease-free after five years). A longer time is required to evaluate the effects of the nine- month hormone treatment these men received. It's well known that the effects of hormones remain long after they're discontinued. Studies have shown that a year or two after the cessation of hormone treatment, some men still have depressed testosterone levels. The low PSA levels after three years could, therefore, be due to lingering testosterone suppression in some of these men. Whether these men still have negligible PSA levels after five years remains to be seen.

If these results hold up, it will be encouraging news for men with high-risk disease. Evidence keeps mounting that adding hormones to EBRT, seeds, or both improves outcome for many men. How long to use hormones is an open question.

HELPFUL HINTS

• Consider using seeds alone for low-risk cancer. Studies show seeds to be as effective as surgery or EBRT for low-risk prostate cancer.
• Consider using seeds combined with hormones (I recommend at least 8-12 months) for intermediate-risk disease, although IMRT, if available, may be preferable.
• One option for high-risk disease may be a combination of seeds, EBRT, and hormones.

Key References

D'Amico A et al. Five-year biochemical outcome after radical prostatectomy, external beam radiation therapy, or interstitial radiation therapy for clinically localized prostate cancer. Proceeding of the 40th Annual ASTRO Meeting. 1999; *Abstract* 2147.

Stone N and Stock R. Prostate brachytherapy: treatment strategies. *J Urology* 1999; 162: 421.

Crook J et al. Systematic overview of the evidence for brachytherapy in clinically localized prostate cancer. *CMAJ* 2001; 164: 975-987.

Why Seeds Alone Are Insufficient For Intermediate-and High-Risk Prostate Cancer

Why does brachytherapy yield good results in men with low-risk cancer, but not for more aggressive disease? The answer may lie in the rate that the dose of radiation is delivered. Seeds, especially radioactive iodine, deliver the radiation slowly over time. Laboratory experiments on cancer cells indicate that, especially for more aggressive cancers, the dose rate is significant. Why? Because poorly differentiated cancer cells divide more rapidly than well-differentiated ones. Prostate cancer cells die when the accumulated dose is sufficient to disrupt cells that are trying to divide. With the slow-dose release of iodine seeds, there may not be enough radiation build-up in the faster dividing cancer cells to kill them when they divide. Adding hormones may sensitize these cells so that they're more responsive to the effects of radiation. Then they may be more likely to die when attempting to multiply. Hormones may also have a direct lethal effect on cancer cells. For these reasons, I-125 should not be considered for intermediate- or high-risk disease.

Radioactive palladium (Pd-103) delivers its radiation three times as fast as I-125. If seeds are used for intermediate-risk cancers, Pd-103 is preferable to I-125. Its faster dose rate is more likely to kill rapidly dividing cancer cells. It's most effective when combined with hormonal therapy.

Palladium-103 can be effective even if the cancer has penetrated the capsule of the prostate. Studies that exam-

ine surgically removed cancer specimens show that in 90%-
99% of cases, capsular penetration is limited to 4 millimeters (mm) or less. Pd-103 has an effective range of up to 5
millimeters. Its radiation output can, therefore, reach most
cancers that have penetrated the capsule, but have not
spread farther.

For low-risk cancer, Pd-103 and I-125 are both effective
in reaching cancer cells that may have penetrated the prostate capsule. Dr. Davis, Dr. Pisansky, Dr. Bostwick, and their
group at the Mayo Clinic found that in more than 100 men
with low-risk prostate cancer, the maximum amount of capsular penetration was a scant 0.6 mm. This is within easy
reach of both I-125 and Pd-103. So in low-risk cases, seeds
can be depended upon, if properly placed, to reach virtually
all cancers that have penetrated the prostate capsule.

Interestingly, recent studies have shown that Pd-103 seeds
used alone are equally effective as Pd-103 seeds combined
with EBRT. If this becomes well established, there will be no
reason to risk the additional side effects, costs, and inconvenience of adding EBRT to Pd-103 seed implants. Combining Pd-103 with hormones may be a more promising combination.

Key References
   Sohayda C et al. Extent of extracapsular extension in localized prostate cancer. *Urology* 2000; 55: 382-386.
   Davis B, Pisansky T, et al. The radial distance of extraprostatic extension of
prostate carcinoma: implications for prostate brachytherapy. *Cancer* 1999; 85:
2630-2637.

Side Effects of Seed Implants

Brachytherapy is becoming an increasingly popular option for men with low- to intermediate-risk prostate cancer.
Many men prefer this option, because it can be over and
done with in just a day, it's much easier on men than surgery,
and it's far less time-consuming than EBRT. Given the fact
that it's equally effective as surgery or EBRT in low-risk cases

and as effective when combined with hormones in intermediate-risk situations, seeds are often an attractive choice. In the modern PSA era, more and more men are having their prostate cancer diagnosed early, at a time when seeds are most effective.

Contrary to popular belief, however, seed implantation is not free from side effects. Although men may go home the same day as the procedure, urinary side effects are common within the first 60 days. In a multi-institutional New York study that included Sloan Kettering, 600 consecutive cases of seed implants were reviewed over a five-year period from 1992 to 1997. Seventy-three percent had Pd-103; 27% had I-125. Seventy percent of these treated men developed urinary symptoms after their procedures; 29% had to urinate frequently, but required little or no medication, while 38% had difficulty in starting their urine stream (urinary retention) and required medication to do so. Two percent of the men required tubes in their bladders to drain the urine or a surgical procedure (TURP) to regain their ability to urinate. Men with urinary symptoms prior to seed implants generally had more severe side effects. Also, men with larger prostates before seeds had more symptoms after implant. There was no significant difference in the urinary symptoms produced by I-125 or Pd-103. This is an interesting finding because some brachytherapists consider I-125 to be less toxic than Pd-103.

A fair number of men will have urinary symptoms that persist years after seed implants. In a separate study from the one above, radiation oncologists from Sloan Kettering reviewed the late side effects from I-125 seed implants in 245 patients. They found that 56% of the patients had urinary problems two to four years after seeds were implanted. Twelve men required surgery for urinary retention and 94 men (38%) had symptoms significant enough to require medication. About half the men with late urinary complications improved over the next two to three years to the point where they required little or no medication.

Some men also developed rectal symptoms in this study. Although less than with EBRT, about 13% experienced mild to moderate bowel problems. These generally resolved on their own over one to two years. Another study, also from Sloan Kettering, showed that rectal bleeding may be a problem for some men after seeds. In this group of 109 men, about 19% experienced the discharge of bright red blood from the rectum after I-125 seed implants. In about a third of these cases, the bleeding stopped without treatment between 9 and 48 months after it started. Half the cases required steroid enemas and roughly 15% (three men) required laser treatments to stop the bleeding. Although 15% of men with bleeding required laser therapy, this is less than 3% of the men who got I-125 (3/109).

Some groups have reported fewer bladder and bowel symptoms than Sloan Kettering. Just how common these symptoms are amongst men who have gotten seeds is debatable. I'd be a bit cautious in blindly accepting assurances that there are few, if any, side effects from seeds.

As for sexual complications, the Sloan Kettering study and others show that about 60% of men who were potent prior to receiving seeds remained potent four years later. As with EBRT, potency loss with seeds is gradual. In this study, 80% of potent men were still potent two years after seeds, but only 60% were potent after four years. How much of this additional loss is due to treatment is debatable. Since prostate cancer studies involve a late-middle-age and elderly population, loss of potency will naturally occur in some percentage of men. How much is due to treatment and how much is due to age is difficult to determine. Viagra helps restore potency to many of these men.

Men who receive brachytherapy combined with EBRT may have an increased risks of developing bladder cancer, according to a new study of about 1,000 men presented at the AUA Annual Meeting on April 26, 2003. According to lead physician Dr. Lee Schachter, nearly 1% of men treated with brachytherapy combined with EBRT contracted bladder cancer in a median time of 2.5 years from treatment. This incidence is well over twice the expected incidence in the general population. Ninety percent of these reported bladder cancers were non-invasive.

New sophisticated techniques are currently being developed to enhance the precision of seed placement real-time during the procedure. These may improve the effectiveness while reducing the side effects. As with IMRT for external beam radition, these new dynamic seed-implant techniques will take brachytherapy to a new level.

Key References

Gelblum D et al. Urinary morbidity following ultrasound-guided transperineal prostate seed implantation. *Int J Radiat Oncol Biol Phys* 1998; 42 (supp): 220 (abstract 1023).

Hollister T, Zelefsky M et al. Late toxicity of transperineal 125 Iodine implantation of the prostate for clinically localized prostate cancer. *Int J Radiat Oncol Biol Phys* 1998; 42 (supp): 220 (abstract 1024).

D'Souza D and Zelefsky M. Seed implant brachytherapy for prostate cancer. *CMAJ* 2001; 165: 1003-a.

Schachter L et al. Bladder cancer after brachytherapy for prostate cancer. American Urological Association 2003. Annual Meeting, Chicago, Illinois; April 26-May 1, 2003 (abstract 277).

Viagra (Sildenafil) for Impotency From Seeds

Viagra has made a major difference in men with impotence related to seed implants. In one study, 80% of men who lost potency responded favorably to Viagra. This success ratio is comparable to that achieved with bilateral nerve-sparing radical prostatectomy. Sildenafil has eliminated much of the worry about impotency in potent men receiving brachytherapy.

Key Reference

Merrick G et al. Efficacy of sildenafil citrate in prostate brachytherapy patients with erectile dysfunction. *Urology* 1999; 53: 1112-1116.

Brachytherapy as Salvage for Failed Radiation

Seed implantation is now being tested as a fall-back procedure (salvage) for failed EBRT. So long as there are no signs of distant metastases, small trials show promise. Dr. Beyer at Arizona Oncology Services in Scottsdale, Ariz., reported that 53% of 17 men were biochemically (PSA) free from cancer five years after salvage brachytherapy. Men with PSAs of 10 ng/ml, or less, did significantly better than men with PSAs of greater than 10 at the time of salvage (67% vs. 25% cancer-free at five years). While these results are promising, more and larger studies are needed to get a better fix on the use of this potentially attractive salvage option.

Key Reference

Beyer D. Permanent brachytherapy as salvage treatment for recurrent prostate cancer. *Urology* 1999; 54: 880-883.

High-Density Radiotherapy (HDR)

HDR brachytherapy uses temporary seed implants rather than permanent ones. Iridium-192 (Ir-192) is used in this treatment, rather than I-125 or Pd-103.

HDR uses high-technology computer design to tailor a radiation dose to the exact shape and size of the prostate. In addition, the radiation can be calibrated to deliver a higher dose to the area of the tumor. In this way, HDR can be designed to suit each individual case of prostate cancer, much like IMRT. HDR is most effective when combined with an endorectal MRI or other precise imaging techniques.

HDR has higher energy and a higher dose rate than permanent seed implants. This is an advantage when treating more aggressive tumors. HDR is usually combined with EBRT. This combination results in very few instances where the tumor comes back in the prostate.

With HDR, hollow tubes are inserted into the prostate and Ir-192 seeds are placed at intervals inside these tubes. Both the tubes and the seeds stay in place for two to three days. As soon as they're removed, the man can go home. There are no permanent seeds left in the patient.

HDR is not currently widely available. I asked one knowledgeable radiation oncologist whom he would go to if he had prostate cancer and chose this route. He came out with an unqualified opinion: "Dr. Alvaro Martinez at William Beaumont Hospital in Royal Oaks, Michigan." There are other qualified HDR therapists. Andy Grove, the CEO of Intel, selected a doctor in Seattle. Dr. Nisar Syed at Long Beach Memorial Hospital in Long Beach, Calif., is also experienced in HDR. In Australia HDR is offered at the Peter MacCallum Cancer Institute in Melbourne.

Brachytherapy Summary

• Brachytherapy alone is suitable for men with low-risk prostate cancer (PSA 10 or less, Gleason score 6 or less, and clinical stage T2a or less). In this group, it's as effective as surgery or external beam radiation therapy. More than 90% five-year cure rates as measured by PSA have been reported.

• Palladium-103 seeds plus hormones is an option for men with intermediate-risk cancer (PSA 10.1-19.9) and/or Gleason score 7 and/or clinical stage T2b). Recent studies indicate that EBRT in addition to Pd-103 seeds may not increase effectiveness.

• Seeds can reach most cancers that have penetrated the prostate capsule, especially in the low-risk group.

• Urinary symptoms after seed implants are common. Late symptoms can occur two to four years after seed implantation. Beware of claims that trivialize the side effects of seeds.

• Bright red rectal bleeding can also occur after seeds. It usually clears up by itself or with the help of steroid enemas.

• Impotency can occur in about 40% of potent men. When it does, about 80% will respond favorably to Viagra.

10

CRYOTHERAPY (CRYOSURGERY)

Cryotherapy is a relatively new technique for treating prostate cancer. It works by freezing the entire prostate, including the cancer. It's sometimes used as a primary treatment and sometimes as a salvage treatment after surgery or EBRT.

Until recently, there have been two significant problems with cryotherapy. First, it's been hard for therapists to accurately freeze the entire prostate. This increases the risk of recurrence. Secondly, side effects, notably incontinence and impotency, have been unacceptably high. For these reasons, many medical centers have been shying away from using cryotherapy.

The acknowledged master of cryotherapy is Dr. Fred Lee. Dr. Lee is a prostate cancer survivor. In my opinion, this increases his credibility. When his cancer recurred locally after radiation, he had salvage cryosurgery. Today, he is free from cancer.

Dr. Lee has perfected a technique that markedly improves the long-term outcome of cryosurgery. Called "targeted cryosurgery," it provides accurate freezing of the entire prostate, while dramatically reducing side effects. Targeted cryosurgery is 3½ times more likely to freeze the whole prostate than standard cryosurgery. What's more, though this better coverage would seem more likely to damage surrounding healthy tissues, side effects are actually reduced.

How is this possible? The procedure for cryotherapy involves the placing of "cryoprobes" into the prostate. These probes are then cooled to the point where they freeze and kill both normal and malignant cells. The standard technique uses five cryoprobes, and freezes by using liquid nitrogen. Afterwards, the probes are removed.

Targeted cryotherapy, as pioneered by Dr. Lee, uses six to eight cryoprobes and freezes by using liquified argon gas instead of liquid nitrogen. Liquid argon provides more precise temperature control than liquid nitrogen. This permits better targeting and makes it possible to destroy the entire prostate. During the procedure, a catheter is placed inside the urethra. Warm fluid circulates through this catheter, protecting the urethra from damage. This markedly reduces the risk of urinary complications. At Crittenton Hospital in Rochester Hills, Minnesota, where Dr. Lee and his cryosurgery colleague Dr. Duke Bahn work, only about 4% of patients require medication for incontinence after cryosurgery. This compares with up to 60% in less experienced hands. Again, you can see why the doctor performing the procedure makes a big difference.

Impotency is still a problem, although an expected one. To be certain all the cancer is frozen, the area where the nerves necessary for erection attach to the prostate is usually frozen. This improves the cure rate from cryosurgery. Unfortunately, even in Dr. Lee's hands, 85% become impotent from the procedure. However, about half of these men experience at least a partial return of sexual function with Viagra.

How effective is targeted cryotherapy? In the August 2002 issue of *Urology*, Dr. Bahn and Lee reported their 7-year outcomes using targeted cryotherapy in 590 patients. In these cases it was used as a primary treatment instead of surgery, radiation, or seeds. The men were divided into low-, intermediate-, and high-risk cancer groups. About 16%, 30%, and 54% of the cancers were low-, intermediate-, and high-risk respectively.

At an actuarial follow-up of 7 years from targeted cryotherapy, 61% of both the low- and high-risk men had PSAs of 0.5ng/ml or less; 68% of the intermediate group also had this PSA level. Considering all men with a PSA of 1.0ng/ml or less, 87%, 79%, and 71% of the low-, intermediate-, and high-risk groups respectively met this standard.

If one applied the ASTRO standard as used to evaluate radiation therapy, i.e. 3 consecutive increases in PSA means the treatment failed, 92%, 89%, and 89% of the 3 respective groups would be considered free of cancer, although I think it's fair to say that over time some of these men will most probably have recurrence.

Pointing to the fact that not all these men had been cured, 13% of the men still had cancer when biopsied after freezing. However, and this is interesting, after a mean follow-up of more than 5 years after retreating them with a second cryotherapy, 91% were disease free by the ASTRO standard. Side effects were modest and there were no serious complications.

In the hands of Dr. Bahn and Dr. Lee, these results compare favorably with results from radiation, especially considering that the majority of men were in the high-risk category. Other groups report less efficacious results with far greater and more serious side effects with "standard" (non-targeted) cryosurgery.

If it were me, I would only consider cryosurgery at Crittendon. Period. And I would insist on Dr. Lee, or Dr. Bahn, personally. If I were to have a local recurrence of my cancer after other therapies, I would give this treatment serious consideration. It's far less invasive than surgery, takes only an hour or two, so I could go home the same day, and has fewer complications (in Dr. Lee's hands), especially less incontinence. No scar. No blood loss. Nice package.

One disadvantage of cryosurgery is that it's usually not covered by insurance. It costs about $13,000.

Key References

Lee F, Bahn D et al. Cryosurgery for prostate cancer: improved glandular ablation by use of 6 to 8 cryoprobes. *Urology* 1999; 54: 135-140.

Bahn D, Lee F et al. Targeted cryoablation of the prostate: 7-year outcomes in the primary treatment of prostate cancer. *Urology* 2002; 60: 3-11.

11

HORMONE THERAPY/ ANDROGEN BLOCKADE

It's an indisputable fact that androgens stimulate the growth of prostate cancer. Prostate cancer is extremely rare in eunuchs and in men who have a deficiency in 5-alpha reductase, the enzyme that converts testosterone to the much more potent androgen DHT. Low-fat high-fiber diets rich in soy, a plant-derived mildly estrogenic (phytoestrogen) food, and lots of green tea may influence sex hormone metabolism in Asian men (see page 322), and these Asians have considerably less clinically significant prostate cancer.

Additionally, it has been shown that both castration and Proscar (potent androgen reducers) increase levels of insulin-like growth factor binding protein-3 (IGFBP-3). IGFBP-3 appears to have a direct inhibitory effect on the growth of prostate cancer cells. Also, two population studies observed a reduction in the risk of prostate cancer in men with high IGFBP-3 levels (for a full discussion of IGFBP-3, IGF-1 and related factors see page 278). Reducing androgens is an important aspect of prostate cancer control and treatment.

Key References

Aquilina J et al. Androgen deprivation as a strategy for prostate cancer chemopre-vention. *J Natl Cancer Inst* 1997; 89: 689-696.

Pollak, M. Insulin-like growth factors and prostate cancer. *Epidemiol Reviews* 2001; 23: 59-66.

What Is Hormonal Therapy?

A hormone is a substance produced by the body that helps regulate its function. Androgens are male sex hormones. They increase sexual desire (libido) and influence a number of secondary masculine characteristics, such as increasing body hair, muscle mass, and bone density. A lesser-known effect of male hormones is the stimulatory impact they have on the growth of prostate cells, both normal and cancerous.

Prostate cancer cells thrive in an androgen-rich environment. The two hormones that stimulate prostate cancer cell growth the most are testosterone and dihydrotestosterone, commonly referred to as DHT. DHT is formed by the action of an enzyme, 5-alpha reductase, on testosterone. Although testosterone significantly increases the growth rate of prostate cancer cells, DHT increases this growth rate 5 to 10 fold! Besides stimulating growth, these powerful hormones also deactivate a suicide program in prostate cancer cells. So removal of these two hormones from the system both stops the growth of prostate cancer cells and triggers their built-in suicide program. This process of programmed cell death is called apoptosis (a-pop-TOE-sis). You'll see it often when reading about prostate cancer. But the bottom line is this: Shut off the androgen spigot and prostate cancer cells die or, as new studies show, at least become dormant. It generally takes about 9 months for the population of cancer cells affected by the absence of androgens to die or "go to sleep."

Hormonal therapy is designed to either remove these androgens from the system or to render them ineffective in stimulating prostate cancer cell growth and inhibiting apoptosis. As you know, testosterone is produced by the testes. This accounts for 90% of all male hormones. The other 10% is made in the adrenals, small glands perched on top of each kidney.

The most immediate and direct way to cut off testosterone production and its conversion to the more potent DHT is to remove the testicles. Until a little over 10 years ago, removal of the testes was commonly combined with radical prostatectomy when surgical findings were unfavorable. An uncle of mine had this done at the Mayo Clinic about 13 years ago for prostate cancer of predominately diploid cell type (favorable) that was found to have spread to his lymph nodes at the time of surgery. His biggest complaint today at age 80 is that he's slowing down too much to get around the paddle tennis court effectively. As for his prostate cancer, his PSA is undetectable. Not a trace.

Known as orchidectomy (or orchiectomy), surgical castration is a simple procedure that permanently shuts down testosterone production. A number of studies show that men who undergo orchiectomy do better long-term. The problem is that the mere thought of losing their testicles makes most men cringe. They often think they're "losing their manhood," permanently and irrevocably.

Modern medicine now manufactures drugs that are equally effective to surgical castration at shutting down testosterone production. They're administered by injections every 3 to 4 months. Unlike surgical castration, this "chemical castration," also known as "medical castration," is often reversible. If the drugs are not used too long, after their use is discontinued most men will eventually regain normal, or near normal, testosterone production. Obviously, this greatly mitigates the adverse physical and psychological effects of testicular removal. Even when testosterone production needs to be permanently shut off in men with advanced disease, most men choose chemical control to surgical castration.

You may be wondering why any man would opt for surgical castration over getting a shot 3 to 4 times a year. Some elderly men choose surgery because they're past having sexual activity. The surgery is easy, convenient, and less expensive than the quarterly injections. Younger men generally opt for the shots.

By the way, thanks to Viagra, a number of men with either form of castration are capable of sustaining erections sufficient for sexual intercourse.

The class of drugs used for medical castration is known as luteinizing hormone-releasing hormone (LH-RH) agonists. They interfere with naturally occurring signals from the pituitary gland that "tell" the testes to make testosterone. In short order they bring testosterone levels down to those achieved with surgical castration. Two drugs are now widely available for this purpose: Lupron (leuprorelin) and Zoladex (goserelin). They're equally effective.

Blocking the Effects of Androgens Without Cutting off Production—Anti-Androgens

Another method of controlling androgenic hormones is the use of drugs that block the impact of these hormones on cancer cells without cutting off their production. At the cellular level, androgens must latch on to a specific site on the cell known as a receptor. The hormone molecule binds to this site in a manner similar to a key fitting a lock. Although many binding sites exist on the surface of cells, only one configuration is designed to wed with testosterone or DHT. This site is called the androgen receptor.

But modern medicine has created a synthetic imposter—a molecule that the receptor "thinks" is an androgen, but is, in fact, inert and without effect. Given in sufficient quantity, this molecule will saturate the androgen-binding sites with a high degree of affinity. Locking on tight to the receptor, these man-made "anti-androgens" prevent testosterone and DHT from latching on to the cancer cells. There are plenty of sex hormones circulating around, but there's no place for them to land. The beauty of this medical subterfuge is that the person taking the anti-androgen still has normal testosterone levels and all that comes with it, but the cancer cells are deprived their growth stimulation and suicide prevention programs.

Besides blocking the effects of testosterone produced by the testes, anti-androgens also block the 10% of male hormones produced by the adrenal glands. The two widely used anti-androgens are Casodex (bicalutamide) and Eulexin (flutamide). The recent trend is for Casodex to be used more frequently than Eulexin, due to generally fewer side effects and patient tolerance for high doses.

Proscar

Proscar is a drug that works by blocking the conversion of testosterone to DHT by interfering with the enzyme, 5-alpha reductase, responsible for this conversion. It is effective in greatly reducing DHT levels. Since less testosterone is being converted to DHT, testosterone levels tend to increase when Proscar is taken. Proscar is the same medicine (Propecia) that some men take to help stop the balding process. Baldness is related to high DHT levels. As you might expect, there's a correlation between baldness and prostate cancer.

The use of Proscar to help treat prostate cancer is controversial. Although it significantly decreases DHT levels, it raises testosterone levels. Since DHT is a much more potent androgen than testosterone, intuitively this seems like a good trade-off, but this has yet to be proven. Although some clinicians swear by Proscar, others are adamantly opposed to its use. Medical studies to clarify this issue are in progress. Personally, I take 5 mg of Proscar (1 tab) daily. In my view, the potential benefits outweigh the possible risks.

Complete Androgen Blockade (CAB)

The debate rages about the best way to accomplish a reduction in androgens. By far the most popular combination used by most medical oncologists is Lupron and Casodex (or Eulexin). This CAB combination effectively eliminates both testosterone production and the effects of the adrenal androgens. As discussed, some oncologists also add Proscar to the mix.

Although CAB, either with or without Proscar, is clearly effective, it generally has more undesirable side effects, such as diarrhea, nausea, hot flashes, and forgetfulness, than either an LH-RH agonist alone, or surgical castration. Unless it's clearly more effective, CAB is not routinely warranted due to its increased toxicity. Is it more effective than an LH-RH agonist or castration? A review of the medical literature by Dr. Mario Eisenberger and his group at Johns Hopkins indicates that it probably isn't. In a recent article in the *Journal of Urology*, the Hopkins group reviewed and analyzed data from 27 clinical trials using various combinations of androgen blockade. Only three showed a statistically significant benefit to adding an anti-androgen (Casodex or Eulexin) to orchiectomy or an LH-RH agonist. Their review of the data also revealed a decrease in the quality of life in men on CAB when compared to medical, or surgical, castration alone.

Adding to the argument for using only an LH-RH agonist or undergoing orchiectomy are the previously discussed works of Dr. Messing in surgery, and Dr. Bolla in radiation. Both of these doctors reported increased life expectancy when they combined long-term use of an LH-RH agonist with surgery or radiation. Neither used an anti-androgen or Proscar. Although the final answer is not yet in on whether CAB is worth the additional side effects, at this perspiring moment, the pendulum is swinging back toward using either medical or surgical castration alone. You'll get plenty of argument about this, however, from some very well informed doctors who are convinced that CAB is the way to go. The jury is still out.

Using Anti-Androgens

The anti-androgens Casodex or Eulexin are taken orally. Casodex is taken only once a day; Eulexin must be taken three times a day. Casodex seems to have fewer side effects than Eulexin. Diarrhea and liver damage as measured by elevated blood levels of transaminases, chemicals released into the blood by damaged liver cells, are seen more often in men taking Eulexin (any liver damage is usually reversed by stopping the drug). For this reason and its easier once-daily intake, Casodex is now used more often by medical oncologists.

High-Dose (150-mg) Casodex Therapy

We've examined the case for using an LH-RH agonist like Lupron alone without Casodex or Proscar. What about using only Casodex without Lupron? Astra Zeneca, a large British pharmaceutical company, addressed this issue in the largest clinical trial ever mounted in prostate cancer. Eight thousand men scattered internationally were given 150 mg of Casodex daily after having had surgery, radiation, or watchful waiting for early prostate cancer. It now appears, according to informed sources, that this trial may have failed to show an increase in life expectancy. Although a number of doctors in the United States, and a greater number in Europe, still use high-dose Casodex as part of their treatment plan, the results of the Astra Zeneca trial may not show a significant benefit in extending the lifespan of the men using it.

Are you confused? Perhaps a review is in order.

• Hormones are helpful for men with locally advanced, intermediate, or high-risk prostate cancer, when combined with a definitive treatment such as surgery or radiation.
• How long to take hormones varies with the circumstance. Aggressive cancers should be treated for 2 to 3 years.
• Men with lymph node involvement found during radical prostatectomy

(or by lymph node biopsy prior to radiation) should stay on an LH-RH agonist indefinitely (Lupron or Zoladex) or be surgically castrated. Current evidence indicates that adding an anti-androgen like Casodex may not add any protection against cancer progression and may increase side effects.

• Casodex blocks the effects of all androgens whether produced in the testes or the adrenal glands by interfering with their ability to bind to prostate cancer cells. It does not alter testosterone levels.

• New clinical trials indicate that high-dose Casodex (150mg) used alone (monotherapy) does not significantly increase life-expectancy in men with low-risk prostate cancer.

• Proscar blocks the conversion of testosterone to the more potent DHT. While reducing DHT levels, it increases testosterone levels. Studies are in process to evaluate Proscar's benefits both as an adjunct to other hormones and for maintenance after hormonal therapy. At this point experts disagree on when and if it should be used.

Key Reference
Laufer M et al. Complete androgen blockade for prostate cancer: what went wrong? *J Urology* 2000; 164: 3-9.

Who Should Use Hormones?

This is one of the hottest topics is the treatment of prostate cancer: Who should use hormones, which hormones, and for how long? More and more studies are showing that blocking the production of male hormones (androgen blockade) is helpful for many men, especially when combined with surgery, radiation, and in some instances, seeds.

Some oncologists are treating men with complete androgen blockade, using a combination of Lupron, Casodex, and Proscar for 12-13 months. Then the men are maintained on Proscar alone. Although I considered this option particularly attractive because it left my prostate gland intact, I rejected it. The available data left me with serious doubts as to whether this program would cure my cancer. Also, the results of this regime have not been published in a journal subject to peer review by other doctors. More studies are necessary.

I could find only two studies that touched on what complete androgen blockade without additional treatment might do. The first, by Martin Gleave from Vancouver, B.C., gave patients eight months of hormones prior to surgery. PSA values declined to less than 0.2 ng/ml in 84% of the cases. There were, however, considerable individual differences: 28% of the men reached this level within three months; an additional 42% reached it between the third and fifth months; 20% more attained undetectable PSAs between the fifth and eighth months. At the time of surgery, 10% of the patients had no sign of prostate cancer when their prostates were carefully examined by the pathologist. So, it's probable that 10% of the men in this study were cured by hormones alone.

Another clinical trial was reported in 1998 by Dr. Kollermann and colleagues. This group reasoned that since the response to androgen blockade is variable, they would wait until the PSA reached undetectable levels before operating. Although the average time they waited was about six months, the range was between three and 22 months. In this group 28% had prostates free of cancer at the time of surgery.

These results are impressive. They show that in some patients, hormones alone seem sufficient to cure prostate cancer. If I'd known that I would be one of these lucky 10%-28% who are cancer-free after hormones, I would definitely have chosen this route. Likewise, if I'd known that by taking the hormones longer, say two years, my chances of being cured would be 80%, I'd have also selected hormones. If I'd known that, although I might have residual viable cancer cells around, their growth could be controlled with Proscar for many years to come, hormones alone would have been for me.

But I didn't know any of these things. Although a 10%-28% probable cure rate was interesting, a 72%-90% chance of harboring active cancer cells was a far greater risk than I was willing to take. And though it seemed likely that I could shorten those odds by using androgen blockade longer and perhaps adding Proscar, I had no idea by how much. Ultimately, I decided to combine 3-D conformal radiation therapy with 27 months of hormones. Thirty-six months of hormones would probably increase my chance of cure, but the additional 9 months would also increase my chance of permanent inability to produce testosterone. I want to stress, however, that based on medical studies, life expectancy is only increased for sure in most men with three years of hormones plus radiation. In choosing 27 months, I'm gambling. I'm trading off some probable life-extending benefits for improved quality of life. Time will tell if this was wise.

To review, the only study that shows an increased life expectancy by combining hormones with radiation used an LH-RH agonist for three years, plus radiation. The next closest study, in terms of time of hormone use with this combination, employed hormones for $10\frac{1}{2}$ months. This study showed excellent local control (freedom of cancer in the prostate), but no benefit in extension of survival. Somewhere between $10\frac{1}{2}$ and 36 months, survival benefits accrue. Since we don't know exactly when yet (studies are in progress), all we can currently say is that three years of hormones when combined with radiation increases survival.

It also increases the risk of permanent testosterone suppression. At two years, hormones leave 29% of men with testosterone at permanently castrate levels. Although I've seen no published data at three years, it's obviously higher. I chose 27 months of androgen blockade because I thought it provided the best balance between increased life expectancy (probable, but unproven) and maintaining the ability to produce testosterone (60%-70%). My testosterone levels and sexuality have now returned to normal.

I would love to see the results of a prospective randomized study comparing androgen blockade alone with external beam radiation, or surgery. Such a study is currently underway. The Canadian Urologic Oncology Group is conducting a trial for men with Gleason grade 7 or higher, PSA equal to or greater than 20ng/ml, and stage T2 or greater. The men will be randomized to receive either complete androgen blockade alone (CAB), or CAB and radiation. This study should tell us how much radiation therapy adds to CAB in this high-risk group. The results should be interesting indeed.

LH-RH Agonist Injections

Lupron and Zoladex are given by injection. Lupron can be injected either into a big muscle (such as the gluteus maxiumus) or just under the skin in a fatty part of the body, like right next to the belly button. Speaking from personal experience, the subcutaneous injection is less painful than the intramuscular one. This is especially true if the drug is injected slowly, meaning over about one minute. A subcutaneous injection uses a smaller needle than an intramuscular one.

Zoladex is a small pellet. It's routinely deposited just beneath the skin next to the belly button. It uses a large-bore needle, but the doctor will first use a local anesthetic, such as Novocaine or Lidocaine, so you won't feel the larger needle. Deadening the skin with a local anesthetic creates a little more discomfort than a subcutaneous Lupron injection, but neither is major.

Lupron is available in both a one-month and a three-month "depot" (slow-release) form. I suggest using the one-month form initially to evaluate the severity of any side effects, then switching to the three-month form. A four-month depot formulation may be available by the time you read this. One-year depot injections are currently being developed.

Bottom line: If you're getting an LH-RH agonist, I suggest discussing subcutaneous Lupron injections with your doctor. They're equally effective and less painful than intra-muscular Lupron or subcutancous Zoladex pellets. If you're taking aspirin, stop for about 7-10 days prior to the shot to avoid bruising.

Avoiding "Testosterone Flare"

Another use for Casodex or Eulexin is to prevent "test-osterone flare" when Lupron or Zoladex are about to be used. The initial response to these LH-RH agonists is a sudden *increase* in testosterone levels. Although temporary (within two to four weeks, testosterone levels plunge to castrate lev-els), this increased testosterone level can cause a flare-up in prostate cancer-related symptoms. This is both undesirable and dangerous.

It has become standard procedure to give men at least 7 days of an anti-androgen before starting Lupron or Zoladex. This is the only prudent course. Some doctors, such as Dr. Bolla, give their patients 28 days of an anti-androgen to pro-vide an additional margin of safety. It's surprising, therefore, that some patient surveys reveal that only 18% of men start-ing hormonal therapy were told about testosterone flare by their doctors.

Using Hormonal Blockade Only to Treat Prostate Cancer?

Are there any situations where hormonal blockade by itself might be considered? I think there are. For example, hormones are an option for men who have slow-growing tu-mors with Gleason scores of 6 or less and low PSAs and have ruled out surgery and radiation due to unacceptable poten-tial side effects. This option might be especially appealing for older men, for whom the side effects from hormones of decreased libido and impotency may be less of an issue. Hormones could be given for 6-12 months (I recommend 12), then stopped, and the PSA monitored. If there was a good response (PSA dropped to undetectable levels), then it starts rising again, the cycle could be repeated (see "Intermittent Androgen Suppression"). Using Proscar for maintenance after hormones is also an option, although there is no conclusive proof yet of its efficacy; some doctors have found that using Proscar prolongs the interval that men can be off hormonal threapy (see "Proscar Maintenance"). Especially if combined with appropriate lifestyle changes, this intermittent hormone blockade might keep the cancer at bay for many years with manageable side effects. If the cancer changes character and becomes more aggressive, surgery or radiation are still available options at that point. Much of this discussion is still conjecture, because a definitive study comparing CAB, or an LH-RH agonist alone with watchful waiting, has not yet been published.

Another group of men that might benefit from hormones alone are those where complicating medical problems increase the risk of surgery or radiation. Examples of this include men with diabetes, colitis, or severe hemorrhoids.

Also, elderly men too old for surgery who have rejected watchful waiting as an alternative and fear complications from radiation but want their PSAs down might consider hormonal blockade.

Hormones and PIN

As previously discussed in the chapter on risk factors, high-grade PIN is thought to be a "pre-cancerous" condition. When hormones are given to men prior to surgery, pathologists have observed that PIN is reduced or eliminated. Some prostate cancer experts are intrigued with the possibility that hormones, by eliminating high-grade PIN, may protect some men at high risk of developing cancer. African-American men have more high-grade PIN than Caucasians. This high-risk population might particularly benefit from a course of hormones.

Combining Hormonal Therapy with Radiation

Although hormonal therapy alone, or in combination with Proscar, is a bit too speculative at this stage for me, I'm impressed with a number of recent studies that show that hormones improve the efficacy of radiation and surgery.

Evidence is mounting that CAB or an LH-RH agonist alone combined with radiation are more effective than radiation alone. To me it's compelling. Here's why:

Study 1

The Radiation Therapy Oncology Group (RTOG) conducted a randomized trial of 977 high-risk patients: 468 received radiation alone; 477 received radiation plus two years of CAB started during the last week of radiation therapy. The group that got only radiation was treated with hormone therapy if their cancer recurred. The chart shows the results for the first eight years:

	Radiation Only	Radiation + CAB	Probability
Local recurrence	37%	23%	<.001
Distant metastases	37%	27%	<.001
Disease-free survival	25%	36%	<.001
5-year overall survival	71%	75%	No significant difference
8-year overall survival	47%	49%	No significant difference

When the various sub-groups were broken down, the investigators found that men with Gleason scores of 8-10 did have significantly improved overall survival (P=0.036) when

CAB was added to radiation. Other men with lower Gleason scores didn't. While this study shows highly significant improvement in the rate of local recurrence, distant metastases, and disease-free survival, it shows an absolute survival advantage for only the small sub-set of men with very aggressive tumors. Please observe that in this study hormones were not started until radiation was completed. It's possible that hormones are more effective when started prior to radiation. As we've seen, there's laboratory evidence that hormones may sensitize prostate cancer cells to the effects of radiation. Further studies are warranted.

Study 2

In 1997 Dr. Laverdiere and his group reported on 121 patients with T2-T4 prostate tumors randomized to receive: external beam radiation alone; radiation preceded by three months CAB; or CAB for three months before radiation, during radiation, and for six months after radiation. This last group had a total of around 10½ months of CAB. All groups received 64 Gy of radiation, a low dose by today's standards. All patients had prostate biopsies 12 months and 24 months after radiation. The following chart tells the story.

Percentage of Positive Biopsies for Prostate Cancer		
	12 months	24 months
Radiation Only	62%	65%
Radiation plus 3 months CAB (prior to radiation)	30%	28%
Radiation plus a total of 10-1/2 months CAB (prior to, during, and after radiation)	4%	5%

The difference here is striking. Not only did CAB reduce the incidence of local recurrence, but a longer course of CAB *dramatically* reduced this risk. Even adjusting for as much as 23% false negative sextant biopsies (biopsies that miss existing cancer), as reported in the literature, these results are still impressive. PSA levels were also significantly lower at 12 months, with longer CAB patients showing the lowest values. At 24 months, however, PSA levels were not significantly different between those men who received three months of CAB and those who received 10½ months. Both groups were significantly different from the radiation only group, however. Despite these better PSA readings two years out, there was not a significant difference in survival expectations. Since survival is the key end-point in all cancer studies, it can't be said that CAB did anything more than reduce local recurrence at 24 months.

Open questions include the additional protection that higher doses or radiation might provide, and what effect longer hormone use might add.

Study 3

This landmark study was conducted by Michel Bolla, M.D., a French professor of radiation oncology at University Hospital in Grenoble, France. It appeared in the July 1997 issue of the prestigious *New England Journal of Medicine*—and immediately raised the eyebrows of many radiation oncologists. Doctors who might have been reserving judgment on the efficacy of hormones combined with radiation were convinced by this study that adding hormones is clearly better than radiation alone for men with locally advanced prostate cancer.

In this randomized prospective study of men with locally advanced prostate cancer (intermediate- and high-risk patients), 190 patients received external beam radiation alone; 195 patients were given CAB for one month, then goserelin (Zoladex) alone for an additional 35 months—a total of three years of hormonal therapy with only an LH-RH agonist, plus protection against "flare." In this group, radiation was started at the same time as hormones. All men in this trial received a total of 70 Gy of radiation divided into equal daily doses, five days per week for seven weeks. Note that these investigators used CAB for only one month to inhibit the sudden increase in testosterone levels, which often show up when LH-RH agonists like goserelin are administered. Using an anti-androgen, like Casodex or flutamide, is standard practice before using an LH-RH analog.

Here are their five-year data:

	Radiation Alone	Radiation + Three Years Zoladex
Overall survival at 5 years	62%	79%
Free of disease at 5 years (for surviving patients)	48%	85%

Both of these comparisons are statistically significant. This study is extremely important because it shows that hormone therapy, even without an anti-androgen, when given long-term with radiation prolongs life in men with locally advanced disease. This is the first well-conducted trial that has shown extended life expectancy for the entire group of men with locally advanced cancer. The RTOG study (Study 1) improved survival only in men with Gleason scores of 8 and higher. The Laverdiere study (Study 2) showed that 10½ months of CAB dramatically reduced the chances of the cancer returning to the prostate, but did not show improved survival.

So where does this leave us? What we now know is that in cases where locally advanced disease is suspected by using the Partin tables, hormone therapy should be combined with radiation. This reduces the chance of local recurrence of the cancer, decreases the odds of distant metastases (primarily to bone), and, most importantly, increases life expectancy. What is still unknown is how long hormone therapy must be given to achieve all of these objectives. Dr. Bolla selected three years of hormones because in breast cancer, which has been extensively investigated and has many shared characteristics with prostate cancer, three or more years of hormones works best.

It's also noteworthy that Dr. Bolla used only an LH-RH agonist for all but the first month of treatment. Combined with Dr. Messing's findings, this lends strong suport to the case for using an anti-androgen like Casodex only to avoid the cancer flaring up at the beginning of hormonal therapy.

More studies are required to establish the minimum time necessary to obtain the desired results with prostate cancer. The ideal combination of radiation dose and hormone duration has not yet been established. At the time of this writing, only Dr. Bolla's work shows increased life expectancy—three years of an LH-RH agonist plus 70 Gy of radiation. Higher radiation doses might logically allow for shorter hormone use, but again, there's presently no data on this.

There are good reasons to reduce the time on hormones as much as possible, so long as the results are not compromised. For one thing, hormones have side effects for most men. These can include loss of sex drive, impotency, hot flashes, irritability, forgetfulness, mood swings, weight gain, breast enlargement and/or tenderness, and osteoporosis (bone loss). Additionally, the longer a man is on hormones, the more likely he is to have his production of testosterone permanently stopped. After two years of CAB, about 29% of men lose their ability to make testosterone. At three years this figure is much higher. Since return to normal sexual function is a high priority for many men, prolonged use of hormones is fraught with risks that might permanently compromise lifestyle. How much is enough remains to be determined.

For a discussion on the use of hormones in recurrent prostate cancer, refer to the section "Advanced Disease."

Hormones and Surgery

In the chapter on surgery we discussed the use of three months of hormones prior to surgery. As you may recall, while this dramatically reduced the incidence of positive margins found at surgery, it provided no survival benefits. We also discussed Dr. Ed Messing's work, which showed that continued immediate use of a LH-RH agonist, or orchiectomy, significantly increased life expectancy in men found to have lymph-node metastases at the time of surgery.

But what about other men using hormones after surgery? Is it warranted? If so, when? These issues were addressed by Dr. Thomas Seay and his associates at the Mayo Clinic. They tested the effects of hormones and/or radiotherapy after surgery both for men in whom the cancer had penetrated the prostate capsule, and in men whose cancer was confined to the gland itself. Treatment during or after surgery or radiation is referred to as "adjuvant" treatment. Treatment prior to surgery or radiation is called "neoadjuvant." Dr. Seay's group examined the effect of adjuvant hormonal treatment on local recurrence in

> **HELPFUL HINT**
>
> Men with positive surgical margins, seminal vesicle involvement, or lymph-node metastases found at surgery treated with adjuvant therapy within 3 months of surgery do as well in terms of their cancer returning in the prostate area as men with organ-confined disease who do not receive adjuvant therapy.

the area of the surgically removed prostate. Men documented by the pathologist to have cancer that had escaped the prostate (pathologic grade T3), including all men with positive surgical margins, seminal-vesicle involvement, or lymph-node metastases, did significantly better with adjuvant therapy right after surgery. What really surprised the researchers, however, was that men with pathologic stage T3 who received adjuvant therapy also did significantly better (less local recurrence) than men whose cancer was totally contained within the prostate (pathologic stage T2).

This confirms the fact that a significant number of men with organ-confined cancer at the time of surgery do eventually have recurrences. The ones at highest risk, as shown by a prior Mayo Clinic study that tracked PSA after surgery, are men with high pre-operative PSA, high Gleason scores, and non-diploid tumors. It might be prudent, the Mayo investigators concluded, for men in this group to consider 8-12 months of hormones after surgery. As with radiation, the optimal time period for adjuvant hormonal therapy has not yet been established.

Guide to Adjuvant Therapy

Category 1—Men with organ-confined tumors, but high (greater than 20) initial PSAs, Gleason score of 7 or higher, and non-diploid tumors, or men with well-localized positive surgical margins should consider 8-12 months of hormonal therapy (I think 12 months is preferable). Some oncologists would use hormones for two years.

Category 2—Men with multiple positive surgical margins consider adjuvant external beam radiation therapy and 8-12 months of hormones.

Category 3—Men with seminal-vesicle or lymph-node involvement should consider on-going male-hormone suppression indefinitely using either an LH-RH agonist or orchiectomy. We know from Dr. Messing's work that many men found to have lymph node involvement at the time of surgery do well long term on this regimen. From this we can conclude that hormonal therapy not only reduces local cancer recurrence, it also reduces distant metastases and saves lives. Many of the men on continuous hormone therapy continue to have no sign of disease (undetectable PSAs) 7 years after surgery and the start of hormones.

Hormone Therapy to Become More Frequent?

Although hormonal therapy is not yet routinely prescribed

immediately after surgery for men with a high risk of cancer recurrence based on surgical findings, their early use after surgery is becoming more common. It's true that half the men with positive surgical margins will remain free of cancer long-term without any treatment and the side effects of hormone use must be weighed against the potential benefits.

I was on CAB for the first year, then switched to Lupron only (after Dr. Bolla's work was published) for an additional 15 months, a total of 27 months of hormonal therapy. Having a Gleason 7 tumor with perineural invasion puts me at significant risk for recurrence, despite having received 73.8 Gy of EBRT. In the course of writing this book, I spoke with scores of prostate cancer experts. My personal situation often came up in these talks. The range of opinions as to whether or not I should be on hormones varied from none at all to three years. All but two experts recommended up to one year, with six to eight months being about the average recommendation. Only two doctors suggested two to three years of hormones, despite the fact that the only study in the literature to show an increase in life expectancy of hormones and radiation (Dr. Bolla's), used three years of hormones. Side effects from hormones may be part of the reason for the clinicians' caution.

With Dr. Bolla's results staring me in the face, why didn't I stay on hormones for the full 3 years? It was a close call. If I'd had a Gleason 4+3 instead of a Gleason 3+4, I would have opted for the full 3 years. Because my Gleason 7 was the less aggressive 3+4 type, after thorough discussions with valued experts, I decided that 27 months was probably sufficient. I decided that the possible additional cancer-controlling benefits of longer treatment were outweighed by the lifestyle benefits of a possible return to normal of my testosterone levels. The longer I stayed on hormones, the greater the chance of permanent testosterone shutdown. My testosterone has now returned to normal and I have had full return of my sexual functions. It's more than 4-1/2 years since my cancer was discovered and 4 years since I started treatment. My PSA is 0.3 ng/ml (on Proscar maintenance) and stable.

So far, it appears as though the decision I made was a good one. I must point out, however, that if my overriding objective was to have the greatest chance of survival, even if it meant permanent loss of testosterone, I would have gone for 3 years of hormones. If I were 10 years older, I might have selected 3 years of hormones. These decisions are complex and will vary from man to man, depending on outlook. Understanding all the facts allows for reasoned individualized decision-making.

Key Reference
Seay T et al. Local control of localized carcinoma of the prostate: impact of adjuvant therapy after radical retropubic prostatectomy. *J Urology* 1996; 155 (supp): 560A.

Side Effects and How to Minimize Them

A variety of side effects can occur when androgens are abruptly cut off. Some develop soon after starting hormone therapy, while others occur only after prolonged use. While it would be ideal to have the beneficial effects of hormonal therapy without symptoms, the side effects of androgen blockade are often more a nuisance than incapacitating. As with all prostate cancer treatments, the attitude of the patient makes a big difference. Men who are resolved to deal with any symptoms with a positive problem-solving attitude will generally be less bothered than men who are convinced they're going to suffer. Both these orientations often become self-fulfilling prophecies—those who believe they can take whatever comes in stride do just fine; those who think they're bound to have a hard time are often miserable. Time works in favor of men with acute symptoms, since some troubling symptoms usually diminish as time passes. Nutrition, exercise, supplements, and medications can also help substantially.

Hot Flashes

Hot flashes (a.k.a. hot flushes) are similar to those experienced by women going through menopause. About 75% of women have menopausal hot flashes, of whom a third have episodes severe enough to significantly alter their quality of life. It's about the same for men on hormones: 75%-80% have hot flashes and roughly a third of these will get severe hot flashes.

Hot flashes are characterized by suddenly feeling very hot. The skin turns red and profuse sweating ensues. These episodes can be not only unpleasant, but also embarrassing. They may occur at inconvenient times, like at a business meeting or a social gathering. They may be misinterpreted as due to nervousness, or illness.

Hot flashes are usually controllable. Over time, they typically diminish in both frequency and severity. About two-thirds of men on hormones either don't have them at all or they're mild enough not to be a worry. Younger men are more prone to hot flashes than older men and symptoms are more often severe. These men often require help (see below).

I noticed that when I was on hormones, I rarely felt warm. Either I felt normal or I was burning up. Events that may trigger hot flashes are:

- Drinking very hot beverages. Better to drink warm drinks.
- Dressing—wearing confining clothes
- Drinking coffee, tea, or alcohol
- Eating spicy foods, like chilis
- Niacin supplements
- Viagra
- Poorly ventilated space, especially bedroom or car
- Moderate to intense exertion—mild exertion generally is not associated with hot flashes
- Electric blanket or too many covers
- Sunbathing
- Bright lights—can affect actors, surgeons, politicians, TV personalities, etc.

Megace

The hot-flash antidote of choice for many physicians is Megace. Megace is a progesterone-like drug that seems to adjust the body thermostat, which has been thrown out of kilter by the sudden reduction in testosterone levels. Low doses of 20-40 mg twice a day are generally prescribed. Megace provides effective relief for most men.

The problem with Megace, in my opinion, is that it's a potent appetite stimulator. In fact, it's often used with cancer patients to increase their appetites. To compound matters, one of the side effects of hormones is weight gain (see below). Obviously, a drug that significantly increases appetite makes weight control more difficult.

Also, it has been reported that, in some cases, Megace is associated with a sudden rise in PSA levels. This seems to be directly attributable to Megace, because the PSA rapidly returns to pre-Megace levels as soon as the drug is stopped. For this reasons some prostate cancer specialists won't prescribe this drug.

When I started CAB, I got moderately severe hot flashes about every 1½ hours, including during sleep. I started taking Megace and the hot flashes were significantly reduced, both in intensity and frequency. But I was ravenous and started gaining weight. I reviewed the literature on how to deal with hot flashes. I found successful substitutes for Megace and was able to control both the hot flashes and my weight without being concerned about rising levels of PSA.

Soy and Genistein

Clinicians I've spoken with tell me that a number of men notice a reduction in the severity of their hot flashes when they change their diet to include more soy products. Soy contains phytoestrogens (plant estrogens) that have a weakly estrogenic effect and may diminish hot flashes. A randomized trial in post-menopausal women did not show a significant effect for a diet high in soy in reducing hot flashes. Yet

Asian women have significantly less menopausal hot flashes than Western women. Only 20% of Asian women get them. Why? Although the reason has not been firmly established, diet is suspected. So far, though, this theory has not been supported by medical evidence. So despite the impression of some oncologists that soy seems to help, this still needs to be confirmed by trials.

Perhaps the diminution of hot flashes that many men experience can be explained by a placebo effect. If the doctor believes something will work and convinces the patient of it, up to 40% of patients will be helped, even if the medicine or, in this case the food, is inactive. This is why "double-blind studies," in which neither the doctor nor the patient knows if he's getting the drug being tested or a placebo, are necessary for proper proof of efficacy beyond the placebo effect.

I don't want to minimize the placebo effect. For those 40% who improve with a placebo, the improvement is just as real as if they were taking the drug. The power of the doctor-patient interaction should not be underestimated. "Good bedside manner" produces better overall results.

Soy's most active ingredient, isoflavone genistein, is available as a supplement (see "Nutrition"). Whether soy or genistein are proved to alleviate hot flashes will depend on the results of future clinical trials. I consume at least 50 grams of soy protein daily. Some men with prostate cancer consume 100 grams a day. This matches the soy intake of the Okinawans, the longest-lived people in the world. If it's helping with the hot flashes, that's a bonus. The main reason I eat soy products is due to their multiple possible beneficial effects on the cancer itself and for their cardiovascular benefits.

Red Clover

The flowers and leaves of the red clover plant are another rich source of phytoestrogens. Like soy, red clover contains the isoflavones genistein and daidzein. It also has high levels of the isoflavones biochanin and formonetin. Some studies indicate that biochanin may directly inhibit the growth of prostate cancer cells. Due to its estrogenic effects, red clover has been known to cause infertility in sheep that feed in fields filled with it. In man, where red-clover supplements represent only a small portion of food intake, the weak estrogen-like effect may reduce hot flashes. Again, though, this has yet to be tested in a clinical trial.

Red-clover extract is available in capsules and tinctures. Red-clover sprouts are also available in some health-food stores. Seeds are readily available too for those who like to do their own sprouting (four to six days).

Other Progesterone-like Drugs

Besides Megace, other synthetic progesterones may be helpful in reducing hot flashes. Provera (medroxyprogesterone) is available in 5-mg tablets. A half to one tablet per day is often effective. Natural progesterone is also available as a cream. A 1% progesterone cream can be found at most health-food shops. Compounding pharmacists can make a more effective 3% progesterone formulation. For this you'll need a doctor's prescription. This extra-strength formula is also available without prescription from some supplement companies, like Life Extension in Hollywood, Florida. To control hot flashes you may need this 3% cream. You apply

---

STOP THE PRESSES

Evidence just released indicates that about 10% of prostate cancer cases are stimulated by progesterone in a manner similar to the way they're stimulated by androgens. This is precisely the reason why clinical trials are necessary. This new finding probably also explains why some men experience a rapid rise in their PSA level on Megace. By the time you read this, big institutions may be able to test for sensitivity to progesterone. If your disease is not sensitive to progesterone, it is probably okay to use Megace or progesterone creams. But if your cancer is stimulated by progesterone, or if you don't know your progesterone-sensitivity status, my advice is to use other means to control hot flashes.

it on the abdomen, the butt, or the inside of arms or legs; it's good to change the area of application each day to avoid skin irritation.

There may be an added advantage to using a natural progesterone cream. Studies show that progesterone inhibits the enzyme 5-alpha reductase, which converts testosterone to the more active DHT in the prostate. This is similar to Proscar. But Proscar has no impact on hot flashes. With natural progesterone you may be getting two desirable effects.

One synthetic progesterone-like product, which unfortunately is not available in the United States, is cyproterone acetate (Androcur). Besides being an effective remedy for hot flashes, it also functions as an anti-androgen, similar to Casodex or Eulexin. With this drug you have the best of both worlds, if you select CAB. It's available in Canada, Australia, New Zealand, and Europe.

Low-Dose Anti-Depressants

The use of low dose anti-depressants, like venlafaxine or sertraline (Zoloft), represents a breakthrough in the treatment of hot flashes. Up to now the only viable drugs have been hormonal. We've already discussed the PSA increase and appetite stimulation that is sometimes seen with Megace. For those reasons, most doctors would feel more confident with a non-hormonal solution. Genistein and red clover have weak enough estrogenic effects so as not to be a concern, but they don't work for everyone.

Enter the Mayo Clinic. In a pilot study of 16 men, 10 had a greater than 50% reduction in hot flashes after four weeks of small amounts of an anti-depressant called venlafaxine. Severe hot flashes were reduced from an average of 2.3 per day to less than one a day. Sertraline (Zoloft) seems to work equally well. The dose required to reduce hot flashes is half of the lowest dose used for depression—25 mg of either drug once a day. This is good news for men on hormones. For many these will provide a safe solution to an annoying problem. At this dose, side effects should be mild or non-existent. Of course, this use needs to be further fleshed out in a larger study before it will get the full stamp of approval of the medical community.

I took 25 mg of Zoloft, and one standardized, 500-mg, red-clover-extract tablet daily. I also consumed lots of soy. That's it. Although I still had several hot flashes a day, they were mild. I no longer woke up at night in a sweat. I believe it's possible for many men on hormones to control their hot flashes without the use of potent progesterone-like products. It's also much easier to control your weight on this regimen, and considerably safer.

Sexual Problems

Loss of sexual desire (libido) is ubiquitous with hormonal therapy; very few men are able to continue having erections and ejaculations when called upon without the help of drugs. For the many others who were previously impotent, the availability of sildenafil (Viagra) has meant the return of an active sex life.

A common misconception is that Viagra increases sexual desire. It does not. Viagra works by inhibiting the enzyme phosphodiesterase type 5. This enzyme normally causes smooth muscle in the penis to contract. By inhibiting it, the smooth muscle in the penis relaxes, allowing blood to flow into the penis during sexual stimulation. Note that increased blood flow will not happen without stimulation. So you need a willing and active partner to make the magic work! Since you'll rarely, if ever, be in a love-making mood, your sexual partner must be informed and understanding for Viagra to be effective.

HELPFUL HINT

Buy the 100-mg Viagra tabs and break them in half if 50 mg is enough for you. Score them with a knife and break in two. You'll save a lot of money.

Since Viagra reduces blood pressure temporarily, it should not be used with nitrates, like nitroglycerine. The combination can cause severe hypotension (low blood pressure) and should be avoided. The dose of Viagra for most men is 50 to 100 mg. It seems to work for impotency from many prostate cancer-related causes, including external beam radiation, seeds, surgery, and hormones. The effects are dose-related. If 50 mg doesn't work for you, 100 mg might. Please note that in men taking ketoconazole (Nizoral), the action of sildenafil may be amplified. For these men, 25 mg is often enough. It should only be taken under a doctor's care. Studies have shown that sildenafil improved the frequency, duration, and hardness of erections. It should be taken about an hour before sexual activity.

Besides being a boon to men with erectile dysfunction (ED), Viagra may help alleviate depression. In a study reported by psychiatrist Matthew Menza in 1999, men taking Viagra for three months had significant improvement of ED compared with men taking a placebo. They also had significantly better scores on the Hamilton rating scale, a test for depression. In three months, 48 out of 66 men who were randomly assigned to the sildenafil group had significantly improved erectile function, versus 10 of 70 men taking a placebo. At the beginning of the study the average score on the Hamilton rating scale was 175 for the treated men; after three months it dropped to an average of 6. (The lower the score, the fewer the symptoms of depression.) There was not a big difference in the before and after level of depression in the placebo group.

The investigators don't know whether the drug has a direct effect upon depression or whether the depression improves with improved sexual function. I suspect the latter, but whatever the reason, the conclusion seems clear—Viagra significantly improved both erections and mood in this group of men. Unless there's an absolute contraindication for taking sildenafil (such as nitrates), side effects are usually mild. Mild headache (which I get when I take it) is common; stuffy nose and red slightly itchy eyes also frequently occur. Flushing is not unusual, especially for men on hormones. Less frequent side effects include a bluish visual tinge and indigestion. All of the above effects are temporary. They wear off in about three to four hours. If you're having ED from any treatment for prostate cancer, I urge you to discuss a trial of Viagra with your doctor. It's safe and effective.

Sublingual (under tongue) new drugs for ED, including oral phentolamine and apomorphine, are now being tested in clinical trials in the United States. Apomorphine, known as UPRIMA, is already available in Europe, Australia, and New Zealand. New drugs for ED should be available in the U.S. by the time you read this. Improved second-generation phosphodiesterase type 5 (PDE-5) inhibitors are being developed. One of these, Cialis, is now available in New Zealand and should be available in the United States by the end of 2003. It works as little as 16 minutes and lasts up to 36 hours, providing users with far more sexual flexibility than Viagra. Other drugs with different mechanisms are also under development. Many men with seemingly insoluble ED are now being helped by these new agents. The situation will continue to improve.

Other Side Effects

Here's a quick look at other possible side effects from hormone therapy and what to do about them. Notice that nutrition, exercise, and supplements may help to reduce or eliminate many of them.

• Osteoporosis—Bisphosphonates, exercise and active vitamin D; see the "Bisphosphonate" chapter.

• Weight gain—Switch to low-fat vegan vegetarian diet. Include fish if you wish. Walk regularly. Build up to two miles a day.

• Mood swings or memory loss—Stay active; yoga, meditation, and breathing exercises should help. A weekly massage is also helpful. Gingko biloba, a supplement that may increase blood flow to the brain, may also be useful.

• Fatigue—Proper nutrition and exercise.

• Muscle loss or weakness—High-resistance weight training; yoga; swimming.

• Increased cholesterol and triglycerides—Low-fat vegan diet, (plus or minus fish), exercise, soy consumption.

• Breast enlargement—A short course of radiation to the breasts will stop this symptom before it begins. This should be considered by men preparing for long-term hormonal therapy. The radiation must be done at the start of treatment. It won't work once breast enlargement has already occurred.

• Increased urinary frequency (especially at night)—Often doesn't require treatment. If severe, Hytrint may reduce frequency. Avoid liquids after 6 p.m.

Conclusions

• Hormonal therapy combined with EBRT improves outcome for locally advanced prostate cancer when compared with EBRT alone. Large randomized studies have shown both significantly less local cancer returns at five years and fewer distant metastases.

• Only three years of hormones combined with EBRT has, so far, been shown to increase life expectancy. It's possible that a shorter duration of hormones (18-27 months) may be equally effective, but there's presently no study that confirms this. The optimum time for hormone use with EBRT has not yet been determined.

• Three months of hormones prior to radical prostatectomy results in significant increases in organ-confined cancer and fewer positive margins at the time of surgery. However, no survival benefit has been found. Only 28% of men reach a PSA nadir after three months of hormones.

• Longer use of hormones prior to surgery may improve outcome. Eight to 12 months of hormones results in higher rates of organ-confined disease and fewer positive margins than three months of hormones. Ninety-one percent of men had undetectable PSAs two years after surgery. In 10% of the men receiving hormones for eight months, and 28% of men who stayed on hormones prior to surgery until their PSA bottomed out (3 to 22 months), no cancer at all could be found in the removed prostate.

• Phase III trials are now underway in Canada to determine the optimal length of time of hormonal therapy prior to surgery. A Canadian group is also comparing hormones plus EBRT to hormones alone.

• Hormonal therapy given to men after surgery for 8-12 months significantly reduces the chance of local recurrence in men at high risk.

• Immediate long-term use of hormones in men found to have cancer in their lymph nodes at the time of surgery significantly improves overall survival, distant metastases, and undetectable PSAs seven years after surgery.

• Side effects from hormonal therapy are common. Most can be minimized by lifestyle changes, medication, and supplements.

Hormonal therapy might be a viable option as the only treatment for men with low-risk cancers. Although the optimal treatment term has not been determined, most practitioners would recommend 12 months for this purpose. Some would add 5 mg of maintenance Proscar indefinitely to reduce DHT levels in the prostate. DHT is ten times as potent as testosterone in stimulating prostate cells to divide.

• A short course of hormonal therapy may prevent high-grade PIN from developing into prostate cancer. While this might nip a "pre-cancerous" lesion in the bud, this has not been sufficiently studied.

12

BISPHOSPHONATES

What They Are and How They Work

Most men (80%-85%) with metastatic prostate cancer eventually have bone involvement. Men often survive a long time despite these bony metastases. The mean survival time is 4 years. Prostate cancer cells have a great affinity for bone. They stick to the bone matrix and a symbiotic relationship ensues. Bone cells release factors that stimulate the growth and proliferation of the cancer cells. In turn, the cancer cells stimulate bone turnover and new bone formation. All experts on prostate cancer would agree that finding a way to keep it from spreading to bone would be a major breakthrough. Although such a "magic bullet" currently does not exist, a class of drugs called "bisphosphonates" has the potential to reduce the affinity for bone that prostate cancer cells exhibit. Studies are now under way to try to determine why prostate cancer cells are attracted and stick to bone, eventually growing into colonies of malignant cells.

Bisphosphonates inhibit the adhesion of prostate (and breast) cancer cells to bone matrix, according to a study published in *Cancer Research* in 1997 by a French group led by Dr. Bossier. In this study tumor cells treated with bisphosphonates lost their stickiness to bone. Interestingly, bisphosphonates did not affect the adhesion of normal cells, called fibroblasts, to bone. The authors concluded: "Bisphosphonates may be useful agents for the prophylactic treatment of patients with cancer that is known to preferentially metastasize to bone."

A study published in the *New England Journal of Medicine* in 1998 showed that a high-risk group of 302 women with breast cancer who received the bisphosphonate clodronate early in their disease had a statistically significant decrease in the incidence of metastases to bone. In fact, only half as many women in the treated group got bone metastases in the three-year test period, compared to the untreated group. Those in the treated group whose cancer did spread to bone developed only half as many metastases as the untreated group. Surprisingly, the number of soft-tissue metastases (liver and lung) were also significantly lower in the treated group. Most importantly, *overall life expectancy* was significantly increased in the treated women. Only six women in the treated group died during the observation period. Twenty-two women in the untreated group died during this same period. The odds of this happening by chance are less than 1 in 1,000! Based on the data in this study clodronate, or other newer bisphosphonates, has now become standard treatment for women with breast cancer in conjunction with conventional hormonal treatment or chemotherapy.

So where does this leave us with prostate cancer? As of this writing we don't yet know, but a number of clinical trials are ongoing. The most extensive clinical trial in progress is a Phase III multi-institutional trial. Within a year or two, we should know a lot more about whether bisphosphonates will become as routine in the treatment of prostate cancer as they have for breast cancer.

There are good reasons to believe that these drugs will work. Two kinds of cells are active in bone metabolism—osteoclasts and osteoblasts. Osteoclasts break down bone; osteoblasts add new bone. Bone cells completely turn over every 100 days or so. Normally, the activity of these two types of cells is in balance; in other words, bone cells that dissolve bone and those that replace it turn over at an equal rate. In breast cancer, the osteoclasts are stimulated to dissolve bone by the release of a peptide by the tumor cells. In prostate cancer, osteoblasts are stimulated to lay down new bone. This is why breast cancer bony metastases are characterized as osteoclastic, while prostate cancer metastases are classified as osteoblastic. In both cases, bone metabolism is out of balance.

New evidence indicates that there appears to be a significant amount of bone breakdown as well as new bone formation in men with bone metastases, since tests show that markers of bone breakdown are increased in these men. Additionally, it has recently been shown that androgen-ablating hormonal therapy also increases bone turnover. From these two important findings it can be inferred that although prostate cancer bony metastases are predominately osteoblastic in nature, there is a significant osteoclastic component in the disease process.

Bisphosphonates inhibit osteoclasts. They dramatically reduce bone resorption. Precisely how they do this is still being worked out. But according to Dr. Mundy of the University of Texas Health Science Center, the mechanism may be a combination of inhibiting the formation of new osteoclasts and speeding up the death rate of mature osteoclasts. However they do it, the net result is that bisphosphonates, by their effect on osteoclasts, reduce bone turnover and, more importantly, reduce the amount of tumor present in bone. Additionally, Dr. Matthew Smith recently reported in the *New England Journal of Medicine* that pamidronate, a bisphosphonate, prevents bone loss in men on hormonal therapy.

You may be thinking that this is all well and good, but bisphosphonates work on osteoclasts and prostate cancer is osteoblastic. This is true. However, the cancer cell produces a substance called urokinase plasminogen activator (uPA), which stimulates osteoblast activity. For osteoblasts to lay down new bone, they require calcium. A drop in calcium may stimulate the osteoclasts to dissolve bone to keep calcium levels in balance, according to a theory postulated by Dr. Stephen Strum, a recently retired medical oncologist and prostate cancer specialist. When the osteoclasts go to work, they release growth factors, just as in the breast cancer model, that help the cancer cells proliferate.

Furthermore, it has been shown both biochemically and histologically (histology is the study of tissue structure) that this abnormal osteoblastic bone formation is preceded by activation of osteoclasts. Moreover, it's this osteoclastic activity that appears to be associated with bone pain in men with prostate cancer. If this is so, then bisphosphonates should reduce bone pain in these men, and they do. In one study there was a 76% decrease in bone pain in men that received intravenous injections of the bisphosphonate olpadronate (Aredia) daily for five days. This response was sustained if the men continued to take oral olpadronate after their intravenous course.

In another study, alendronate (Fosamax) reduced bone pain in 11 out of 12 patients. The investigator, Dr. Adami, concluded, "Administration of large doses of bisphosphonates is one of the most cost-effective palliation treatments for patients with prostate carcinoma with bone metastases, both as first-line therapy and in the long term. With appropriate doses, a large proportion of patients can be maintained free of bone pain until death."

The bottom line is this: By reducing bone turnover, bisphosphonates seem to play an important role in curtailing the synergistic interplay between prostate cancer cells and bone cells. This considerably reduces bone pain in many men. New animal studies using the new more potent bisphosphonate zoledronic acid (Zometa) show a decrease in bone metastases. This, combined with the proven results in breast cancer, bodes well for the possible future use of bisphosphonates in preventing, or delaying, the spread of prostate cancer to bone.

Bisphosphonates, Hormones, and Osteoporosis

The use of bisphosphonates has been well-established in the prevention of osteoporosis in men taking hormones for more than six months. With androgen deprivation there's increased bone turnover and bone loss, according to Dr. Celestia Higano, a medical oncologist at the University of Washington. She studied 16 normal men who started complete androgen blockade. She found that they all lost bone density on hormonal therapy. The average loss was 4% in the lumbar spine in nine months. This is a faster rate of loss than that suffered by post-menopausal women.

An Australian study noted an even faster rate of bone loss—an average of 7% annually. It's estimated that each one to two years of androgen deprivation doubles the risk of bone fractures due to osteoporosis. One to two years later this risk doubles again, and continues to double every couple of years. Men on long-term hormonal therapy are therefore at substantial risk for complications of osteoporosis. Bisphosphonates significantly reduce this risk. In fact, some men may actually increase their bone density by using bisphosphonates, while on complete hormonal blockade (see Michael Milken's story in "Putting It All Together"). Combining this medication with weight-bearing exercise probably improves its effectiveness.

Taking Bisphosphonates
As a Preventive Measure

Side effects from bisphosphonates are minimal, consisting mostly of minor gastro-intestinal symptoms in some men. Given this fact, Michael Milken posed this intriguing question to a panel of experts on prostate cancer: "If there are no known serious side effects from bisphosphonates, and they might prevent, or slow down, the spread of prostate cancer to bone, why wouldn't you take bisphosphonates if you have prostate cancer and can afford it?" Some members of the panel responded that as yet there's no scientific proof that bisphosphonates inhibit the spread of prostate cancer to bone. They would prefer to wait until the results of studies currently in progress are finished.

The physicians' caution is understandable. There could be long-term side effects that are not apparent currently. Since we don't have firm scientific evidence of bisphosphonates' efficacy, their use for this purpose may be premature. This is a reasonable, prudent scientific position.

But for the man who has prostate cancer now, especially if his PSA is rising, he can't wait. Although the panel members were not entirely comfortable with it, the consensus was that, under these circumstances, they could understand the rationale for taking bisphosphonates.

In my opinion, the risk/reward ratio clearly favors taking bisphosphonates, if you have recurrent prostate cancer (rising PSA after definitive local therapy) or are on hormonal therapy. Also, if you're relying on lifestyle changes alone (watchful waiting) to combat your disease, this medication might provide some additional protection, though it hasn't been proven. At the time of this writing, bisphosphonates are not covered by insurance. They cost about $80 per month. Hopefully, by the time you read this, there will be enough hard evidence to cover their use in health plans. Otherwise, you'll have to weigh the potential benefits against the cost and potential risk. I take them and plan on continuing to do so until I'm reasonably sure that my cancer will not recur. I take one 70-mg Fosamax tablet weekly.

Having said all of this, the jury is still out on whether bisphosphonates will ultimately be proven to reduce bony metastases in men with prostate cancer. A counter-argument can be made that since bisphosphonates inhibit and kill osteoclasts, this could lead to more osteoblast activity, which could make the prostate cancer worse. This is precisely why clinical trials are so important: to resolve issues such as these. For now, we can only conclusively say that bisphosphonates reduce bone pain in the wide majority of men with painful bony tumors and help prevent osteoporosis.

Nutritional Factors That May Be Helpful in Avoiding Osteoporosis

The following may be especially useful for men on hormones:

• Green leafy vegetables are rich in vitamin K. High levels of vitamin K are associated with a reduced risk of hip fractures.

• An English study shows that women who drink tea have higher bone density that those who don't.

Key References

Adami S. Bisphosphonates in prostate cancer. *Cancer* 1997; 80: 1679-1679.

Pelger R et al. Effects of the bisphosphonate olpadronate in patients with carcinoma of the prostate metastatic to the skeleton. *Bone* 1998; 22: 403-408.

Coleman R. Skeletal complications of malignancy. *Cancer* 1997; 80: 1588-1594.

Boissier S et al. Bisphosphonates inhibit prostate and breast carcinoma cell adhesion to unmineralized and mineralized bone extracellular matrices. *Cancer Res* 1997; 57: 3890-3894.

Diel I et al. Reduction in new metastases in breast cancer with adjuvant clodronate treatment. *N Engl J Med* 1998; 339: 357-363.

Smith M et al. Pamidronate to prevent bone loss during androgen-deprivation therapy for prostate cancer. *N Engl J Med* 2001; 345: 948-955.

Padalecki S. Androgen deprivation causes bone loss and increased prostate cancer metastases to bone: prevention by zoledronic acid. Ninth Annual Prostate Cancer Foundation Retreat, September 20-22, 2002; poster 63.

13

PC-SPES: A COMPLEMENTARY HERBAL REMEDY

Complementary Medicine: An Overview

For years a running battle has been waged between traditional and alternative medicine. When I was in medical school, the attitude conveyed by my instructors was this: "What you don't learn here has little if any validity." Criticism from the medical establishment of vitamins, supplements, and herbs has been based on a paucity of well-designed studies. Questions arise about standardization, quality control, and false or misleading representations by unqualified people working in health-food stores.

To a large extent, these concerns seem justified. For example, in a test of ginseng preparations, potency varied widely; 25% of the products analyzed had no ginsenosides in them. Another example: Some Chinese-grown astragulus, an herb with possible immune-enhancing qualities, has high levels of selenium, and while some selenium seems to reduce prostate cancer, too much can be toxic. Although it's unlikely for a man taking astragulus to reach toxic blood levels of selenium, it's conceivable if he takes large amounts of a high-selenium astragulus preparation, along with supplemental selenium. It would be helpful if the selenium concentration of astragulus formulations was specified. But there is no requirement to do so. Standardization and quality control from batch to batch would, in my opinion, greatly benefit the herb and supplement industry.

The medical community, on the other hand, has carried its distaste for alternative remedies too far. For many years, it has resisted a mounting body of evidence on the positive effects of vitamins and antioxidants. Even today, not all doctors would embrace the efficacy of vitamin E in reducing heart disease. Low-dose aspirin is more palatable to most doctors for this purpose. Actually, both are effective. New evidence shows that they work synergistically—that is, they're more effective taken together than the sum of each of their individual activities.

Some doctors seem to viscerally recoil at the mere mention of non-medical therapies. Although as many as 60% of cancer patients use herbal remedies, they are reluctant to discuss this with their medical practitioners. In fact, surveys show that up to 70% of patients using alternative medicines don't tell their doctors! Why? Because they fear the doctor's probable response, which, in all likelihood, will be critical. Patients have learned not to broach the subjects of vitamins, supplements, and herbs to avoid being lectured or put down. Since they believe what they're taking may be having a beneficial effect, the result of the doctor's disapproval can lead to conflict. Rather than go through this, they simply keep complementary augmentations to their medical program to themselves.

Yet another good example of this "alternative phobia" came from first-hand experience. A few years ago my mother was diagnosed with lung cancer. It had spread widely beyond the lungs. The regional lymph nodes in her chest, pancreas, adrenal glands, and bones were all involved. A distant lymph node just below the clavicle was also involved, a particularly ominous sign.

The medical oncologist was pleasant, honest, and well-informed. After long discussions with the doctor, in which I participated, my mother chose a course of chemotherapy with an agent that has relatively minor side effects. At the same time, at my suggestion, she began an aggressive complementary anti-cancer program of nutrition, exercise, herbs, supplements, massage, and meditation. The doctor told her the chance of a short remission with the chemotherapeutic agent she had selected was 25%.

Her response surprised everyone. Within three months, there was no discernible cancer in her adrenal glands, pancreas, bones, or distant lymph node. Her primary lung cancer and thoracic lymph-node involvement had shrunk by 50%. The doctor told me this was one of the best responses he'd ever seen. Then I broached the ineffable. I started to tell him about her complementary anti-cancer program. He politely cut me off, saying, "Whatever she's doing she should keep doing."

I asked, "But don't you want to know what it is?"

"No," he responded emphatically, "it would only be anecdotal and of no use. It would probably confuse me."

I sat there feeling nonplussed. Were I in his position, curiosity alone would have dictated an explanation. Yet this talented physician closed down all discussion.

His objection is accurate. Of course it's anecdotal! It applies to only one case, my mother. But it's no more anecdotal than the effect of the chemotherapeutic agent in this particular case. The oncologist was quite impressed with how *it* worked! I think there's a good chance that, based on this particularly good result, he will be more likely to use this form of chemotherapy on other lung cancer patients—just as he's likely to quickly forget that my mother had been supported by a strong complementary program.

Couldn't she be just one of the 25% that responds to this regimen? She could be. Of those that do respond, her response was in the top 1%, according to the oncologist. This makes the overall odds of this response 1 in 400. Still possible, due to chance, though unlikely. My guess is that her lifestyle changes made a difference in improving the effectiveness of the chemotherapy. It makes sense that cancer patients with a strengthened immune system are more likely to be able to better combat cancer.

What's necessary to bridge the gap between traditional medicine and complementary medicine? Controlled randomized prospective medical studies. But these take money. Lots of money. Who will fund them? Certainly not the drug companies, which have a vested interest in seeing them fail. Since naturally occurring substances cannot be patented, there is no financial motivation for a commercial company to finance such research. This has restricted high-powered studies.

Recently, however, a couple of developments have emerged that may help bring traditional and complementary medicine closer together, especially in prostate cancer. First, the National Cancer Institute is financing studies on natural products that may have anti-cancer benefits. Secondly, a private foundation, Michael Milken's Prostate Cancer Foundation (formerly CaP CURE), has funded nutritional research and studies on herbal remedies for prostate cancer. One of these, PC-SPES, has attracted the attention of some top mainstream specialists in prostate cancer. Regrettably, it was recently found to be contaminated with DES and other drugs, but new studies show it works differently than DES.

Ideally, complementary and conventional medicine should work together. They are not at odds with each other. In combination, their effect can be synergistic. To accomplish this goal, more good studies are required to better define the benefits of non-medical interventions. Equally important, doctors must become educated on useful complementary strategies. This is beginning to happen.

Traditional Chinese Medicine (TCM) and PC-SPES

There are currently more than 700 TCM anti-cancer recipes, according to Dr. Shaomeng Wang in a poster presented at the Prostate Cancer Foundation Retreat in September 2002. From these recipes, about 8,000 small molecules can be isolated that have more than 100 targets in cancer therapy. One such small molecule has a potent effect on the Bcl-2 family of proteins that are often observed in men with hormone-resistant prostate cancer. In the laboratory this powerful small molecule, isolated from TCM, causes hormone-resistant prostate cancer cells to self-destruct. It also seems to work synergistically with the chemotherapeutic agent Taxotere in inhibiting the action of Bcl-2 and related proteins. BL-193, as this new small molecule is called, when combined with Taxotere caused complete disappearance of 50% of prostate tumors in mice. It can be taken orally and has been found to have very few side effects in humans. Clinical trials will commence soon at the University of Michigan Cancer Center for men with hormone-refractory prostate cancer.

It's my belief that TCM will provide useful adjuncts to Western medicine in future comprehensive cancer treatment programs.

Key Reference
Wang S. Design of Bcl-2 and Bcl-xl small molecule inhibitors as an entirely new class of therapy for prostate cancer. Poster presentation # 98; Ninth Annual Prostate Cancer Foundation Scientific Retreat. September 20-22, 2002.

PC-SPES—Prologue

PC-SPES is a Chinese herbal formulation that gained popularity as an herbal treatment for prostate cancer. It showed great promise, because clinical trials demonstrated that it had activity in both hormone-dependent and hormone-independent prostate cancer. Recently, it has come to light that certain batches were contaminated with drugs, such as diethylstilbesterol (DES), an estrogen; indomethicin, an anti-inflammatory; and warfarin, an anti-coagulant. Since PC-SPES has significant estrogenic activity and DES is an estrogen, DES was thought to be the most significant of these drug contaminants. PC-SPES has now been taken off the market.

As I was debating whether to delete the ensuing chapter,

a new study financed by the Prostate Cancer Foundation (formerly CaP CURE) was published in the November 6, 2002, issue of the *Journal of the National Cancer Institute*. This new study, authored by Dr. Peter Nelson and his colleagues at the Fred Hutchison Cancer Research Institute in Seattle, Washington, demonstrates how PC-SPES and DES affect the expression of different genes in prostate cancer cells. The genes that are activated by exposure to PC-SPES turn out to be different from those activated by DES.

Two of the most significant classes of gene changes when prostate cancer cells were exposed to PC-SPES were genes relating to the response of the cells to androgens, including the androgen receptor, and genes involved in the formation of microtubules. Both sets of genes were down-regulated. A decrease in the androgen receptor means that the cancer cells were less susceptible to the mitotic and growth effects of androgens. Microtubules are essential for cell division. By severely down-regulating the genes responsible for their creation, PC-SPES markedly decreases the cancer cell's ability to divide and multiply. The net effect of these genetic down-regulations is an inhibition of prostate cancer cell growth.

It's noteworthy that DES doesn't inhibit the androgen receptor and doesn't have the same effect on microtubules as PC-SPES. Therefore, despite the inescapable and unfortunate fact that some lots of PC-SPES were clearly contaminated, it has now been shown conclusively that PC-SPES and DES have different mechanisms of action in prostate cancer cells.

Due to this just-released study and the fact that there are a number of men with advanced prostate cancer who are in long-term remissions with PC-SPES, I've decided to include the ensuing chapter, even though the formula is not currently available in the United States.

The National Institute of Health is becoming involved in the study of PC-SPES and new batches (which will be thoroughly tested for any drug contaminants) have been ordered from China.

I believe that PC-SPES will get resurrected and become

an important part of the arsenal of treatments for prostate cancer.

Another interesting finding in Dr. Nelson's study is that the combination of PC-SPES and the chemotherapeutic drug Taxol actually decreased the tumor response when compared to either agent alone. *PC-SPES should not be used with Taxol or Taxotere.* This finding once again supports this important point: You must tell your doctors about complementary or alternative medicines, herbs, or vitamins that you're taking, since they may either interfere with or enhance the effects of prescription medications.

Key References

Bonham M et al. Effects of the herbal extract PC-SPES on microtubule dynamics and paclitaxel-mediated prostate tumor growth inhibition. *J Natl Cancer Instit* 2002; 94: 1641-1947.

Nelson P. Identity of clinically relevant active pathways of complementary and alternative prostate cancer therapies. Ninth Annual Prostate Cancer Foundation Retreat, September 20-22, 2002.

What Is PC-SPES?

PC-SPES is an herbal formula that combines seven Chinese herbs and one American herb. It's the creation of chemist Sophie Chen, Ph.D., and Allan Wang, M.D. Here are the eight herbs with a brief description of each.

• Dendranthema (chrysanthemum)—A calming herb, with cooling properties. Helps eliminate toxins from the body.

• Isatis indigotica—Contains beta-sitosterol and indirubin, both of which have anti-cancer effects.

• Glycyrrhiza glabra (licorice)—Anti-inflammatory and anti-cancer effects. Reduces serum testosterone levels. Also stimulates the immune system. Contains quercetin, which is thought to have anti-tumor properties.

• Ganoderma lucidum—Derived from a hard umbrella-like mushroom that grows on certain trees. Ganoderma has anti-tumor properties and immune-system-modulating effects. Evidence indicates that it may increase natural killer (NK) cells, immune system cells known to be active in fighting cancer.

• Panax pseudo-ginseng—Know as an "adaptagen," this herb may help with stress reduction. It also has immune-system-stimulating properties. Like ganoderma, it stimulates the activity of NK cells.

• Scutellaria baicalensis (scute)—Has anti-bacterial and anti-tumor effects. Contains baicalin, baicalein, and wogonin, all of which have been shown to have independent, dose-dependent, anti-proliferative effects on cancer cells. Scute significantly reduces the growth of bladder cancer in mice. These effects were reported in the June 2000 issue of the journal *Urology*. Japanese researchers from Osaka City University Medical School, led by Dr. Ikemoto concluded, "These results suggest that Chinese herbal medicines may become an attractive and promising treatment for bladder cancer." Baicalin, the most potent ingredient, may also upregulate (increase) the expression of the p27 tumor suppressor gene.

• Rabdosia rebescens—Has anti-tumor actions. May help reduce side effects from other cancer treatments, such as chemotherapy.

• Serenoa repens—This is the only Western herb in PC-SPES. It may have an effect on inhibiting 5-alpha reductase, reducing the conversion of testosterone to DHT, although studies conflict on this.

Does PC-SPES Work?

Normally, an herbal preparation like PC-SPES wouldn't get off the ground in conventional medical circles. Without available funding for proper clinical trials, it would be destined to remain mired in the murk of other herbal remedies. At best, it would be rejected as peripheral. At worst, it might even be branded as dangerous. But thanks to funding from the Prostate Cancer Foundation it has, for the most part, escaped this fate.

Dr. Eric Small, a respected medical oncologist at the University of California-San Francisco and his team, have subjected PC-SPES to the same rigorous standards used to test any new medicine—controlled clinical trials. They studied 70 men, 33 of whom had never had hormonal therapy. These 33 men fell into 2 groups. The first group of 22 men had been treated with either surgery or radiation, but had a rising PSA, indicating that their treatment had been unsuccessful. The second group, 11 men, had never had hormones, and was using PC-SPES as their initial treatment for prostate cancer.

When testing the usefulness of any new drug for prostate cancer, a criterion that is used to measure effectiveness is a drop in PSA of 50%, or more. In the 33 men who had never received hormones, 22 who had either surgery or radiation and now have a rising PSA (meaning the primary treatment failed), and 11 using PC-SPES as their first primary treatment, all had a drop in PSA of at least 50%. And 58% of these men reached undetectable PSA levels. In addition, Dr. Small's team documented at least a 50% decrease in the size of the prostate tumor in 15 out of 20 men tested. So far, only man has developed hormone-resistant disease while on PC-SPES.

The balance of the men in this study had hormone-independent prostate cancer, meaning their cancer no longer responded to androgen deprivation. PC-SPES worked in this group too. This surprised investigators who believed that the effect of PC-SPES came from its estrogenic properties. Men in this group had rising PSAs, despite castrate testosterone levels from hormones. With PC-SPES, 57% had a drop in PSA of at least 50%. Even men who had received so-called second line hormonal therapy with ketokonazole (Nizoral), and whose PSA was again rising after this treatment failed, responded to PC-SPES. 56% of these men had a PSA decline of at least 50%. This compares favorably to most current chemotherapeutic regimens, and has fewer significant side effects. If these results are confirmed, PC-SPES should be seriously considered before chemotherapy. Another alternative would be to use it in conjunction with chemo (but not with Taxol or Taxotere).

Still to be determined is how long PC-SPES will be effective for each of these categories. I'm also interested in following the progress of those men that are using PC-SPES as their primary treatment.

Dose of PC-SPES

PC-SPES comes in capsules. There are 333 mg of the formula in each. It does not require a prescription. Dr. Small gives the men in his trials one capsule three times a day for the first week. During the second week they take two capsules three times a day. From then on they take three capsules three times a day.

Some men who have gotten excellent responses from PC-SPES, outside of Dr. Small's studies, have experimented with reduced doses. Some take six per day and reduce this gradually to three per day when their PSA bottoms out. Optimal doses for various uses in prostate cancer have not been firmly established. Generally speaking, the more advanced the cancer, the higher the required dose. The men experimenting with dose reductions are using their PSA response as a guideline. If their PSA begins to inch up after a dose reduction, they increase their dosage. It appears that the minimal maintenance dose is three capsules per day. Lesser amounts are probably ineffective.

Using PC-SPES for PSA Maintenance After Hormones

Dr. Aaron Katz is an assistant professor of Urology at Columbia Presbyterian Hospital in New York City. He has actively used PC-SPES in some men who have prostate cancer. His main approach has been to lower a man's PSA to at least 4.0 ng/ml with complete androgen blockade. He then stops the hormones and puts his patients on three capsules of PC-SPES daily. He has had excellent results in stabilizing

PSAs at low, or undetectable, levels using this low-dose program. At this dose, side effects are also minimized.

Dr. Katz stresses that, in his opinion, PC-SPES should not be used as a replacement for conventional treatment, but rather as a complementary treatment. Used sequentially with hormones, as Dr. Katz often does, PC-SPES can help reduce the side effects of hormones. It may also have a direct effect on apoptosis in prostate cancer cells. Based on Dr. Small's trials, cancer cells that are no longer dependent on androgens to grow may also be killed by the actions of PC-SPES. This is a good complement to the effects of traditional hormone therapy, which works only on androgen-dependent cancer cells.

Another traditional cancer treatment that PC-SPES may complement is radiation. In a report published in the *International Journal of Oncology*, Dr. Darzynkiewicz and his team from the New York Medical College in Valhalla, New York, observed that PC-SPES sensitized lymphoma U937 cancer cells to the effects of radiation. One and a half Gy of radiation did not increase apoptosis in these cells. But incubating these cells in PC-SPES first resulted in programmed cell death (apoptosis) in 22% of the cells. When these PC-SPES-treated cells additionally were subjected to 1.5 Gy of irradiation, apoptosis increased to 32% of the cells. When the radiation dose was cranked up to 5.0 Gy, apoptosis was observed in 46%.

Lymphoma cells are not prostate cancer cells. Additional laboratory and animal studies need to be conducted to confirm PC-SPES's sensitizing effect on prostate cancer cells. Then, if the results are positive, human trials are necessary. If proven to sensitize prostate cancer cells to radiation, PC-SPES will have achieved another complementary link in the treatment of prostate cancer.

Side Effects From PC-SPES

The side effects from PC-SPES increase with the dose. At the therapeutic dose of nine capsules daily used in Dr. Small's studies, the following side effects were observed:

- Loss of libido in virtually all men.
- Loss of potency in all men who were potent prior to treatment.
- Breast enlargement and/or tenderness in virtually all men.
- Hot flashes in 33%.
- Leg cramps in about 33%.
- Slight nausea or diarrhea in 33%.
- 15%-20% had an allergic reaction (alleviated by Benadryl).
- Two out of 70 men had blood clots in their legs or lungs.

How to Reduce the Side Effects of PC-SPES

Although nothing can be done about the loss of libido, some men regain potency with Viagra. Since more than 90% reach castrate levels of testosterone while on high-doses of PC-SPES, loss of libido and potency is to be expected. Although no studies have been done on the use of Viagra in men taking PC-SPES, one would logically expect the results to be similar to those experienced by men on hormones. Many men can, therefore, expect a positive response.

Breast enlargement and tenderness seem to be the side effect that troubles PC-SPES users most. A short course of painless localized radiation to the breasts before starting PC-SPES eliminates this problem. If you plan on taking six or more PC-SPES per day, I urge you to consider this preventive treatment. More and more doctors who use PC-SPES are recommending this to avoid annoying breast-related side effects. Tamoxifen may also reduce breast-related symptoms.

Hot flashes are far less common with PC-SPES than with hormonal therapy. If they require treatment, please refer to the "Hot Flashes" section of the Hormonal Therapy chapter.

I would try nutritional modifications, such as increasing soy and red-clover intake, first. If this is not enough, try adding a low-dose anti-depressant.

The slight nausea and diarrhea usually require no treatment. Lomotil to control diarrhea may be required in some cases.

Allergic reactions can be controlled by taking Benadryl.

Leg cramps are reduced, according to reports from men who have had this symptom, by drinking V-8 juice daily. This is a good idea in any event since it's high in lycopene (see page 297).

The only potentially serious side effect from PC-SPES is blood clots. These can cause swelling and pain in the legs. They may break off and be carried to the lungs. Dr. Small has noted, however, that men with advanced prostate cancer naturally have an increased rate of these vascular mishaps. Nevertheless, Dr. Small routinely prescribes the blood thinner Coumadin for PC-SPES users.

Some doctors may recommend aspirin to thin the blood for men taking PC-SPES. But Dr. Small points out, "Aspirin won't do anything for men on PC-SPES. With PC-SPES, clotting problems, if they occur, do so in the venous system. Aspirin works on the arterial system, not the venous system."

How PC-SPES Works

Now that there's sound evidence that PC-SPES helps reduce prostate cancer, questions arise as to what compounds in this herbal mixture are having an effect and why. Chinese medicine is based on the premise that herbs can be combined to act synergistically to restore balance and harmony to the body. Acting together, they're more potent than any component acting individually. PC-SPES is a synergistic formulation that not only has a direct anti-proliferative effect on prostate cancer cells, but also decreases inflammation and stimulates the immune system. The effects are interactive and amplify each other.

Western medicine works on a different premise. It is more cause-and-effect oriented. As such, the question in the minds of Western researchers is, "What is the *active* ingredient of PC-SPES?" This may be difficult to ascertain, because PC-SPES has multiple, synergistic, biological actions. Let's examine some of these effects.

• Hormonal effect—The action of PC-SPES that has been most discussed is its effect on testosterone. At a dose of nine capsules a day, testosterone levels drop in virtually all men who have normal levels when beginning PC-SPES. In more than 90% of these men, it drops to levels comparable to CAB or orchiectomy. In fact, before Dr. Small's work showed an independent non-hormonal action, critics of PC-SPES labeled the formula as a "poorly understood, non-standardized, hormone treatment with potentially serious side effects" (deep-vein blood clots). Certainly androgen reduction is one of the ways PC-SPES works, but that's not the whole story. Some users report a rise in their testosterone levels six months or more after starting PC-SPES.

• Bcl-2 oncogene reduction—As you'll probably recall, the bcl-2 oncogene protects cancer cells from apoptosis, their natural way of dying. This destructive gene is often switched on (upregulated) in advanced disease. If cancer cells in the prostate biopsy stain positive for bcl-2 overproduction, it's a bad prognostic sign. PC-SPES switches off (downregulates) bcl-2. In a lab experiment on lymphoma cells, there was 33% less detectable bcl-2 within 48 hours of their exposure to an extract of PC-SPES at concentrations comparable to those achievable in men taking the formula. Lower levels of bcl-2 means that prostate cancer cells are likely to die as programmed. PC-SPES may also increase the susceptibility of the cancer cells to other treatments, like radiation or chemotherapy.

• Decreased proliferation of cancer cells—PC-SPES slows down the growth rate of cancer cells in the laboratory. It arrests their development at a stage in their growth cycle called G-1. PC-SPES has this effect on a variety of cancer cells tested, including both androgen-sensitive and andro-gen-independent prostate cancer cell lines.

• Reduces the ability of prostate cancer cells to form colonies—One of the ways cancer cells grow and spread is by their ability to clump together and form colonies. You may recall that a cancer cell circulating alone is vulnerable to attack by the body's immune defenses, like NK cells or T-4 lympho-cytes. If cancer cells can join together and form a colony, they are less vulnerable. They can also release growth factors that promote the development of blood vessels (angiogenesis). This provides the budding colony access to sources of nutrition. The result is a thriving site of metastatic cancer. In the lab, cancer cells treated with PC-SPES have difficulty forming colonies. Androgen-independent prostate cancer cells (known as PC-3) were the most sensitive to PC-SPES of the 9 different cancer cell lines tested for colony formation, in experiments conducted at New York Medical College. Preventing prostate cancer cells from forming colonies should slow down the development of metastatic disease.

• Decreases the amount of the androgen receptor—For testosterone and other androgens to stimulate the growth of prostate cancer cells, they must have a way to attach to the cancer cell. Like a space ship attaching to a space station, specific sites exist in the nucleus of prostate cancer cells that can receive and lock in androgens. The quantity of these androgen-binding sites is controlled by a gene called the "androgen receptor (AR)." When this gene is turned on (upregulated), more androgen receptors are formed; when it's downregulated, fewer ARs result. The fewer ARs there are, the less effect testosterone and other male hormones can have in stimulating prostate cancer cells to grow. In the lab, PC-SPES reduces the amount of AR in the nucleus of pros-tate cancer cells, presumably by downregulating the AR gene.

• Decreases the binding of male hormones to the andro-gen receptor—In addition to reducing the amount of the AR in prostate cancer cells, PC-SPES also decreases the ability of testosterone and other hormones to attach to those ARs that remain. Studies show that the ability of androgens to bind to the androgen receptor is reduced by 2.5 times after prostate cancer cells have been treated with PC-SPES. The combination of a reduction in the amount of the AR and the reduced binding ability of androgens work together to minimize the proliferative effects of male hormones on prostate cancer cells.

• Anti-inflammatory effects—As previously discussed, inflammation may play a role in the development of prostate cancer. Two herbs in PC-SPES in particular, scutellaria and glycyrrhiza, reduce inflammation.

• Antioxidant effects—Antioxidants are discussed in detail in Chapter 18. Oxidation can damage DNA. Anti-oxidants can reduce or prevent this DNA damage. PC-SPES contains saponins, flavonoids, and polyphenols, all effective antioxidants.

• Drop in PSA—One of the most striking effects of PC-SPES is a significant drop in PSA levels in many men who try it. Androgen-responsive prostate cancer cells treated in the lab with PC-SPES for four to six days had a 60%-70% decrease in PSA production. It's not clear whether PC-SPES has a direct effect on the gene responsible for PSA production (by downregulating it), or whether the effect of PC-SPES is indirect. Reduction in the amount of AR, an arrest of prostate cancer cell growth in the G-1 phase, and an increase in apoptosis of prostate cancer cells should all have an indirect effect in reducing PSA levels.

This debate, as to whether PC-SPES has a direct effect on the PSA gene or an indirect effect due to its action in subduing prostate cancer cells, is not merely theoretical. Men with advanced disease want to know whether the formula is reducing their cancer or just lowering their PSA. Based on laboratory data, animal experiments, and objective human response as quantified by Dr. Small and others, I think it's safe to conclude that PC-SPES retards the development of and kills prostate cancer cells.

PC-SPES and Metastatic Prostate Cancer

We know from patient feedback and Dr. Small's findings that PC-SPES can sometimes produce dramatic clinical responses in some men with metastatic prostate cancer who've become refractory to hormonal therapy. Dr. Raj Tiwari and his associates at the New York Medical College tested the effectiveness of PC-SPES on a particularly deadly line of prostate cancer cells known as MAT-LyLu. These cells are known both for their rapid proliferation and resistance to most forms of treatment.

PC-SPES was fed to some rats as part of their diet. Control rats received no PC-SPES. Ten thousand live MAT-LyLu prostate cancer cells were injected into the skin of each animal. Tumors formed at the site of this injection in all rats that were not given PC-SPES. Later, all these rats had metastases to their lungs.

Rats fed PC-SPES were divided into two groups. One was fed the formula equal to 0.025% of their total diet; the second group got twice this amount, 0.05%. About three weeks after the cancer cells were injected into the PC-SPES-fed animals, an effect was observed in a dose-dependent manner. That is, rats with diets composed of 0.05% PC-SPES responded better than rats getting 0.025%. Specifically, rats receiving the lower amount had a 20% decrease in tumors that could be felt in the skin where the cancer cells had been injected. Animals that got the higher dose had a 40% decrease in palpable tumors at the injection site. While all the rats without PC-SPES in their diet got skin tumors, some of the animals that got PC-SPES didn't develop a detectable tumor mass at the injection site. The rats that had no skin tumor at the injection site also had no lung metastases. But rats that were on the PC-SPES diet, and still developed cancer that could be felt in the skin, also developed lung metastases. This would indicate that some rats responded to PC-SPES, while others did not.

Interestingly, this parallels the clinical experience in men taking PC-SPES. Some get dramatic responses, while others seem to have no response at all, according to Dr. Mittleman, one of the lead investigators in the above rat study. Perhaps there are differences in the immune response to the herbs. Some men's immune systems may be compromised from prior treatments, like chemotherapy. Conceivably, this could impair their response to PC-SPES. This is supported by the finding that PC-SPES seems to lose effectiveness in men who have active infections. When the immune system is fighting an infection, it seems incapable of also responding to stimulation from herbs. With chemo, the immune system is often compromised and may similarly be unable to respond to stimulation. The manufacturer recommends stopping the herbs at times of acute infections, even colds and flus.

Another possibility is that PC-SPES might be more active in men in whom the bcl-2 oncogene is switched on. According to Dr. Howard Scher at Sloan Kettering, 70% of men with androgen-independent metastatic disease have an overexpression of bcl-2. Are these the same men who respond to PC-SPES? By down-regulating bcl-2, these men might have dramatic PSA responses. It would be interesting to test cancer tissue from PC-SPES responders for bcl-2 to examine this hypothesis. At this point, these potential mechanisms are mere conjecture.

One last point before leaving this study. The researchers calculated that rats eating a diet with 0.05% PC-SPES were ingesting an amount approximately equivalent to nine capsules a day, the recommended therapeutic dose for men with advanced disease. Rats ingesting a 0.025% PC-SPES diet were getting the equivalent of about four capsules. The authors believe that doses lower than 0.025% may not have a significant impact on tumor development and lung metastases in rats. Extending this to man, doses less than three to four capsules daily may be ineffectual. Until more is known to establish the minimum dose required to produce an effect, it is probably wise not to use less than three capsules per day, if you're taking PC-SPES.

On the other hand, doses higher than nine capsules per day should be used with extreme caution to avoid estrogen-like side effects, like deep-vein thrombosis. Although there may be cases when up to 12 capsules a day may be taken for a short time under close medical supervision, for most men nine capsules a day is sufficient to induce a response in those likely to respond. Doses higher than 12 capsules per day should never be used. This is another case where too much of a potentially good thing may be harmful.

Prostate cancer experts concur: The behavior of this cancer involves a balance between factors that lead to cell death and survival. When this balance tips in favor of prolonged cancer-cell survival, the cancer grows. The greater this imbalance, the more dangerous the cancer. The nature of the prostate cancer in each individual is constantly changing. To control the disease, it's imperative to restore the balance between cell life and death. Perhaps, in the Chinese tradition, PC-SPES helps restore this balance in some men. Over time, we'll hopefully discover the reasons for the drastically different response observed in men using PC-SPES.

Potential Uses

For men with low-risk disease who elect to use lifestyle changes as their primary treatment and defer definitive therapy (surgery, radiation, etc.), PC-SPES might be used to reduce the PSA level and, perhaps, shrink the tumor. For this purpose, six per day is probably sufficient, declining to three per day when the PSA bottoms out. Close PSA monitoring every one to three months is recommended. Remember, PC-SPES used in this manner should be part of an overall lifestyle strategy, rather than as a substitute for these lifestyle changes. This use has not yet been verified in clinical trials.

As a complement to hormonal therapy, if intermittent androgen blockade is being used, PC-SPES might be used during the periods off hormones. Three capsules daily are what Dr. Katz uses for this purpose.

Due to its apparent reduction in bcl-2 gene expression, PC-SPES may weaken prostate cancer cells so that they respond better to other treatments, like radiation or chemotherapy. Consider using PC-SPES to complement these therapies. Please note, however, that this use is based on a conclusion that has not yet been documented by clinical trials.

As a second-line hormonal treatment to be used with men when CAB is no longer effective, PC-SPES could be used either before or after ketoconazole. More than half the men who no longer respond to ketoconazole have a greater than 50% decline in their PSA on 9 capsules of PC-SPES per day. Dr. Mittleman has shown that PC-SPES is active in rats against the highly metastatic prostate cancer cell line MAT-LyLu. This is significant, because this cell line is resistant to most treatments.

Summary and Caveats

PC-SPES may be an effective complement to conventional treatment for certain men with prostate cancer. It may not be appropriate for other men. If you're planning to use PC-SPES, it's important that you tell your doctors; if they're not familiar with the product, you will have to educate them. One reason it's important to tell them is that they may attribute a drop in PSA to another treatment. Believing that this is what's working, your doctor may up the dose, which could be counterproductive. Another reason is that if side effects develop from PC-SPES, your doctor will correctly understand their source and not misinterpret them. It's always best to work in close consultation with your doctor on all aspects of your prostate cancer program. PC-SPES is no exception.

Eastern medicine relies on a combination of ingredients that work together and amplify each other. In this case, the whole may be greater than the sum of its parts. The combination of herbs is more effective than any one component, even if that single ingredient is taken in much larger amounts. Avoid the temptation of noticing one or more of the eight components in PC-SPES in your local health-food shop and taking it (them) thinking that you'll get a similar effect. You won't.

PC-SPES is classified as a nutritional supplement. Due to previously mentioned contamination problems, it is currently unavailable in the U.S. Hopefully, it will be reintroduced shortly with tighter controls.

PC-SPES should be used in conjunction with proper nutrition, exercise, and stress-reduction programs. It should be considered as part of an overall lifestyle program rather than an end in itself.

It has not been proven that PC-SPES alone can cure prostate cancer. Although there is sound reason for enthusiasm for this product, there is no basis to conclude that it cures prostate cancer.

The amount of PC-SPES should be gradually increased to desired levels. In Dr. Small's studies, men started with three capsules a day for the first week, increased to six capsules per day for the second week, and leveled out at nine capsules a day at the beginning of the third week.

PC-SPES is not cheap. When available, the cost was $108 for 60 capsules. This works out to about $325 per month for men taking six capsules daily, and nearly $500 per month for men taking nine capsules a day, like those in Dr. Small's trials. PC-SPES is not currently covered by medical insurance.

Key References

Ikemoto S et al. Antitumor effects of Scutellariae radix and its components baicalein, baicalin, and wogonin on bladder cancer cell lines. *Urology* 2000; 55: 951-955.

Halicka D et al. Apoptosis and cell cycle effects induced by extracts of the Chinese herbal preparation PC-SPES. *Int J Oncol* 1997; 11: 437-448.

Hsieh TC et al. Effects of PC-SPES on proliferation and expression of AR/PSA in androresponsive LNCaP cells are independent of estradiol. *Anticancer Research* 2002; 22: 2051-2060.

Lu X et. al. PC-SPES inhibits cell proliferation by modulating p21, cyclins D, E and multiple cell cycle-related genes in prostate cancer cells. *Cell Cycle* 2003; 2: 59-63.

Tiwari R et al. Anti-tumor effects of PC-SPES an herbal formulation for prostate cancer. *Int J Oncol* 1999; 14: 713-719.

Presentation by Eric Small, M.D. on clinical trials of PC-SPES in hormone-naive and androgen-independent cases of prostate cancer. Presented at the 1999 Prostate Cancer Foundation Prostate Cancer Retreat, Lake Tahoe, Nevada.

14

ADVANCED DISEASE, RECURRENCE, AND METASTASES

Overview

In 2002, about 30,000 American men died of prostate cancer. This is down from the 42,000 who died in 1997. Part of this is probably due to earlier cancer detection in the PSA era and part to improved treatment.

Between 1986 and 1992, 11% of Caucasians and 20% of African-Americans had metastatic prostate cancer at the time of their initial diagnosis. These percentages have dropped with widespread PSA testing. In 2002, men with metastatic disease when first diagnosed are relatively uncommon in the United States.

How Cancer Metastasizes

For a cancer to grow in a place distant from its primary location requires a series of steps. Cells must break off from the main tumor, travel safely to their new location, establish themselves, and multiply. This process is more difficult than you might think. Isolated tumor cells are fragile. They can be killed by immune-system cells, such as NK cells and T-4 lymphocytes. They can also be affected by proteins formed by genes that may suppress metastases. One such "metastasis-suppressor gene" is found on chromosome 11 in women. It suppresses the formation of breast cancer metastases, not by preventing a breast cancer cell from reaching a target organ, but by preventing it from growing once it gets there. Given the similarities between breast and prostate cancer, it's reasonable to assume that similar genes will be found in men.

Similarities Between Breast Cancer and Prostate Cancer

• Breast tissue and prostate tissue have the same embryonic origins.
• The incidence of both breast cancer and prostate cancer among ethnic groups is similar.
• Both breast cancer and prostate cancer are classified as "hormonal cancers"—cancers influenced by hormones.
• Men with a family history of breast cancer are at an increased risk for prostate cancer.
• Breast tissue can produce PSA. In breast cancer an elevated PSA is a *favorable* prognostic sign; in prostate cancer it is a poor prognostic indicator. No tissue other than prostate produces as much PSA as breast tissue. Other tissues that produce PSA make only minute amounts.
• Dietary factors, such as high-fat diets, are associated with both breast cancer and prostate cancer.
• Some of the most promising chemotherapeutic agents in prostate cancer are also active in breast cancer (Taxol and Taxotere).
• Both breast cancer and prostate cancer are influenced by "oncogenes" and "cancer-suppressing genes."
• The primary target for metastases of both breast cancer and prostate cancer is bone.

In prostate cancer, we know that cells break off from the primary tumor early in the disease. Using a new sensitive assay, they can be found in the bone marrow in 50%-70% of men at the time of radical prostatectomy. They can also be found, nearly as frequently, in the blood. Using an enrichment technique that sharpens the accuracy of the assay, cancer cells are found in the peripheral blood in 73% and in the bone marrow of 82% of men at the time of surgery. Allowing for errors in sampling, virtually 100% of patients have prostate cancer cells in the blood and bone marrow, even when

both clinically and pathologically the cancer appears confined to the prostate. The fact that 70%-80% of these men
are cured of their cancer by surgery attests to the difficulty
circulating cancer cells have in finding their way to a new
home, surviving, and growing. Fortunately.

The primary target for the migrating prostate cancer cell
is bone. Proteins in the bone matrix called integrins hook up
with specific binding sites on the prostate cancer cell that
hold it tightly. This allows the cancer cell to take up resi-
dence in the bone matrix. Another bone protein known as
osteonectin helps the prostate cancer cells spread and invade. Not only do these cells have a particular affinity for
bone, some are able to survive in bone for many years in a
dormant state. This is why in some men, recurrences can
occur five to eight years or longer after surgery or radiation.
Dormant cells are probably immune to chemotherapy, which
depends on cell division to do its work.

How do prostate cancer cells survive? If we can understand this completely, perhaps we can devise preventive treatments. They survive by producing chemicals that stimulate
their growth and immortality. They also produce substances
that act on normal cells, inducing them to perform tasks that
benefit the cancer cells.

Both prostate and breast cancer cells seem particularly
well-suited to influence bone cells. Dr. Gregory Mundy from
the University of Texas at San Antonio presented just such
an interaction at the September 1999 meeting of the American Association for Cancer Research in Colorado. As reported
by Dr. H. Steven Wiley, Dr. Mundy's work shows how breast
cancer cells can produce a substance called parathyroid hor-
mone-related peptide (PTHrP), which can stimulate osteoclasts to dissolve tiny pockets of bone. This breakdown of
bone releases growth factors that stimulate development of
the cancer cells. A mutually beneficial relationship is established between the normal osteoclast and the abnormal malignant cell. The stimulated osteoclasts destroy more and more
bone while, at the same time, producing progressively more

growth factors that allow the cancer cells to proliferate. The result can be an established metastatic tumor growing out of control.

A similar symbiotic relationship exists in prostate cancer. As we saw in the section on bisphosphonates, the cancer cell produces urokinase plasminogen activator (uPA), which stimulates osteoblast activity, which in turn helps the cancer cells proliferate.

The prostate cancer cell throws in another diabolical twist. Besides stimulating osteoblast activity, uPA can also split IGF-1 from its binding protein. If you recall the discussion on IGF-1, free circulating IGF-1 is active and elevated levels are associated with prostate cancer. IGF-1 bound to proteins (IGFBPs) is inactive. By tying up IGF-1, IGFBPs are thought to be protective. uPA has the ability to increase IGF-1 levels by detaching it from these binding proteins.

The released IGF-1 not only stimulates osteoblasts, but also switches on the cancer cell to produce more uPA. The result is a vicious circle that greatly enhances the survival and growth of the tumor colonies in bone.

Given all this, 70%-80% of men with low-risk prostate cancer are still cured, despite the fact that most, if not all, have cancer cells in their bone marrow. This is a tribute to the human body's mechanisms that maintain balance and harmony. The immune system and in-built genetic safeguards, such as cancer suppressor genes, seem to overwhelm the cancer cells in many cases, despite their clever little molecular ploys. Our job is to assist these protective mechanisms as much as possible through constructive lifestyle changes.

Key References

Elmajian D et al. Metastatic prostate cancer: An update. *Hospital Medicine* 1997; 33: 48-52.

Wiley S. Molecular aspects of metastasis. Meeting briefs of the American Association for Cancer Research. Sept. 22-26, 1999 Snowmass Village, Colorado.

Strum S. Bone integrity affects the natural history of prostate cancer. *PCRInsights* 1999; 2: 1-6.

Vassella R. Prostate cancer and bone metastasis. Presentation at the 1999 Prostate Cancer Foundation Retreat, Lake Tahoe, Nevada.

Byzova T. Integrins, VEGF, and bone matrix in prostate cancer metastases. Ninth Annual Prostate Cancer Foundation Scientific Retreat. September 20-22, 2002, poster #8.

Advanced Disease—How To Treat It

If at some point you're found to have metastatic prostate cancer, the choice of treatment generally depends on the extent of the metastases. Prostate cancer usually spreads from the area of the prostate to the pelvic lymph nodes. If documented lymph-node involvement is found in tests done as part of the initial work-up for newly diagnosed prostate cancer, but the bone scan indicates no tumor masses in the bones, there are several choices of treatment.

Radiation or surgery, combined with androgen ablation using an LH-RH agonist, or perhaps orchiectomy, can produce long-term remissions. Men in this group should probably remain on a program that maintains testosterone at castrate levels indefinitely. Some doctors recommend only long-term hormonal therapy without the surgery or radiation. However, Dr. Bolla's work combining hormones with radiation in high-risk patients, and Dr. Messing's work combining radical prostatectomy with permanent testosterone suppression for men with known lymph-node involvement, are persuasive. Despite a greater risk of side effects, there's now enough evidence that if it were me, I'd choose combination therapy if I had this level of disease at the outset. I would probably choose radiation plus an LH-RH agonist.

Men whose PSA starts rising again at some later point might benefit from the discussion later in this section on what to do when primary hormonal therapy is no longer effective.

Although with the present level of medical knowledge, cure is unlikely with cancer that has advanced this far, extremely long remissions (in excess of 10 years) are possible.

Ten years from now, we may have a cure for advanced prostate cancer. Many men with metastatic disease have a goal of surviving until a cure is in hand. New therapies may help them in reaching this target (see "New and Future Developments").

How to Approach a Rising PSA After Surgery or Radiation

Sometimes, despite surgery or radiation and the body's containment controls, the PSA begins to rise. Since the prostate has either been surgically removed or effectively eliminated by radiation, normal prostate cell growth is not the cause of this rising PSA. In virtually every case, barring lab error, the cause of a rising PSA after primary treatment is from microscopic spots of cancer growth in the area of the prostate, lymph nodes, or bone. Usually, these minute cancer growths are too small to be picked up by even sensitive tests like the ProstaScint scan. There are generally no symptoms. Were it not for the routine PSA follow-up test, there would be no clue that the cancer had started to progress.

What to do? After resisting the instinctive inclination to panic, you can benefit from a logic-based optimistic approach to the problem. In the pre-PSA era, men didn't know that their disease had progressed until they developed symptoms, such as bone pain. Today, with regular PSA monitoring after primary treatment, patients know that the cancer has recurred at a stage when the cancer is still relatively weak and they're strong. This provides more options.

The first thing to do is to try to find out whether the cancer has returned to the prostate area. An endorectal MRI, possibly combined with a spectroscopic MRI (if available), will help to determine if the cancer has recurred locally. A ProstaScint scan may pick up lymph-node metastases. In many men, however, no observable cancer colonies will be found. What then?

Before deciding what to do, it's best, in my opinion, to determine your objectives. Typically, there's no firmly established treatment plan for this situation. Each man, together with his wife or partner, must carefully weigh the potential benefits of each treatment option against the possible side effects. Is extending survival your overriding objective? How important are quality-of-life considerations, such as maintaining sexual function? Are you willing to trade some possible survival benefits for improved quality of life now?

Some men may decide that survival is the main issue. They may want to stretch the disease out as long as possible, hopefully until a cure is available. They're prepared to deal with the side effects of treatment. Others may want to live a normal life free from the side effects of treatment for as long as possible, resorting to treatment only when the cancer advances to the point where it causes symptoms, or is about to.

It's no wonder that the foremost prostate cancer specialists have diametrically differing approaches to an asymptomatic rising PSA. Their own biases and preferences may inadvertently become part of the equation. Some argue that a rising PSA should be treated immediately, when the cancer burden is still low. Others contend that men should continue to live normal lives, free of treatment, until cancer shows up on the bone scan. They do a bone scan every six months and as soon as they see disease, they recommend treatment. At this point most men have no symptoms from the bone lesions. Doctors advocating this approach correctly point out that it can take many years for bone metastases to develop, years that can be enjoyed free from the side effects of treatment. When treatment becomes necessary, hormonal therapy will likely delay cancer-related symptoms for several more years. But like many aspects of prostate cancer, this course of action may involve trade-offs.

Here are some facts that may help you get around this thorny issue. A large trial randomized 938 men who had either locally advanced prostate cancer or metastases with no symptoms. They received either an LH-RH agonist or orchiectomy immediately or they waited until bone pain from the cancer developed before receiving treatment. The randomly selected group that did not receive treatment until symptoms developed did significantly worse long-term, in terms of complications from the spreading cancer, than men who got immediate hormonal therapy. Blockage of urine from local recurrence of the cancer required surgery (transurethral resection) in 30% of the men who waited to be treated versus 14% who got immediate treatment, a highly significant difference.

Other complications, such as bone fractures from the cancer, blockage of the ureters (the tubes that run between the kidney and the bladder), and metastases to locations other than bone, were all more common in the group that did not receive immediate treatment. Most importantly, in the delayed-treatment group, death from prostate cancer was significantly more common. During the test period, 144 out of 244 men died, compared to 96 out of 256 men in the immediately treated group. Also, men in the delayed-treatment group developed bone metastases significantly faster than did men in the immediately treated group. Unfortunately, this study has been criticized, because some of the men in the deferred group died without receiving any hormones prior to death. How much this impacts the study is an important unknown that can't be resolved.

An earlier study showed a survival advantage for younger men with high-grade cancer when treated immediately. Despite the controversy, the consensus among prostate cancer experts is that, from what we know currently, immediate treatment probably prolongs survival, especially in men under 70, and increases the time free from symptoms of metastatic cancer. On the other hand, men who get immediate hormonal therapy frequently report a decreased quality of life. They will probably have little or no interest in sex, may be unable to have erections (although Viagra helps), may get hot flashes, lose bone density, be fatigued, and may have some cognitive and emotional symptoms, such as loss of memory or irritability. Don't forget, though, aids are available for these potential side effects as described in the chapter "Hormonal Therapy."

Key References

The Medical Research Council Prostate Cancer Working Party Investigators Group: Immediate versus deferred treatment for advanced prostate cancer: initial results of the Medical Research Council trial. *Br J Urology* 1997; 79: 235-246.

Byar D and Corle D. Hormone therapy for prostate cancer: results of the Veterans Administration Cooperative Urological Research Group's studies of the prostate. *Cancer* 1973; 32: 1126-1130.

Rabbani F and Fair W. Androgen deprivation therapy for prostate cancer: An overview. *Infect Urology* 1999; 12: 69-74.

Moul J. Contemporary hormonal management of advanced prostate cancer. *Oncol* 1998; 12: 499-505.

Intermittent Androgen Suppression (IAS)

At this point you might be wondering if there's a middle ground between survival on one hand and quality of life on the other. Recently, just such a treatment has been developed. Instead of using standard continuous hormonal therapy, intermittent androgen suppression (IAS) employs alternating on-off cycles of hormones. Men go on hormones for a period of time, then stop. When their PSA again rises to a predetermined point, they start hormones again. During the off period, symptoms associated with androgen withdrawal usually abate.

Interestingly, IAS was not originally developed as a way to minimize side effects in men undergoing hormonal therapy. It was devised as a way to delay disease progression and possibly increase overall survival. Animal experiments in mice showed that IAS increased the time it took for prostate cancer cells to become androgen-independent (no longer affected by androgen suppression) by *threefold*.

These favorable results in mice led to clinical testing in humans of IAS, beginning in 1992. The results of these trials compare favorably for

> **HELPFUL HINT**
>
> All men on either continuous, or intermittent, androgen suppression therapy should be taking bisphosphonates to minimize osteoporosis and possibly help prevent bone metastases. Active vitamin D (Rocaltrol) is also recommended.

IAS versus continuous hormonal therapy. Although the early human studies do not yet confirm the dramatic results seen in mice, IAS seems no worse than continuous treatment in preventing progression and prolonging survival. In the meantime, there's no question that the quality of life is improved during the period when men are off hormones. The average (mean) time off treatment in trials of IAS is 5-16 months. There are reported cases of as long as four years off treatment. IAS appears to be most effective in men who start treatment early after recurrence when they have no cancer symptoms and low volumes of tumor. It is most effective in men who have a low PSA nadir in response to the initial course of hormones. These are the best candidates for successful IAS.

Although IAS may still be considered to be experimental by some oncologists, most of the top doctors in the field are now using it for selected men with low tumor burdens and low PSA nadirs. Prostate cancer experts do differ, however, as to when to start IAS in men with rising PSAs after primary treatment. Some use a fixed PSA point, like 3-5 ng/ml; some wait for the first radiographic evidence of bone metastases (usually before symptoms develop). Others will recommend starting IAS immediately after they're convinced that local treatment has failed (rising PSA). At this point, there's not enough information available to determine which of these schedules is optimal. *But the current leaning of experts is toward earlier treatment.* The standard length of initial hormone therapy is eight to nine months. Complete an-

---

Late Note: A prospective randomized trial of IAS versus continual androgen suppression was just completed by a group of German researchers. Reported at the April-May 2003 meeting of the American Urological Association (AUA) in Chicago, results confirmed equivalent survival benefits and far better quality-of-life for IAS. Most men who were sexually active before treatment regained sexual function with testosterone levels returning to normal during the period off hormones. This study adds further support to using IAS early in men with recurrent prostate cancer.

drogen blockade (CAB) is used most often. After this course of hormones, men stay off treatment until the PSA rises to 3-5 ng/ml. Then the cycle is repeated. Responses have been documented in up to five on-off cycles lasting many years. IAS should be monitored by a medical oncologist specializing in prostate cancer.

Key References

Theyer G and Hamilton G. Current status of intermittent androgen suppression in the treatment of prostate cancer. *Urology* 1998; 52: 353-359.

Gleave M, Bruchovsky N et al. Intermittent androgen suppression: rationale and clinical experience. Schroeder F (editor). *Recent Advances in Prostate Cancer and BPH*, Parthenon Press, 1997.

Tunn U et al. Intermittent better than continuous androgen deprivation therapy to improve quality of life. AUA 98th Annual Meeting, April 29, 2003 in Chicago, Illinois; abstract 1481.

Proscar During the Off-Period of IAS

Dr. Steven Strum has studied the use of 5 mg of Proscar once a day during the off-period from hormones. He has anecdotally reported a significant increase in the time off hormones in men who take Proscar during this period. In fact, nearly 40% of the men on Proscar were still off hormones four years later. However, I couldn't find a published paper subject to peer-review (scrutiny by other experts) on this subject. These results need to be confirmed by others, but they're encouraging. If borne out, it would appear that a large number of men can enjoy a prolonged period free from both the symptoms of cancer and the side effects of hormones. Dr. Charles Myers has also observed prolonged time off hormones in men on Proscar maintenance and advocates its use during the periods off hormones. (Please note that these clinical impressions have not been confirmed by randomized, prospective clinical trials.)

Parenthetically, I've mentioned in various places in this book the use of Proscar as maintenance therapy after hormonal therapy either alone or combined with another treatment, such as EBRT. Here, too, its use is controversial and experimental.

• As previously discussed, it blocks the conversion of testosterone to DHT. Five milligrams a day reduce the blood levels of DHT by 80%. However, although DHT levels are reduced by Proscar, testosterone levels are increased. The effects of this tradeoff on prostate cancer is still being evaluated.

• Recent evidence indicates that Proscar may have an anti-angiogenic effect by reducing the blood flow to the prostate. Conceivably, this could deprive a tumor of oxygen and nutrients.

Proscar and PSA

Proscar "artificially" reduces PSA by about 50%. By "artificial," I mean that it can lower PSA levels without necessarily reducing cancer activity. For this reason, PSA levels need to be "adjusted" in men taking Proscar. A good rule of thumb is to double the PSA value to get an accurate reading. For men using Proscar during the interval when off hormones during IAS, hormonal therapy should be resumed when the PSA hits 1.5-2.5 ng/ml, instead of 3.0-5.0 ng/ml. Appropriate PSA adjustments will give Proscar users a more accurate assessment of their disease activity.

Some excellent clinicians think it's counterproductive to use Proscar during the off-period of IAS. They point to the need to achieve normal hormonal balance to "resensitize" cancer cells to androgens so that subsequent blockade will be more effective. They fear Proscar may interfere with the establishment of normal hormone balance.

Bottom Line on Proscar and IAS

Although some doctors use Proscar during the off-period in IAS, its use is controversial. Until appropriate studies are done, its use should be considered experimental.

What To Do If Hormonal Therapy Is No Longer Effective

For men who have recurrent disease, there may come a time when the hormone regimen they're using no longer works. In this case, the PSA will keep rising despite treatment. What to do? First, if you're on only an LH-RH agonist, try adding an anti-androgen like Casodex or Eulexin. This may produce a lower level of PSA. If you're already on an anti-androgen, switching from Casodex to Eulexin, or vice versa, might be effective. When switching from Eulexin to Casodex, it's probably more effective to use 150 mg of Casodex daily, instead of 50 mg/day. If none of these steps work to stabilize or decrease the PSA level, discontinue the anti-androgen, but continue the LH-RH agonist. Some men will benefit from what has been labeled the "anti-androgen withdrawal syndrome."

Anti-Androgen Withdrawal Syndrome (AAWS)

The AAWS was first reported in 1993 by Dr. Howard Scher and his group at Sloan Kettering. They observed that some men had significant drops in their PSAs and a reduction in cancer symptoms when anti-androgens were discontinued after they were no longer able to help control a rising PSA. Slightly more than 20% of men with prostate cancer responded to stopping anti-androgens. Although Dr. Scher's original findings were on the effects of Eulexin withdrawal, the AAWS has also been reported with Casodex withdrawal. Generally, the longer a man has been using an anti-androgen, the more likely he is to have AAWS. When it happens, it usually lasts for three to five months. During this time, trials indicate that about 60% of men that have cancer-related symptoms will have reduced complaints.

After AAWS: Secondary Hormonal Therapy

When the PSA starts rising again after the AAWS, or in men in whom anti-androgen withdrawal has had no effect, experts diverge on the next step. Part of the reason for this is the rapid developments in testing new drugs and novel treatments for prostate cancer. Most doctors will recommend a "secondary" hormonal treatment. The most common drug used for this purpose is ketoconazole (Nizoral). Aminoglutethamide (Cytadren) is another possibility. Its action is similar to ketoconazole. Both of these drugs block the production of the three androgens produced by the adrenal glands: DHEA, DHEA-sulfate, and androstenedione. They also partially block the production of cortisol, a necessary non-androgenic steroid. For this reason, hydrocortisone is usually given with these drugs that block adrenal-gland output. Hydrocortisone has also been shown to have a small direct effect on prostate cancer cells, so it may serve a dual purpose.

It should be clear at this point that our objective is to throw roadblocks in the path of the cancer, attempting to slow it down as much as possible. We're seeking remissions with a decent quality of life. Our goal is delay. Hopefully, if we can hold the cancer back long enough, a cure will be discovered. With gene therapy advancing rapidly, and new therapies for advanced disease being developed, this hope is more than just blue sky.

Chemotherapy (Chemo)

Up until very recently, chemotherapy was only used during the advanced stage of prostate cancer with symptoms. It was used primarily to lessen pain from bone metastases. The reason for this limited use? Because no chemotherapeutic regimen had been shown to extend survival. If it doesn't extend survival, then symptom relief is all that's left. Since side effects from chemo are common, it made no sense to use it except to alleviate symptoms more debilitating than these side effects. This differs from breast cancer, where chemo is frequently used as an up-front treatment.

Why the difference? Prostate cancer is often very slow growing. Cancer cells can lie dormant for several years, then suddenly begin to multiply. Chemotherapy is toxic to rapidly dividing cells, which is why a drop in the white and red blood cell (and platelet) count is a common undesirable effect of chemo. These blood cells have rapid turnover, so they're sensitive to the effects of chemo. But prostate cancer cells generally are not turning over quickly enough for a single chemotherapy drug to kill them. Prostate cancer researchers have been experimenting with multiple drug combinations to overcome this problem. Some of these combinations work synergistically. The combined effect is greater than the sum of the individual effects.

Numerous combinations have been tried. But only very recently has a combination regimen been developed that not only relieves pain and produces measurable reductions in the volume of cancer in some men, but also appears to increase survival.

This combination uses three drugs: estramustine (Emcyt), docetaxel (Taxotere), and dexamethasone. The primary anti-cancer effects come from Emcyt and Taxotere; dexamethasone is used mainly to reduce swelling, a frequent side effect of Emcyt.

MPT PSA Response

PSA Decline of:	Percentage of Men showing PSA Decline
50%	60%
75%	40%
to normal	25%

EPT PSA Response

PSA Decline of:	Percentage of Men showing PSA Decline
50%	50%
75%	25%
to normal	7.7% (1 of 13 men)

One medical group has the most experience with this combination: Dr. Daniel Petrylak and his team at Columbia Presbyterian Hospital in New York City. The results of Phase I and Phase II trials look very promising. In this study, 34 men with metastatic prostate cancer no longer responsive to hormonal manipulations were divided into two groups: 1) men with minimal prior chemotherapy or radiation to relieve bone pain (MPT); 2) men with extensive prior chemotherapy or radiation to bone (EPT). The following chart shows the percentage of men in each group that responded with a 50% or greater drop in their PSAs. The median PSA prior to treatment in the MPT group was 62.7 ng/ml. In the EPT group it was 193.5 ng/ml.

I spoke with Dr. Petrylak about these encouraging results. He was most excited not about the positive PSA response, although that was excellent compared to other combination chemotherapy. What intrigued him most was the fact that this regimen *improves overall survival*. According to Dr. Petrylak, the average survival in men with cancer to this extent is six to eight months, using other chemo regimens. Dr. Petylak's trial started in 1996. Out of 34 patients, 6 were still alive in late 1999 at the time of our conversation. The longest survivor at that time was 43 months! The median survival was 23.8 months. This is about three times longer than the usual expectation.

Phase I and Phase II trials in men who no longer respond to hormonal therapy show significantly improved survival. Taxotere has the greatest activity against prostate cancer, but its efficacy is improved with Emcyt. Phase III trials involving hundreds of men in multiple medical centers across the country are now in progress. Dr. Petrylak points out that Emcyt has more serious side effects than Taxotere, such as blood clots in the legs. Further studies are required to establish the minimum dose of Emcyt necessary to get the desired cancer-killing effects. *To date, this chemo combination is the only one that has been proven to increase survival.*

How about side effects? As with all chemotherapy agents,

there were some, but they were tolerable. Nausea occurred in less than one-third of the treated men and vomiting in 12%; 9% developed deep-vein blood clots. The most common side effect was swelling from fluid retention in 65% of the men, but only one man had severe swelling. Slightly less than half the men had an elevation in blood tests that evaluate the function of the liver, but stopping treatment for this reason was uncommon. These tests returned to normal after treatment. Depressed white-blood-cell (WBC) count, frequently a limiting factor in chemotherapy, occurred infrequently. Dangerous levels of depressed WBCs (grade 4) occurred in only two of the 34 men and lasted for less than a week.

Although these side effects may sound horrific, they're relatively minor compared with most other chemotherapy programs. Offsetting them is a decrease in cancer-related pain. At the beginning of this study, 15 men required narcotics for pain control. (The pain from prostate cancer is commonly related to bone lesions. It typically starts as vague aches and pains in the low-back area. It becomes progressively more severe and constant. Beside bisphosphonates, Cox II inhibitors like Celebrex and Vioxx combined with opiates may be necessary. Fentanyl patches may also be effective prior to starting opiates for pain control.) After treatment, eight men (53%) stopped using their pain medication. Exchanging a significant reduction in pain for the relatively minor side effects of this program is a trade most men are happy to make. Add to this the likely extension of life and it makes sense to give this treatment serious consideration.

Dr. Petrylak believes that the role of chemotherapy in prostate cancer is changing. He thinks regimens such as his will be even more effective in men with less cancer. They may be most effective used early in stronger men, perhaps as part of the initial treatment program. As he puts it, "In the near future, chemotherapy will move up-front, as it has in breast cancer, and become part of primary therapy. It will be combined with surgery and radiation, either with or without adjuvant hormonal therapy." Based on the results of his initial studies, I wouldn't bet against it.

This regimen is now attracting attention. Another New York group, from New York University School of Medicine, confirmed Dr. Petrylak's results. In another Phase I trial with Taxotere and Emcyt, 14 out of 17 men (82%), only one of whom had received prior chemo, had a PSA decline of at least 50%, and four men had their PSAs drop to normal (less than 4.0 ng/ml). This supports Dr. Petrylak's belief that this combination may be even more effective when used earlier in healthier men with lower tumor burdens.

Key References

Petrylak D. Chemotherapy for androgen-independent prostate cancer. *Semin Urol Oncol* 2002; 20: 3135.

Petrylak D et al. Phase I trial of docetaxel with estramustine in androgen-independent prostate cancer. *J Clin Oncol* 1999; 17: 958-967.

Kreis W et al. Phase I trial of the combination of daily estramustine phosphate and intermitent docetaxel in patients with metastatic hormone refractory prostate carcinoma. *Ann Oncol* 1999; 10: 33-38.

Other Chemotherapy

No other currently available chemotherapy regimen shows the promise of docetaxel (Taxotere) and estramustine (Emcyt) in extending life expectancy. For this reason, chemo should be considered only as a way to possibly reduce cancer-related symptoms. With this goal in mind, it seems logical to me to select agents with as few noxious side effects as possible, but with a reasonable chance of improvement in pain.

One drug that fits this description is mitoxantrone. It's given in combination with a steroid, usually prednisone. Prednisone by itself is known to have some minor effects on reducing cancer pain. A randomized Canadian study compared mitoxantrone and prednisone with prednisone alone. In this trial Dr. Tannock and his associates found that 29% of men treated with the combination of mitoxantrone and prednisone had significant reductions in bone pain. Only 12% of the randomly selected men that got prednisone alone experienced the same relief.

Symptomatic relief also lasted much longer in the group that got the combination of the two drugs: a median duration of 43 weeks versus 12 weeks. However, there was no overall difference in survival between the two groups.

A reduction in the frequency and severity of pain by a combination of mitoxantrone and steroids, versus steroids alone, was confirmed in a larger study conducted by Dr. Philip Kantoff and colleagues at Dana-Farber Cancer Institute in Boston. This randomized series included 242 men with hormone-refractory prostate cancer (cancer that no longer responds to hormones). While confirming pain reduction, these investigators also found no survival advantage in adding mitoxantrone to steroids. Side effects were "very modest."

Mitoxantrone is well-tolerated. Bone-marrow suppression (low WBC, RBC, and platelets) is rarely severe. For this reason it has become a favorite of a number of medical oncologists. It is the only chemotherapy available in New Zealand as of May 2003 and is government funded.

Some prostate cancer specialists are more aggressive. Dr. Christopher Logothetis of M.D. Anderson in Houston, Tex., believes in hitting the tumor hard early in the disease process. He's a leader in the evolving consensus that it's better to go to war against the cancer earlier rather than later. When the tumor is still weak and the patient is strong, the chances are greater, in his opinion, for a longer-term remission.

His chemotherapy protocol combines two active chemotherapy regimens into one. A Phase II trial of 16 men with advanced disease has been conducted. Dr. Logothetis alternates doxorubicin (Adriamycin) and ketoconazole with vinblastine and estramustine. Response rates to this regimen are high: 75% of the men had a complete, or partial, measurable response to this treatment with pain relief and/or shrinkage of the tumor, while two-thirds had a drop in their PSAs of 50% or more. The median response lasted 8.4 months.

Surprisingly, blood-cell suppression was minimal. The most significant side effects were swelling in the arms or legs (49%) and deep-vein clotting (19%). I must point out that Dr. Logothetis is a master at delivering and monitoring this program. He skillfully uses a combination of drugs that stimulate the production of red and white blood cells, reduce nausea, and minimize blood clotting. Personally, were I to select this treatment, I'd have to go to Houston. I wouldn't trust anyone else.

Dr. Logothetis' philosophy is to aggressively fight the cancer, while controlling treatment risks with modern supportive drugs. While not all medical oncologists approach prostate cancer this way, you'll have difficulty finding anyone who contests the fact that Dr. Logothetis is an extremely knowledgable and capable oncologist. The applicability of his approach depends a lot on the attitude and orientation of the man with prostate cancer. As we've previously discussed, this is a personal decision.

Other chemotherapy combinations that have been shown to reduce cancer symptoms and improve the quality of life in some men are:

Etoposide plus estramustine (Emcyt)

Paclitaxel (Taxol) plus estramustine

Ketoconazole plus doxorubicin

Vinblastine plus estramustine

(Note: The third and fourth combinations above are alternated by Dr. Logothetis in his protocol. Some oncologists use them separately.)

Cytoxan plus 5-fluorouracil (5-FU). Some oncologists may add weekly Taxotere to this combination.

Please remember, however, that while they may provide symptom relief from bone pain, none of the above combinations has been shown to extend life. For this reason, if I were faced with recurring prostate cancer that no longer responded to hormones, I'd choose Taxotere and Emcyt—the Petrylak combo—in an effort to extend survival as well as to reduce pain.

Key References

Tannock I et al. Chemotherapy with mitoxantrone plus prednisone or prednisone alone for symptomatic hormone-resistant prostate cancer: a Canadian randomized trial with palliative end points. *J Clin Oncol* 1996; 14: 1756.

Kantoff P et al. Hydrocortisone with or without mitoxantrone in men with hormone-refractory prostate cancer: results of the Cancer and Leukemia Group B 9182 study. *J Clin Oncol* 1999; 17: 2506.

Ellerhorst J et al. Phase II trial of alternating weekly chemohormonal therapy for patients with androgen-independent prostate cancer. *Clin Cancer Res* 1997; 3: 2371.

Methods of Dealing With Bone Pain

Autopsy studies in men who die of prostate cancer show that in up to 90% of cases, the cancer has spread to bone. Starting with the most common, the order of metastasis to bone is: pelvis and sacrum, spine, femur, ribs, scapula (shoulder blade).

Most men who die of prostate cancer succumb to cachexia. They lose weight and become immobilized due to complications from bone problems, such as spontaneous bone fractures, which are painful, and compressed vertebrae.

One of the major concerns of men with hormone-independent prostate cancer is bone pain. This is a common cancer-related symptom that affects the majority of men at this stage. One of the better options for reducing bone pain is the use of bisphosphonates. Aredia, given weekly intravenously, is probably more effective than oral Fosamax for this purpose. Zoledronate, also administered by IV, is several times more potent that Aredia and seems to be proportionately more effective.

Radioactive Isotopes

Chemotherapy and bisphosphonates are not the only options for relieving bone pain in some men. Radioactive isotopes, such as strontium-89 (SR-89) and samarium-153 (Quadramet), are taken up by bone in the same way as calcium. Given by intravenous injection, they concentrate in areas of high cell turnover, such as the osteoblastic areas effected by prostate cancer. These spots are the source of bone pain.

In clinical trials, partial relief of bone pain was observed in up to 80% of patients using SR-89 and complete pain relief occurred in about 20%. Men also reported an increased ability to get around and a better quality of life after treatment.

The effects of strontium-89 and samarium-153 are similar. Strontium-89 has been available longer and has been used in more trials. Samarium-153 was approved by the FDA in October 1997.

At the 2002 Prostate Cancer Foundation Retreat, Dr. Christopher Logothetis reported on a study showing that SR-89 combined with chemo appears to improve survival in men with advanced prostate cancer.

External beam radiation to painful areas of bone alleviates the pain in approximately the same percentage of men as strontium-89 or samarium-153. This has led investigators to try combining radioisotopes with external beam spot radiation. Although adding the radioisotope strontium-89 did not further reduce pain, it did provide beneficial long-term effects. Over time, men in the combined therapy group developed significantly fewer painful bone metastases than those who received only spot radiation.

Radioisotopes can, to some extent, suppress the development of red and white blood cells and platelets in the bone marrow. This is the main side effect. However, since the isotopes are concentrated in areas of high bone turnover, they remain predominately on the bone surface, and don't penetrate the marrow. For this reason, they can be used after spot radiation.

Caution must be used if chemotherapy is being considered after radioisotopes. Since both can suppress bone-marrow activity, the combination could increase the risks of severe depression of circulating blood cells and platelets; this could lead to infection, anemia, and bleeding tendencies. Oncologists are well aware of this risk and will advise men accordingly.

Endothelin-1

Another possibility is endothelin-1 (ABT-627). In a Phase II trial a significant number of men who randomly received this drug rather than a placebo had less pain. Taken orally, ABT-627 seems to work by decreasing the survival and slowing the growth of cancer cells. This drug is not yet FDA approved, but clinical trials are ongoing. (See "New and Future Developments" for more.)

Key References

Porter A et al. Results of a randomized Phase III trial to evaluate the efficacy of strontium-89 adjuvant to local field external beam irradiation in the management of endocrine resistant metastatic prostate cancer. *Int J Rad Oncol Biol Phys* 1993; 25: 805.

Nelson J et al. Preliminary Phase II results using ABT-627, an endothelin-A selective receptor antagonist, in men with symptomatic hormone-refractory prostate cancer. American Urological Association 95th Annual Meeting; Apr. 29- May 4, 2000. *Abstract* 709.

Kamradt J, Smith D, and Pienta K. Hormone-refractory prostate cancer: National Comprehensive Cancer Network guidelines. University of Michigan Comprehensive Cancer Center Website: www.cancer.med.umich.edu/prostcan

Logothetis C. Advances in prostate cancer therapy. Ninth Annual Prostate Cancer Foundation Scientific Retreat. September 20-22, 2002.

Relieving Pain With Analgesics

It's important, both psychologically and physically, that men be kept free from cancer-induced pain. Pain is one of the greatest fears of men with advancing prostate cancer. Besides the treatments already discussed that reduce pain by reducing the amount of cancer in painful places like bone, a host of available drugs deal directly with the perception of pain. These drugs, known as analgesics, reduce pain without affecting the growth of the cancer.

A 1999 study published in *Cancer* shows that most cancer patients can remain pain-free, or nearly so, while being cared for at home. An Italian study involving 3,678 terminally ill cancer patients used progressive pain-control measures, starting with non-narcotic analgesics and progressing to stronger and stronger narcotics as required. In the week before death, this study reports, 90% of patients had either no pain or mild pain, 9% had moderate pain, and only 1% had severe pain.

Advances in pain control continue. Recently, skin patches of fentanyl, an effective new analgesic that can be used prior to narcotics, have been released. Using these patches can extend the period of normal activity without pain or the use of more powerful drugs.

Many cancer centers now have groups that specialize in pain management. Seek these out. There's no reason in today's medical environment for most men with advanced prostate cancer to suffer.

Conclusion

• Up until a couple of years ago, there was little hope for men with advanced metastatic disease. Fortunately, this is changing. The chemotherapeutic combination of Taxotere and Emcyt provides survival benefits, and a number of combinations provide a greater than 50% decrease in PSA in the majority of men, together with pain relief and improved quality of life.

• Some very exciting compounds are in the pipeline at various stages of clinical development. In the last section of the book, we'll take a look at what's new and what future treatments for prostate cancer are likely to evolve.

15

CHOOSING AMONG TREATMENTS FOR NEWLY DIAGNOSED PROSTATE CANCER

In this section, we've covered the various treatments available for newly diagnosed prostate cancer. How do you make an intelligent decision on which to choose? It depends on your level of disease, your tolerance to potential side effects from treatment, availability of an expert in a particular treatment in your area, and your philosophy. The less aggressive the cancer, the greater your treatment options. Let's break it down.

Group 1: Low Risk

PSA = 10 or less *and*
Gleason score = 6 or less *and*
Clinical stage = T2a or less

Treatment Choices
(In Alphabetical Order)
Active lifestyle changes (nutrition, supplements, exercise, stress reduction)
Brachytherapy (seeds)
Cryotherapy
Hormonal therapy
Radiation therapy (external beam), either alone or with 3 months of hormones prior to treatment
Surgery (radical prostatectomy)—nerve-sparing procedure

Well-Studied Treatments

Recent studies have shown that for this level of disease, surgery, external beam radiation therapy (EBRT), and brachy-therapy are all equally effective, with long-term freedom from metastases at 80%-90%. Adding three months of hormones seemed to improve the efficacy of EBRT (93% free of disease at five years by PSA measurements, according to a study by Dr. Michael Zelefsky at Sloan Kettering), but did not improve the outcome of seeds in this group.

In the opinion of some very fine doctors, such as my own radiation oncologist, Dr. Ken Russell, and Dr. Dan Petrylak, a medical oncologist at Columbia Presbyterian, a logical way to approach this decision is by deciding which potential side effects are most tolerable. These were reviewed earlier. Philosophical considerations like "wanting the cancer out now," objections to invasive procedures, time commitments, ability to travel, and availability of an expert in a particular treatment may also play a role in the choice of treatment.

Newer Less-Studied Approaches

Lifestyle changes—Lifestyle changes, including nutrition, exercise, and stress reduction, are currently being studied by Dr. Dean Ornish in Sausalito, Calif., for men with this level of disease. A low-fat, high-fiber, high-soy, green-tea diet is combined with selected supplements, meditation, and yoga. PSA is closely monitored. It's too early to know the outcome, but the initial response is encouraging.

Some well-known medical oncologists, such as Dr. Charles (Snuffy) Myers in Charlottesville, Virginia, are now using this approach on men with low-risk prostate cancer willing to make the required lifestyle adjustments. Dr. Myers points out that the risk of dying from heart disease often exceeds the risk of dying from this form of prostate cancer. As luck would have it, these lifestyle adjustments reduce the chances of dying from heart disease, so the changes may have a dual function. Dr. Myers says that he can generally identify those men likely to respond to these modifications within 2-3 months. For non-responders, surgery, EBRT, or seeds are all still viable alternatives. Men with low-risk tumors that can't be felt on rectal exam may be particularly good candidates for this approach, since studies at Johns Hopkins show that these men are most likely to still be curable if these conservative measures fail to stop cancer progression. Close supervision by a doctor familiar with this approach to treatment is imperative.

Hormonal therapy—Hormonal blockade for a defined period of time (say one year) has not been rigorously tested. Some doctors claim to have excellent results with "triple therapy," a combination of Lupron, Casodex, and Proscar for 12-13 months. After this, patients are maintained only on Proscar. This approach has not been studied in a well-designed medical trial. Long-term use of 150 mg of Casodex is still being evaluated.

Cryotherapy—This approach should be considered only if impotency is not an issue and only in the best of hands.

What would I do if I had this level of disease (negative DRE)? Fair question. If I had clinical stage T1c, I would give aggressive lifestyle changes a go. With T2a clinical staging, I'd still make the lifestyle changes, but I'd go with three months of hormones, followed by EBRT from a top radiation oncologist (see recommended list). The 93% success rate reported by Dr. Zelefsky and co-workers is about as good as it gets. I want to reiterate, however, that these choices best fit *my* requirements. Other men will differ in their evaluation of what's best for them. Take a hard look at the potential side effects of each treatment, then decide.

Group 2: Intermediate Risk

PSA = greater than 10 but less than 20 *and/or*

Gleason score = 7 *and/or*

Clinical stage = T2b-T2c

(Here the chance of extracapsular extension of the cancer increases.)

Treatment Choices

Radiation combined with hormonal therapy—High-dose external beam radiation therapy with IMRT (if available) plus hormonal therapy before, during, and after radiation for a total of eight months to three years. Since the risk is greater, the treatment needs to be amplified. Using hormones for at least eight months may help kill cancer cells that may have escaped into the circulation. Hormonal therapy has the ability to affect cancer cells throughout the body (systemic therapy). By combining aggressive local therapy with systemic therapy, you have the best chance of cure.

Today, I would want to have at least 78 Gy of EBRT and, if combined with IMRT, at least as high as 81 Gy. Remember, the higher the radiation dose, the greater the chance of eradicating the cancer. However, very high doses, like 90 Gy, may have more late radiation side effects. It's not yet clear what the ceiling is for safe dose intensity. In my view, 81 Gy with IMRT combined with hormones strikes the best balance between efficacy and safety in most cases, based on present evidence. IMRT is currently available at the University of California-San Francisco, Baylor in Houston, and Sloan Kettering in New York City. By the time you read this, its use may be more widespread.

How long to use hormones hasn't yet been established. The only study to show a survival benefit was Dr. Bolla's. Men in this group used Casodex for a month to prevent "hormonal flare" from the temporary increase in testosterone that occurs when Lupron or Zoladex are initiated. After the first month, Dr. Bolla used only Zoladex (though Lupron would be equally effective). In another study, 10½ months of androgen blockade showed excellent local control of cancer in the area of the prostate, but no survival benefit. The optimal time for hormonal therapy seems to be somewhere between 10½ months and three years. Now, we can only guess.

I had "Group 2" level of disease. I chose to use androgen blockade for 27 months. This decision was arbitrary. At two years nearly 30% of men have permanent shut down of testosterone production. Although I could find no data at three years, obviously it's higher. Twenty-seven months seemed like a reasonable compromise to me. However, if cure had been my only consideration, I would have stayed on hormones for three years.

Surgery—Although the chance of extracapsular extension is high, some doctors, including some excellent medical oncologists, might still prefer surgery. Reasons? First, thanks to pathologic re-staging, you'll know where you stand. This information can tell you if further treatment is required. Also, by removing the malignancy, the "disease burden" will be reduced. This may allow your immune system to better fight any remaining cancer. Some clinicians anecdotally report that their surgical patients "seem to do better." Having said this, most doctors do not recommend surgery for men with a high probability of extraprostatic disease. Whether to add hormones or radiation depends on the surgical finding. As we now know, continuous immediate use of Lupron, or orchiectomy, for men with lymph-node involvement found at surgery can result in long-term remission from cancer. This finding makes surgery a more attractive option for men with intermediate-risk disease.

Brachytherapy combined with hormonal blockade—For this level of disease, seeds alone show poor results. However, combined with hormones, Pd-103 seeds have comparable results to EBRT. Hormonal therapy is generally recommended for 12 months. Many doctors will also recommend combining EBRT with Pd-103 seeds. However, recent studies don't show improved results from added EBRT. Based on present evidence, it seems as though adding EBRT to palladium seeds is of questionable value and may increase side effects. Adding hormones, however, is mandatory for this level of cancer. Use the acceptability of potential side effects as a guide to choose between these treatments.

Group 3: High-Risk Disease Caught Early

Gleason score = 8-10 *and*
PSA = 10 or less

Treatment Choices

Surgery—This is an option, despite the fact that anyone in Group 3 has an aggressive cancer. A strong argument can be made to include 8-12 months of androgen blockade in addition to surgery to "mop up" cancer cells that may have escaped the prostate, even if the cancer is found to be confined to the prostate at the time of surgery. I recommend that men with aggressive cancers get an endorectal MRI *before* starting hormonal therapy. If the erMRI indicates that the tumor is still contained in the prostate, surgery becomes a more viable option.

Radiation—High-intensity radiation, preferably with IMRT, combined with hormonal therapy as discussed for Group 2.

Brachytherapy—Not recommended for these aggressive tumors.

Group 4: High-Risk

Clinical stage = T3 *or*
Gleason score = 8-10 *and* PSA greater than 10 but less than 20 *or*
Gleason score = 7 or less *and* PSA greater than 20.
All of the above with no signs of lymph-node or bone metastases.

Treatment Choices

Until recently, high-intensity external beam radiation, (at least 70 Gy as used by Dr. Bolla), plus three years of hormonal therapy, was the clear-cut treatment of choice in this group. With Dr. Messing's work, surgery plus hormonal therapy is now also an option. If lymph-node metastases are found at surgery, permanent androgen blockade using an LH-RH agonist (or orchiectomy) is strongly recommended based on Dr. Messing's study.

For men with seminal-vesicle involvement found at surgery, a combination of post-operative EBRT (64-66 Gy), plus three years of hormonal therapy, is probably the best plan. Positive surgical margins (single) may be treated with EBRT soon after surgery, although this has not been firmly established and some experts disagree. If there are multiple areas of positive margins, hormonal therapy should be added to EBRT.

Brachytherapy should not be considered in this group.

Group 5

Gleason score = 8-10
PSA = greater than 20
Or men with documented lymph-node metastases, but no bone involvement.

Treatment Choice

Here, the treatment of choice is high-intensity EBRT, plus permanent hormonal therapy. Surgery is rarely recommended for men with aggressive cancers with PSAs greater than 10, or for less aggressive cancers with PSAs greater than 20, or with known lymph node metastases.

Group 6: Men with Documented Bone Metastases

Treatment Choices

Hormonal therapy, either permanent or intermittent— Chemotherapy is not generally used before hormonal therapy, although it's an option, either alone or in combination with hormones.

Clinical trials of new treatments, such as vaccines, vitamin-D analogues, or anti-angiogenesis drugs, are also an option. Personally, I would probably select hormonal therapy combined with a potent Vitamin D analog and the bisphosphanate Zoledronate. My objective would be to try to reduce the number and spread of the bone metastases to the greatest possible extent.

If you're in this group and interested, try contacting Dana Farber in Boston, M.D. Anderson in Houston, or the University of Wisconsin in Madison (see "New and Future Developments" for details on animal studies and Phase I trials).

16

PROSTATE CANCER CARE DOWN UNDER

Since I now live in New Zealand, I thought it appropriate to evaluate the standard of care for men living in New Zealand and Australia. Generally speaking, the standard of care is not as advanced as in America. However, there are some very dedicated and knowledgeable urologists and oncologists down under.

In Australia, the leading centers for prostate cancer seem to be the Peter MacCallum Cancer Institute in Melbourne and Sir Charles Gairdner Hospital in Perth. Both these institutions have a number of fine surgeons well-versed in the nerve-sparing procedure for prostatectomy.

The Australian leader in radiation therapy is probably the Peter MacCallum Cancer Institute. It currently offers 3-D conformal EBRT with dose escalation to 74Gy. It's also the only place in Australia that can do IMRT as of the time of this writing. IMRT has been available here since the year 2000. Contact Dr. Keen Hun Tai or Dr. Gill Duchense at 61-3-9656-1111 for details. Other cancer centers only go as high as 66-70Gy for their external beam radiation therapy. If you're in Perth, contact Dr. David Joseph at Sir Charles Gairdner.

In Australia, government funding is now available for radioactive seed implants in men with low-risk prostate cancer. Both of the above-mentioned centers offer this treatment option. Peter MacCallum also offers high-density removable implant therapy for intermediate-risk patients using Iridium-192 implants that are removed after 30 hours of exposure. This provides about 85-88 Gy to the prostate.

In New Zealand, Dr. Andrew Miller in Palmerston North is currently the only radiation oncologist using 74Gy of conformal beam radiation therapy. He has done so for about the past 4 years, is very comfortable delivering this dose, and has only minor rectal side effects. He also has IMRT capabilities and will soon escalate the dose to 76Gy and then succeed it with 78Gy. Dr. Miller is convinced, as I am, that at least 78Gy with IMRT is the appropriate radiation dose for men with intermediate-risk prostate cancer.

In Auckland, Dr. John Matthews is a knowledgeable, dedicated, and hard-working radiation oncologist. Although he currently uses only 66Gy, he has been an active part of clinical trials in combined Australia/New Zealand studies. One large trial that closed about a year ago prospectively and randomly compared 3-5 months of Zoladex (LH-RH agonist) combined with between 64Gy and 74Gy of 3-D conformal EBRT. Results for this 800-man clinical trial for men with low, intermediate, and high-risk prostate cancer will not be available until perhaps 2004 or beyond.

As for chemotherapy down under, I think it's fair to say that it's a bit behind the States. The taxanes (Taxotere and Taxol) have not been approved for government funding in either Australia or New Zealand and won't be, I'm told, until Phase III trials are completed in America. Then there's likely to be an additional 6- to 12-month lag. In New Zealand, completion of Phase III trials in the United States may still not be enough to trigger government funding. The funding authority must evaluate the efficacy of treatment versus other drugs in other diseases. Decisions must be made, some of them difficult ones, on how to allocate budgeted funds amongst promising new drug applications. The doctors I spoke with all agree that this will eventually happen, but the timing is up in the air. Male health has played second fiddle to female health in the New Zealand funding arena. Men need to become more vocal and less stoic, in my opinion, to get their fair share of the available funds.

Emcyt is not available for any treatment in Australia, according to medical oncologist Dr. Guy Toner of the Peter MacCallum Cancer Institute in Melbourne, Australia. Dr. Toner is at a loss to explain why Emcyt is unavailable, but points out that Australia is a small market relative to the United States and the European Union and warrants less attention from drug companies.

The only chemotherapy regimen approved for funding for prostate cancer is the combination of mitoxantrone and prednisone. Clinical trials are currently in progress in Australia comparing this regimen with Taxotere and prednisone. This trial would be an excellent option for Australian men who have stopped responding to hormonal therapy. If you're interested, contact Dr. Toner about this or other clinical trials in Australia.

Australia is also testing some of the new promising treatments for advanced prostate cancer. One such trial, a Phase II trial of Iressa (see "New and Future Developments"), is now well along and results will be reported in May 2003, according to Dr. Toner.

On the nutrition side, Dr. Costello, Professor of Urology at the Royal Melbourne Hospital, is investigating the impact of selenium supplements on prostate cancer prevention. Soil selenium levels are generally low in Australia and New Zealand, so selenium supplementation could make a difference in prostate cancer onset and/or progression.

17

NUTRITION

The role of diet in preserving health is becoming progressively more established in the medical community. Food selection and total caloric intake are now recognized as key ingredients to a longer higher-quality life. The incidence of some of the major killers—heart disease, cancer, and Alzheimer's—are all influenced by diet. Obesity in America has increased rapidly over the past 15 years. Diabetes, a disease highly correlated with obesity, has also increased proportionately. Annual deaths from diabetes-related causes increased 40% from 1985 to 1999. Deaths from diabetes are now nearly equal to deaths from breast cancer!

At this point, it has been well-established that a reduced animal-fat diet with increased consumption of fruits and vegetables will protect you from heart disease. Soy protein, as you will read later in this chapter, seems to be particularly effective at reducing the risks of heart disease, so much so that the stringently controlling FDA has allowed soy-protein manufacturers to add this statement to their products: "Diets low in saturated fat and cholesterol that include 25 grams of soy protein (per day) may reduce the risk of heart disease." Permission such as this is not given lightly by the FDA.

Can diet and supplements really do anything to prevent prostate cancer? Can changes in nutritional habits retard its spread in men that already have the disease? I'm convinced they can. But there is no scientific proof that this is so. Scientific proof would require prospective (not retrospective), controlled, randomized studies of large patient populations for long periods of time. It would require hard evidence that the dietary products or supplements were faithfully being consumed in the specified quantities over the entire time of the study. Short of very regular urine and blood samples, a researcher could not be certain that a study participant was following the prescribed regimen. Such studies are difficult and expensive to mount. They would cost millions of dollars and take at least 10 years to start producing meaningful data. As one top researcher in the field put it: "I'd be dead before I got results from this kind of study."

In light of the lack of medical proof that dietary factors make a significant difference in the incidence or progression of prostate cancer, why am I convinced that they're useful? To understand my conviction, it's helpful to compare science with the justice system in the United States. At a criminal trial, the burden of proof is "beyond a reasonable doubt." At a civil trial, the standard is "a preponderance of the evidence." Scientific proof is analogous to "beyond a reasonable doubt." With diet and supplements, we're not yet there.

But "a preponderance of the evidence" is a standard that's more easily met. I think the evidence of the benefits of nutrition meets this measure. Here's why.

Epidemiologic Studies

The term "epidemiology" as used in the title of this section refers to population comparisons, not the study of widespread disease (epidemics). When prostate cancer is compared in different countries, interesting details emerge. In Asian populations, for example, the incidence of microscopically detectable prostate cancer is similar to that of Western cultures, but these cancers become clinically significant much less frequently than those in Western nations. The extent of this difference is striking. African-Americans have 100 times as much *clinical* prostate cancer as Chinese men. A hundred times! American Caucasians have about 20 times as much clinically significant prostate cancer as Japanese men. It's not that these Asian men don't have cancer in their prostates; they do. It just remains dormant until they die of something else and even when Japanese men get clinical prostate cancer, it tends to be less aggressive.

When Asian men migrate to the United States, within one generation the incidence of clinically recognizable prostate cancer approaches that of Western men. Additionally, the rate of clinically observable prostate cancer has been rising in Japan as Japanese eating habits become progressively more Westernized. From 1950 to 1975, the incidence of prostate cancer increased six-fold!

This pattern of disease expression implicates environmental factors as the main reason why prostate cancer becomes a problem for some men, but remains latent for others. If the difference was all due to genetics, then why would a change in environment so dramatically change the development of clinically significant prostate cancer in Japanese men? Investigators around the globe have attempted to identify the environmental differences that account for this markedly altered disease history. Dietary factors appear to be the most important. A high-calorie diet is one culprit.

Fewer Calories Slow Prostate Cancer Growth

It's been well-established that restricting calories in the diet of laboratory animals prolongs life and reduces cancer. Centenarians (people who live to be 100 or more) in Okinawa consume an average of about 1,200 calories daily. While this seems very low, it should be noted that these elderly people are sedentary and burn fewer calories than active adults. This low caloric intake is almost certainly part of their longevity success.

A recent study done at Harvard Medical School showed a dramatic reduction in the growth rate of prostate tumors transplanted into rats that ate a reduced calorie diet. At the end of the study, a 20% reduction in calories resulted in 62%

lower tumor weight, when compared to tumor weight in rats eating a normal diet. Interestingly, this result did not seem to be related to fat content in the respective diets. So long as calories were controlled, increasing the amount of calories coming from fat did not appear to affect tumor growth.

The average Japanese man consumes about 2,000 calories daily; the average American man devours nearly 3,500 calories per day, almost twice as much. Only a small part of this difference can be accounted for by differences in height and weight. The rest is due to dramatically different eating habits. Too many calories lead to obesity. And obesity is associated not only with a significantly increased risk of prostate cancer, but also of other cancers, heart disease, and diabetes. In fact, most experts I've spoken with agree that, aside from not smoking, calorie reduction is the most beneficial step one can take to increase longevity. Prostate cancer is no exception. As calories go down, the risk of prostate cancer goes right down with them.

How does reducing calories slow the growth of prostate cancer? That's not known. One possible mechanism is a reduction in serum insulin and IGF-1 levels. It has been well-established, both in rodents and primates, that calorie restriction lowers insulin levels in the blood. Fewer calories reduce IGF-1 levels in humans. Exercise also helps lower insulin levels. Lower insulin levels lead to an increase in a hormone called sex hormone binding globulin (SHBG). SHBG binds circulating testosterone. One way that calorie restriction might decrease the growth of prostate cancer, then, is by reducing the amount of circulating testosterone.

Insulin and IGF-1 are also known to have a direct effect on prostate cells. They increase the rate of cell division. This "mitogenic effect," as it's called, may speed up the growth of prostate cancer cells in the transplanted tumors in animal studies. Whatever the mechanism of its action, calorie restriction is strongly associated with a slowdown in the growth and development of prostate cancer. This effect seems to be independent of fat content in the diet.

Calorie restriction is difficult, to put it mildly, for most of us. Researchers are now working on ways to reduce calorie absorption from the digestive tract by perfecting foods that have ingredients that can't be metabolized. When perfected, these will accommodate the joys of eating and satiety without the unwanted calories. Such products may be as near as a year or two away.

What To Eat

Besides putting a lid on calories, a proper diet seems to make a difference in prostate cancer prevention. It also appears to reduce the rate of tumor growth in men that have prostate cancer. Epidemiologic studies indicate that fruits, vegetables, fiber, soy, tomatoes, and green tea are associated with a reduction of prostate cancer. Diets high in fat, especially from red meat and dairy products, correlate with an increase in prostate cancer and prostate cancer mortality. Additionally, cows and chickens are routinely fed hormones to stimulate growth and antibodies to decrease infections. According to CNN, 40% of all antibiotics produced annually go into beef and poultry food. Consuming growth-stimulating hormones can't be good for men with cancer that grows more rapidly when exposed to them.

So what you eat makes a difference. The National Cancer Institute attributes more than one-third of all cancers to dietary factors. It's also something that you can directly control.

Fruits, Vegetables, and Fiber

The National Cancer Institute (NCI) recommends five servings of fruits or vegetables each day to help prevent prostate cancer and to slow its progression. This may sound like a lot, but an apple or orange counts as a serving. If you eat a fruit salad at breakfast containing an apple, orange, strawberries, and kiwi fruit, as I do, you're well on your way to your five servings. A banana in your soy protein drink, a salad, and a couple of vegetable dishes at lunch or dinner and you've more than eclipsed the NCI recommendation.

As for fiber, the NCI recommends 25-35 grams daily. Eating fruits and vegetables provides fiber, so by eating five or more servings a day, you're well on your way to getting your required fiber. An orange or banana has about three grams of fiber. A cup of raspberries has eight grams. Add to this a high-fiber cereal, such as All-Bran, Grape Nuts, or Shredded Wheat, and you'll get an additional 10 grams of fiber per day. By eating a bowl of one of these cereals with a nice fruit salad, you'll be consuming more dietary fiber than the average American eats in an entire day!

Grain dishes—rice, barley, couscous, and polenta—are high in fiber. Brown rice has more fiber than white rice. So do some of the Japanese noodle products, like soba, which is made out of buckwheat. Nuts and seeds are also rich in fiber, but you'll need to consume them in moderation due to the calories in them. Whole-grain, sprouted-grain, and black breads, along with rye wafers, are also excellent sources of fiber. They can be used for sandwiches or between-meal snacks. Read the package carefully and select only varieties that are low in fat. Bread can be a source of "hidden" fats, if not carefully selected.

Beans, peas, and lentils are particularly high in fiber. Beans (legumes) contain more than 10 grams of fiber per cup, and peas have about nine grams per cup. Due to the way they're metabolized, they're an even better source of fiber than whole-grain breads. These foods are also a rich source of beneficial lignans. If you stop eating meat, you'll have much more room for a variety of fiber-rich foods.

Avoid Fatty Foods

Fiber helps the body remove fats by binding fat that has been ingested. This fiber-bound fat is then eliminated. (As an added benefit, fiber increases the transit time of intestinal wastes. This may reduce the risk of colon cancer by more rapidly removing intestinal toxins that can potentially damage normal colon cells.) You can help this process along by reducing your total intake of fats and oils, especially from red meat, dairy products, and partially hydrogenated oils found in packaged foods. Red-meat and dairy products, such as whole milk, butter, and cheese, are loaded with fats. Population studies have shown that the incidence of prostate cancer is highest in countries where fat consumption is greatest. This association also holds true for deaths from prostate cancer. The United States, Canada, and Western European countries have much higher death rates from prostate cancer than China, Japan, Taiwan, and Thailand. Interestingly, dairy products are rarely consumed in Asian countries. Likewise, portions of red meat, when consumed, are small.

A high consumption of fat may lead to obesity. Eighteen percent of the United States population is now considered to be obese, up from 12% as recently as 1991. This is a 50% increase! As Dr. Jeffrey Koplan, director of the Centers for Disease Control and Prevention (CDC) in Atlanta, puts it: "Obesity has spread with the speed and dispersion characteristic of a communicable disease epidemic." According to Dr. Koplan, more than half of all Americans are overweight.

The typical Japanese diet has about 20% calories from fat; Americans have about 36% fat calories on average, down from 40% ten years ago. Although this may appear to be an improvement, it isn't really, because Americans have increased their calorie intake. The total amount of fat consumed has actually increased. Twenty percent of total calories from fat is a good target for prevention of prostate cancer and heart disease. For men that already have prostate cancer, 10%-15% is a better target.

Note that we're discussing the percentage of *calories* from fat, not the percentage of fat by weight. Since gram for gram, fat has more than twice the calories of carbohydrates or protein, 20% of calories from fat is equivalent to less than 10% fat based on weight. When reported on food labels, percentage of fat is based on weight, not calories. One-percent-fat soy milk actually contains in excess of 2% fat based on calories.

Fat is deleterious in a number of ways. Fat contains nine calories per gram; protein and carbohydrates have only four calories per gram. Even the so-called "good oils" still have nine calories per gram. It's really difficult, therefore, to control your caloric intake if you eat lots of fats or oils. Although in the laboratory, experimental animals can be maintained on high-fat diets while limiting the number of calories, it's virtually impossible for men to get 40% or more of their calories from fat and still limit their total calories to the point where they don't gain weight.

Fat, especially animal fat, has been implicated in a number of studies as a risk factor for prostate cancer. A study of more than 47,000 men, all health professionals, done in 1993 at Harvard Medical School showed that men eating a high-fat diet, primarily from red meat, had nearly double the risk of getting advanced prostate cancer as those eating a low-fat diet. These findings were confirmed in May 1999 in a study reported in the *British Journal of Cancer*. This case-controlled study compared 175 men with prostate cancer with 233 controls. Men who consumed the most red meat (those in the top 25% of red-meat consumption) had twice the risk of developing prostate cancer as those men in the lowest quartile. The risk for total fat intake, desserts, and calories was similar: The highest quartile had nearly double the risk in each category as the lowest.

This effect appears to be separate from the caloric risk. In several studies a group of men with high consumption of red meat had a greater risk of getting prostate cancer than a group of men with comparable total caloric intake, but less meat. The relative risk of calories versus fat has not been studied. It's best to control both.

A prospective study on the relationship between dietary fats and prostate cancer survival was conducted at Laval University in Quebec, Canada. Observers studied 384 men diagnosed with prostate cancer for a median time of 5.2 years.

Trained nutritionists interviewed the men about their dietary habits, then divided them into three groups, determined by their fat intake. During the study period, 32 men died of prostate cancer, 9% of the men. The investigators found that saturated fat consumption was significantly associated with the risk of dying from prostate cancer. Those in the top third of saturated fat intake had three times the risk of dying from their cancer, when compared with the third who consumed the lowest amount of saturated fat.

Linolenic and Linoleic Acid

Linolenic acid and linoleic acid are essential fatty acids that must be obtained from dietary sources. The body does not make either of them. But most of us consume far more of these fatty acids than our bodies need.

Meat is rich in a fatty acid called alpha-linolenic acid. In animal studies this fatty acid has consistently been found to stimulate prostate cancer growth. Interestingly, another food replete with alpha-linolenic acid is flax. Flax seed and flax oil are common items in most health-food stores and have been lauded as a nutritional panacea. More than once I've seen flax oil recommended in the popular press for prevention of a variety of cancers, including prostate. Medical evidence does not support this. Although flax products may be beneficial in lowering blood-cholesterol levels while boosting high-density lipoproteins (HDLs), the so-called "good cholesterol," I wouldn't put flax oil into the same body with prostate cancer.

In a 1997 study by the American Health Foundation, observers found that a diet rich in flax oil did not protect mice from the growth of injected prostate cancer cells.

In human studies, flax consumption has been associated with a reduction of some forms of cancer, but not of the prostate. Dr. Charles (Snuffy) Myers thinks it's dangerous. More studies need to be done on what role, if any, linolenic acid-rich flax has in a prostate cancer diet. When in doubt, leave it out.

Polyunsaturated vegetable oils, such as safflower, corn,

and soybean oils, are rich in a fatty acid called *linoleic* acid. These linoleic acid-rich oils stimulate prostate cancer cell growth in the lab and in animals in much the same manner as *linolenic* acid. In fact, they're worse. In mice, prostate tumor growth is enhanced by a diet rich in linoleic acid. One reason for this may be because linoleic acid can be converted in your body into arachidonic acid. As you'll soon read, arachidonic acid is one of the most potent promoters of prostate cancer growth. *All polyunsaturated oils should be avoided.*

The good news is that most vegetables have low overall fat content. By substituting fruits and vegetables for meat, you'll reduce the saturated fat in your diet. The fat in meat is much denser than the fat in vegetables. This means fewer calories in vegetables.

Soy products like tofu are also high in linoleic acid and are generally not low in fat. But soy seems to have other compensating benefits due to its phytoestrogen content. Look for soy products that have the lowest fat levels—lite tofu, low-fat (or non-fat) soy protein isolates, low-fat (or non-fat) soy milk, etc.

What about the "good oils" like olive and walnut? This is an area of conjecture. Much has been written about the "Mediterranean diet." Men living along the Mediterranean Sea have less heart disease and a lower incidence of some cancers, including prostate. Their food is often swimming in olive oil. Does this mean olive oil is protective? Perhaps. A slew of recent studies put olive-oil consumption in a favorable light. It seems to reduce total cholesterol levels, particularly the "bad cholesterol," or LDLs. This may reduce the risk of heart disease, as seen in those people who eat the Mediterranean diet. Diets rich in olive oil have also been reported to do the following:

HELPFUL HINT

Read the label on soy products carefully. You can reduce the amount of fat (linoleic acid) considerably by judicious selection.

- reduce inflammation
- reduce the risk of blood clots
- reduce atherosclerosis
- lower blood pressure
- may reduce the risk of colorectal, breast, and prostate cancer
- decrease arachidonic acid mobilization

Recently, the European Union has countenanced olive oil as the oil of choice for its population. You should too.

Substituting olive oil for lard and saturated and polyunsaturated oils is certainly a positive nutritional change. Palm, cottonseed, and coconut oils contain saturated fats similar to lard. Diets containing high amounts of polyunsaturated oils, such as corn and safflower, have been associated with an increased risk of prostate cancer in laboratory experiments. Olives produce a predominately monounsaturated oil, which is better for health than other oils or fats. But 14% of olive oil is still saturated fat. And a tablespoon of olive oil still has 140 calories! Nutritional experts like Dr. Heber and Dr. Myers conclude that it's best to try to reduce all oil and fat intake, but to use olive oil when oil is required in cooking and salad dressings. Other acceptable oils, all predominately monounsaturated, are walnut, macademia, and avocado oils. The current consensus is that moderate consumption of olive oil is probably beneficial, so long as total caloric consumption is kept under control.

Prostate cancer cells seem to have an affinity for fat. At the 1999 Prostate Cancer Foundation prostate cancer retreat, one investigator told me that unpublished experiments have shown that prostate cancer cells are amaz-

---

HELPFUL HINTS

- Olive oil contains useful nutrients and can be used in moderation, provided that total caloric intake is kept down.
- Macadamia nut oil, walnut oil, or avocado oil can be substituted for olive oil for taste; no other oils should be used either for cooking or in dressings.

ingly efficient at trapping fat molecules and metabolizing them. If a prostate tumor is suspended in saline solution and a spurt of oil is run through the tumor, 80% of the fat is removed by the tumor in a single pass! It makes sense to me to reduce fat intake so that any microscopic colonies of cancer cells will be kept on meager fat rations and their growth will, hopefully, be suppressed.

What Is The Best Diet?

The best diet for the prevention of prostate cancer luckily happens to be the most heart-friendly as well. Doctors Heber, Myers, and Ornish all agree—the optimal diet for heart and prostate is a low-fat vegan diet. A vegan diet is composed of vegetables, fruits, beans, legumes, and grains. Milk, milk products (like yogurt and ice cream), and eggs are not included. All meat and fish are eliminated. Use of oil, any kind of oil, should be minimized, but when required limited to the monounsaturated oils discussed above. Although this diet has not been proven to prevent prostate cancer, it has been proven to lower serum cholesterol levels and protect against heart disease. Epidemiologic and animal studies indicate that this diet also reduces the risk of prostate, breast, and colon cancer, but conclusive proof is not yet in hand.

Does this mean a low-fat vegan diet has no validity? No. It means it's the best available alternative based on present evidence. It will make it easier to control your weight; your serum cholesterol will almost certainly decline (mine went from 180 to 135), and you're likely to be reducing your risk of prostate cancer. Recent data show that adding fish to a vegan diet may provide additional protection against dying from prostate cancer.

Improving on the Low-fat Vegan Diet

Adding soy and green tea to your vegan diet will probably reduce your prostate cancer risk further still. Numerous laboratory, animal, and epidemiologic studies have shown the anti-proliferation potential for these two foods. They are an integral part of the Japanese and Chinese diets.

Cruciferous vegetables should also be eaten regularly. These include broccoli, broccoli sprouts, cauliflower, cabbage, Brussels sprouts, bok choy, kale, chard, radishes, arugula, and watercress. Crucifers contain sulforaphane and indole-3-carbinol. Sulforaphane activates enzymes that have a detoxifying effect on a variety of cancer-causing chemicals. These detoxifying enzymes, called glycosinolates, are potent antioxidants. Sulforaphane is a powerful stimulator for production of glutathione transferases, one of the potent glycosinolates, and other strong detoxifying enzymes.

Indole-3-carbinol has recently been shown to slow down the growth of prostate cancer cells that are no longer sensitive to sex hormones (androgen independent). These are the type of cancer cells that men have when they no longer respond to hormonal therapy. Not only did indole-3-carbinol slow the growth of these aggressive cancer cells, it helped to re-establish the built-in suicide program. This was accomplished by increasing the protein production of the cancer-protective genes p21 and p27 (up-regulation), while down-regulating the expression of the Bcl-2 cancer-promoting gene. Reduction of Bcl-2 is a primary goal in the treatment of prostate cancer.

A gene known as GSTP-1 appears to be lost early in the prostate cancer process. It's inactivated by a process called hypermethylation. Heterocyclicamines from animal fats cooked at high temperatures may accelerate the deactivation of GSTP-1. Loss of GSTP-1 seems to be one of the earliest-observed gene changes in prostate cancer, according to investigations at Johns Hopkins led by Dr. William Nelson. Its function is lost in 65% of men with PIN and 94% of men with localized prostate cancer. Glycosinolates in crucifers may help protect GSTP-1 from the effects of carcinogens like heterocyclicamines. Antioxidants, such as selenium, may also be protective in men in the lowest 25% of selenium blood levels. Selenium supplements in this group may help preserve GSTP-1 function. Selenium blood levels decrease with age, increasing the risk of GSTP-1 inactivation and raising the risk of prostate cancer.

Key Reference

Nelson W. GSTP-1 inactivation and prostate cancer progression. Ninth Annual Prostate Cancer Foundation Retreat, September 20-22, 2002.

It's little wonder that the January 5, 2000, issue of the *Journal of the National Cancer Institute* reported a 41% reduction in the risk of prostate cancer among men eating three or more servings per week of crucifers, compared to men eating one serving or less weekly. In this study, statistical adjustments were made for total vegetable intake so that the reduced risks were specifically isolated to consumption of crucifers. Interestingly, increasing total vegetable consumption also decreased the risk of prostate cancer in this study. Men who ate 28 or more servings of vegetables (all kinds) per week had 35% less risk of developing clinical prostate cancer than men who ate 14 servings or less. The study's authors, from the Fred Hutchison Cancer Research Institute in Seattle, Washington, concluded, "High consumption of vegetables, particularly cruciferous vegetables, is associated with a reduced risk of prostate cancer."

What if you, like ex-president George Bush, hate broccoli? Researchers at Johns Hopkins University found a solution: broccoli sprouts. Three-day-old broccoli sprouts have 10-100 times as much glucoraphanin, a sulforaphane derivative, as the whole vegetable! What's more, for those of us too lazy to grow our own sprouts, tablets containing extracts from these 3-day-old sprouts are readily available and not expensive. Fresh sprouts are also available in selected stores, marketed under the name "BroccoSprouts." These are the same sprouts patented by doctors at Johns Hopkins. Look for them in your local market or health-food store.

In experiments in rats, this extract proved highly effective in decreasing the incidence and development of breast cancer. The researchers concluded: "Small quantities of crucifer sprouts may protect against the risk of cancer as effectively as much larger quantities of mature vegetables of the same variety." Although I eat lots of crucifers, I still take broccoli-sprout tablets when I travel. They are not harmful and may reduce the risk of recurrence of my prostate cancer. I routinely add broccoli sprouts to my salads when I'm at home. Broccoli sprouts are readily available in supermarkets throughout New Zealand.

The Case for Fish

If a low-fat vegan diet is optimal for prevention of prostate cancer (and heart disease), where does this leave fish? The answer is controversial. Fish is rich in menhaden oil. Several studies in mice have shown that a diet rich in menhaden oil significantly retards the growth of transplanted prostate tumors when compared with corn oil (linoleic acid) or flax oil (linolenic acid), both of which stimulate tumor growth. Although both fish oil and flax oil are rich in omega-3 fatty acids, they seem to affect tumor growth differently in mice. A study by Connolly, Coleman, and Rose, reported in 1997 in *Nutrition and Cancer*, showed that genetically identical mice with prostate cancer seemed to benefit from menhaden oil. Mice fed a diet of 18% menhaden oil and 5% corn oil had a 30% reduction in prostate tumor growth, when compared to mice fed 18% flax oil and 5% corn oil, or 18% corn oil and 5% flax oil.

Why the difference, since both flax and fish oils are rich in omega-3 fatty acids? Flax oil is high in alpha-linolenic acid. The two main fatty acids in fish oil are EPA and DHA. Alpha-linolenic acid can be converted in the body to EPA and DHA, but this isn't an efficient process. In the mice being studied, some of the linolenic acid was metabolized to EPA, although not to the same extent as in fish oil. This was not the case for DHA. In fact, DHA levels were lower in the flax oil-fed mice than in the corn oil-fed group! Other studies have shown that DHA, but not EPA, may inhibit an enzyme called protein kinase C. When this enzyme is deactivated in prostate cancer cells, they die more readily, like a normal prostate cell. Their genetic program to die is switched back on and they undergo apoptosis (programmed cell death). This may be part of the reason why fish oil was so much more effective than flax oil in reducing the tumor mass in these mice. Another reason might be that EPA and DHA reduce inflammation, which has been associated with cancer growth.

What about humans? Does eating fish help reduce the risk of prostate cancer? Here the evidence is far less clear. A 1996 study by Dr. Godley and colleagues showed a positive association (increased risk) between linoleic acid (corn, safflower, soy oils) and prostate cancer, as did the Connolly study. They did not, however, find that increased tissue levels of EPA or DHA reduced the risk of prostate cancer. On the other hand, a 1996 study in England reported reduced risk of prostate cancer from eating fish regularly.

A recent New Zealand study done in Auckland and reported in the *British Journal of Cancer* compared the levels of EPA and DHA in the red blood cells of 317 men with prostate cancer and 480 age-matched normal men. The study revealed that men whose EPA and DHA levels were in the top 25% had 41% and 38% less risk of getting prostate cancer respectively, when compared to men in the lowest quartile of EPA and DHA levels.

Dr. Giovannucci at Harvard showed a relationship between total fat consumption and the risk of prostate cancer. He found that high alpha-linolenic acid, predominately from animal fat, was the major culprit. Although fish fats contribute to total fat intake, this study found no effect, either positive or negative, on the risk of prostate cancer from high fish consumption.

A recent preliminary study by Dr. June Chan at the University of California-San Francisco, however, shows that fish consumption four or more times a weeks seems to significantly reduce the risk of progression of prostate cancer in men who already have it. Preliminary results show a 50% reduction in death from prostate cancer in the high-fish-consumption group. These results, presented at the 2001 Prostate Cancer Foundation Retreat, have not yet been published and more cases are still being studied. Dr. Chan believes that this work is still too preliminary to draw conclusions and to recommend frequent fish eating for men with prostate cancer.

New data just released by Dr. Giovannucci does show what appears to be protection from prostate cancer by fish consumption (see "New and Future Developments—Nutrition").

Are you confused yet? You may be thinking, "Don't bug me with linolenic acid and DHA. Just tell me what to eat."

Okay. My considered opinion is that including fish in your diet is fine. I am a prostate cancer survivor and eat fish regularly. I concentrate on fish high in the beneficial fatty acids DHA and EPA. These include wild salmon (not farm-grown), sardines, mackerel, anchovies, tuna, cod, swordfish, and halibut. Why do I avoid farm-fed salmon? The DHA and EPA in salmon comes mainly from eating other fish that have fed on DHA- and EPA-rich algae. Farm-raised fish are fed pellets lacking these fatty acids. Although farm-fed fish have plenty of fat, this fat lacks the high concentration of DHA and EPA of wild fish. When eating high-caloric food like fatty fish, it's important to extract full nutritional benefit. Without high levels of DHA and EPA, farm-raised fish aren't worth the caloric investment.

There's no question that whenever you substitute fish for red meat, you're doing your heart and prostate a favor. Substituting white-meat chicken (cooked without its skin—remember, chicken skin cooked at high temperatures is one of the richest sources of cancer-causing heterocyclic amines) or turkey breast for red meat would also be an improvement. These changes do not necessarily need to be made overnight. Depending on your personality, you may choose to make them gradually, as a process. You may otherwise wish to make a radical dietary change and stick with it. Knowing the operative principles should help.

What should vegans do to obtain adequate amounts of DHA and EPA? The answer, according to nutrition experts like Dr. Myers and Dr. Heber, does not lie in guzzling flax oil. Here a supplement is probably the best answer. If you're a pure vegan (no animal-derived food whatsoever), algae-derived DHA capsules are available, although you'll need about 15 capsules daily to get the anti-inflammatory benefits. DHA can be converted to EPA by the body. If you have no moral problem with consuming fish-oil capsules, these are also readily available and are a less costly way to get active amounts of EPA and DHA. If no fish is eaten, 1,000-mg capsules are available and should be taken twice daily. Men who do eat fish regularly can take less, or none at all, depending on the amount of fish being consumed. (For sources of algae-derived DHA and pure fish oil capsules, see Appendix IV).

By the way, fish consumption has also been associated with a reduction of a variety of degenerative diseases, including heart disease, stroke, arthritis, Alzheimer's, and other cancers. This is, in large part, due to its anti-inflammatory effects. Studies indicate that fish oil inhibits the production of inflammation-causing prostaglandins.

At this time, it's unclear whether a pure low-fat vegan diet or a vegan diet with added fish, is optimal. Either, however, is a highly constructive alternative to what most men currently eat.

More Fat (Not) to Chew On

Besides minimizing (or eliminating) red-meat consumption, you should eliminate the use of polyunsaturated oils and saturated fats. Although red meat is the main source of saturated fats, other sources include egg yolks, butter, coconut oil, and palm oil. Cooking oil should be reduced to minimal levels. The only cooking oil that should be used is olive oil. This is available as a spray, which will help you limit the amount used. Olive oil should also be the main oil used in salad dressings, although macadamia nut, walnut, or avocado oil can be substituted for taste. A delicious salad dressing can be made by mixing soft tofu and a little olive oil with lemon juice, spicy mustard, and fresh garlic. Balsamic vinegar can be substituted for lemon juice, if you prefer the taste.

Reducing oils and red meats will also help you reduce calories. I want to stress that calorie reduction is the single best thing you can do to reduce the risk of degenerative diseases such as cancer, heart disease, stroke, diabetes, and arthritis. Some experts believe that fat intake is not important so long as you're able to keep your calories low (2,000-2,200/day). Animal studies confirm this.

What is the relative value of reducing fats to reducing calories? The answer is not clear. It's probable that both calorie reduction and fat reduction have independent beneficial effects for men with prostate cancer, although fats high in DHA and EPA appear to be protective. Dr. Heber sums it up as follows.

• Fat and oils provide about 140 calories per tablespoon. This means that a mere 15 tablespoons would make up an entire day's diet! Obesity is a major risk factor for cancer and heart disease, so decreasing overall fat intake makes sense. I haven't lost anybody yet to fatty acid deficiency, so 20% (of calories) from fat or less is great, with fat being used to enhance taste where necessary.

• Fruits and vegetables have a natural balance of n-3 (linolenic) and n-6 (linoleic) fatty acids, as well as monounsaturated n-9 fatty acids, so increasing fruit and vegetable intake would be positive.

• Eating low-fat fish rich in n-3 fatty acids is okay, but a vegetarian diet balanced in linolenic and linoleic acid would probably be just as good, and perhaps better.

• Much more research is needed in this area, and [Dr. Heber's group is] planning to include this area as a major emphasis in [its] work at UCLA.

Diet is a complex subject. It's difficult, if not impossible, to isolate one food source from the overall diet. Diet may also be influenced by lifestyle. For example, a man who is 20 pounds overweight may eat lots of red meat, rich desserts, and dairy products. He may drink excessively, hate vegetables, and be under considerable stress. He may exercise infrequently and have a sedentary job. To say that his increased risk of getting prostate, or colon, cancer is from eating red meat is simplistic. A combination of dietary and lifestyle factors is likely involved in his increased risk of cancer. Yet a study looking at red-meat consumption would show an association in this man between his red-meat intake and his risk of developing prostate cancer.

"Epidemiologic studies do not provide cause and effect information," states Dr. Heber. "They indicate a dietary or eating pattern. For example, the associations between red meat and colon cancer say more about the overall diet and lifestyle of the red-meat eater than they do about any chemical contained in the red meat." Practical changes in patterns of eating and exercise are desirable.

How Fats May Stimulate Prostate Cancer Growth

None of the mechanisms by which dietary fat may increase prostate cancer risk have been proven. It's a complex area. Factors that may make a difference include the type and quantity of fat consumed, the interaction of ingested fatty acids with antioxidants, such as vitamins and minerals, changes in fat

---

HELPFUL HINTS

• Overall fat consumption should be reduced to about 20% of consumed calories.

• Calorie reduction is probably the single most important step you can take to increase longevity and the quality of life in old age.

• Some fats are beneficial, especially those containing the fatty acids DHA and EPA found in deep-water fish. Fat consumption should be limited to these and the monounsaturated oils—olive, walnut, macadamia nut, and avocado.

• Reducing calories should always be the paramount consideration, so that intake of even the beneficial oils, like olive oil, should be controlled for optimal health. Each tablespoon has 140 calories.

induced by cooking, and the effects of various fat mixtures on cells in the body.

While these areas are actively being studied, conclusions are hard to come by. We now know that heating saturated fats by cooking animal food, especially at high temperature, produces chemicals called heterocyclic amines, which are directly toxic to cells. This causes damage to cellular DNA. Other theories are more subtle. One that has received a lot of recent attention is the effect of dietary fats on insulin, growth factors, and hormones in the body. Gram for gram, fats have more than twice the calories of protein or carbohydrate and are a significant contributor to obesity, a disease that has reached epidemic levels in the United States.

Obesity and Prostate Cancer

Eating disorders are rampant in the U.S. According to Dr. Heber, half the population doesn't eat a single piece of fruit a day. Only 20% eat the five daily servings of fruits or vegetables recommended by the National Cancer Institute.

Obesity is a much bigger problem than not being able to button your trousers. It causes significant hormonal changes. Insulin levels are increased and diabetes is a common result. Diabetes-related deaths in America have increased 40% over the past 15 years and are now approaching deaths from breast cancer.

Besides diabetes, obese people have a significantly higher risk of heart disease and prostate cancer. They secrete a chemical, called adipocytokine, that leads to inflammation and oxidative changes that increase the risk of prostate cancer, arthritis, atherosclerosis, and other chronic debilitating diseases.

One hormonal change prevalent in obesity is changes in an insulin-related hormone known as insulin-like growth factor-1 (IGF-1). IGF-1 has received considerable attention in recent years in association with the development and spread of prostate cancer.

Key Reference

Heber, D. Investigation of plant-based diets and calorie restriction effects on prostate cancer. Ninth Annual Prostate Cancer Foundation Retreat, September 20-22, 2002.

IGF-1, IGFBP-3, and Prostate Cancer

IGF-1 stimulates prostate cancer cell growth. Although obese men tend to have high levels of IGF-1, men of normal weight can also have elevated IGF-1 levels. I know, because I'm one of those. In the bloodstream, IGF-1 can circulate freely or bind to a protein called IGF binding protein-3 (IGFBP-3). The relationship of IGF-1 to IGFBP-3 and their respective effects on prostate and breast cancer are a hot topic in cancer research. IGF-1 is a powerful stimulator of prostate cancer cell growth and also interferes with apoptosis. Elevated IGF-1 levels increase the risk of prostate cancer development and also increase the chances of localized prostate cancer becoming more aggressive and spreading beyond the prostate. In a prospective study, men in the highest quartile of IGF-1 levels had more than 4 times the risk of prostate cancer than men in the lowest 25%.

IGFBP-3, on the other hand, is a highly beneficial protein. Not only does it neutralize circulating IGF-1 by "mopping" it up, new studies show that it also has a direct inhibitory effect on the growth of prostate cancer cells. In fact, it has just been discovered that one of the main ways vitamin D works against prostate cancer is by increasing IGFBP-3 levels.

All evidence now points toward lowering IGF-1 levels and raising IGFBP-3 levels as one of the more important steps a man can take in preventing prostate cancer. For men who already have prostate cancer, this interplay is even more important. Moving toward a plant-based diet, decreasing calories, and increasing exercise levels all reduce IGF-1 levels and raise IGFBP-3 levels. Increasing vitamin D levels appear to raise IGFBP-3 levels. Silymarin or silibinin supplements may also raise IGFBP-3 levels and decrease IGF-1. For a more complete discussion of this important topic, see pages 418-423.

Key References

Chan JM et al. Plasma insulin-like growth factor-1 and prostate cancer risk: a prospective study. *Science* 1998; 279: 563-565.

Chan JM et al. Insulin-like growth factor-1 (IGF-1) and IGF binding protein-3 as predictors of advanced-stage prostate cancer. *J Natl Cancer Instit* 2002; 94: 1099-1105.

Feldman D. Pathways mediating the growth inhibitory actions of vitamin D in prostate cancer. Ninth Annual Prostate Cancer Foundation Retreat, September 20-22, 2002.

Sex Hormone Binding Globulin (SHBG)

We men have a hormone circulating in our blood called sex hormone binding globulin (SHBG). SHBG binds testosterone in the blood, reducing the levels of free testosterone. Low dietary fat intake leads to increases in SHBG; high fat intake reduces SHBG levels. In 1996, a study conducted at Harvard Medical School by Gann et al. showed a significant increased risk of prostate cancer as the level of testosterone increased. Men with levels in the top 25% of those tested had a two to six times greater chance of getting prostate cancer than men whose testosterone level was in the lowest 25%.

The opposite effect was observed when SHBG was measured by these investigators. The higher the SHBG level, the lower the risk of prostate cancer. Men whose SHBG levels were in the top 25% had a 54% less chance of getting prostate cancer, compared to men in the lowest 25% for SHBG.

The Gann study was prospective, involving 222 men who subsequently developed prostate cancer and 392 controls matched for age, smoking, length of follow-up, etc. Although this was a seemingly well-designed investigation, not all researchers have reached the same conclusion. It cannot be said with any certainty that increased testosterone levels, or low SHBG levels, cause prostate cancer. But the Gann study shows a strong association between these blood factors and prostate cancer. So, although the evidence is not conclusive, it seems beneficial, as far as prostate health is concerned, to maintain relatively high blood levels of SHBG. That means, once again, a low fat intake.

What factors regulate SHBG levels? Major influences include insulin and insulin-like growth factors. As insulin levels in the blood increase, SHBG levels decrease. Obese men often have high insulin and low SHBG. Diet and exercise can lower insulin levels and raise SHBG levels. A 1998 study done at UCLA Medical School monitored the effects on insulin and SHBG levels produced by a three-week diet and exercise program in 27 obese men. The men exercised by walking 30-45 minutes daily and participating in a supervised exercise class. They ate as much as they wanted, but fat was limited to 10% of calories. Protein comprised 10% -15% of calories and complex carbohydrates provided the balance. Carbohydrates were primarily in the form of vegetables, fruits, legumes, and grains. Animal consumption was limited to 85 grams of chicken or fish per week (about three ounces).

At the end of the three weeks, insulin levels had decreased by 43% and SHBG levels had increased by 39%.

Key References

Kolonel L, Noumra N, Cooney R. Dietary fat and prostate cancer: current status. *J Natl Cancer Inst* 1999; 91: 414-428.

Giovannuci E et al. A prospective study of dietary fat and risk of prostate cancer. *J Natl Cancer Inst* 1993; 85: 1571-1579.

Ghosh J, Myers C Jr. Arachadonic acid metabolism and cancer of the prostate (editorial). *Nutrition* 1998; 14: 48-49.

Gann P et al. Prospective study of plasma fatty acids and the risk of prostate cancer. *J Natl Cancer Inst* 1994; 86: 281-286.

Myers CE Jr. *Eating Your Way to Better Health*. Rivanna Health Publications, Inc. 2000; 10-23.

Wang Y et al. Decreased growth of established human prostate LNCaP tumors in nude mice fed a low-fat diet. *J Natl Cancer Inst* 1995; 87: 1456-1462.

Cohen J et al. Fruit and vegetable intakes and prostate cancer risk. *J Natl Cancer Inst* 2000; vol. 92: 61-68.

Fahey J et al. Broccoli sprouts: an exceptionally rich source of inducers of enzymes that protect against chemical carcinogens. Proceedings of the National Academy of Science. 1997; 94: 10367-10372.

Norrish A et al. Prostate cancer risk and consumption of fish oils: a dietary biomarker-based case-control study. Br J Cancer 1999; 81: 1238-1242.

Connolly J, Coleman, M, Rose D. Effects of dietary fatty acids on DU 145 human prostate cancer cell growth in athymic nude mice. Nutrition and Cancer, 1997, 29: 114-119.

Stark A and Madar Z. Olive oil as a functional food: epidemiology and nutritional approaches. Nutrition Reviews 2002; 60: 170-176.

Reed M et al. Dietary lipids; an additional regulator of plasma levels of sex hormone-binding globulin. Journal of Clinical Endocrinology and Metabolism, 1987; 64: 1083-1085.

Tymchuk C et al. Effects of diet and exercise on insulin, sex hormone binding globulin, and prostate-specific antigen. Nutrition and Cancer. 31: 127-131.13.

Koplan J Deitz W. Caloric imbalance and public health policy. Journal of the American Medical Association, 1999; 282: 1579-1581.

Gann P et al. Prospective study of sex hormone levels and risk of prostate cancer. Journal of the National Cancer Institute. 1996; 88: 1118-1126.

Chan J. Presentation at the Ninth Annual Prostate Cancer Foundation Retreat, Washington, D.C., Sept. 20-22, 2002.

18

ANTIOXIDANTS

When exposed to oxygen, many metals rust. This process is known as "oxidation." As we age, oxidative processes in our bodies cause us to "rust." Charged particles, called free radicals, are formed by oxidation and can damage DNA and increase the risk of prostate cancer.

Neutralizing free radicals reduces the risk of prostate and other cancers. Micro-nutrients found in fruits and vegetables act as antioxidants, another good reason to eat these foods regularly. Some commonly known vitamins (C, D, E, A, and beta-carotene) are antioxidants. Other antioxidants include lycopene (primarily from tomato products), selenium, polyphenols (from green tea and red wine), curcumin (from turmeric), and silymarin (from artichokes and milk thistle).

Vitamin C

Vitamin C is a water-soluble antioxidant. It has been widely studied, receiving much attention in newspapers and magazines. It protects us from damage to our DNA from free radicals and stimulates our immune system.

Many studies have shown the association of optimal amounts of vitamin C with a decrease in the incidence of a variety of cancers, including prostate cancer. It's ironic that the man whose name is most associated with vitamin C, two-time Nobel Laureate Dr. Linus Pauling, succumbed to prostate cancer. He was in his 90s when he died, however.

Since vitamin C is water soluble, it's easily excreted from the body. The minimum effective dose is about 1,000 mg, divided into two equal doses of 500 mg. Studies have shown that 1,000 mg is the minimum amount that saturates the blood completely, and you'll often hear recommendations for higher amounts, up to 10 grams per day or more. Higher doses may be advisable in some cases. Even if you eat the five servings of fruits or vegetables, as recommended by the American Cancer Society, which few Americans do, you would only consume roughly 200 mg of vitamin C daily.

Vitamin C intake not only correlates with a reduced risk of cancer, its ingestion is also associated with a reduced risk of heart disease. A study published in the *American Journal of Epidemiology* in 1996 showed a 62% lower risk of heart disease in people who consumed 700 mg or more of vitamin C daily, as compared with those whose daily intake was 60 mg or less. By the way, 60 mg is the Recommended Daily Allowance (RDA). Based on the literature, this amount seems insufficient for optimal health.

People who have cancer tend to have lower blood levels of vitamin C than healthy people. Increasing the amount of vitamin C in cancer patients may help prevent or slow tumor growth. Sometimes megadoses, as recommended by Dr. Pauling, in amounts of 10 grams per day or more have been suggested for people with advanced cancer. Some investigators report excellent results in reducing metastases using these large doses. More studies are required to determine optimal doses of vitamin C for men who have been treated definitively with either radiation or surgery.

For men with prostate cancer who have chosen watchful waiting and those in whom cancer has recurred, 1,500 mg in three divided doses seems appropriate. Note that megadoses may increase the risk of kidney stones in some people. Diarrhea is also common at high doses and should be used as an indicator that dose reduction is in order. Although they may possibly benefit some high-risk advanced-cancer patients, doses of this magnitude should be carefully monitored by your doctor. Please note that it has not been proven that high doses benefit these men and some researchers conclude, based on their studies, that any vitamin C supplementation should be avoided because it may nourish the cancer as well as the immune system. Unless you're eating a predominantly plant-based diet, it seems to me that modest vitamin C supplementation is, on balance, a reasonable approach.

Vitamin E

Vitamin E was discovered in 1922. Most of us think of it as a single compound, but it's actually composed of 8 different compounds, 4 tocopherols and 4 tocotrienols. While all are fat-soluble antioxidants, their effects on inflammation and cancer cell growth differ. Also, their interaction and effectiveness when combined with other nutrients vary. As you'll read below, most of the early work on vitamin E was done on alpha-tocopherol. Indeed, this vitamin E component is what is generally supplied in vitamin E supplements. Recently, the vitamin E component known as gamma-tocopherol has been shown to play a prominent role in the prevention of prostate cancer and heart disease.

Vitamin E is measured in IU, or International Units. One IU is the same as one milligram.

Over the past few years our understanding of the effects and interaction of the various vitamin E components has become more differentiated, although far from complete. Gamma-tocopherol is the rising star in the vitamin E world, especially in relation to prostate cancer risk. Gamma-tocopherol, found in high concentrations in seeds and nuts, is the main source of vitamin E in the U.S. diet. Although this is the most predominate form of dietary vitamin E, the average American consumes only 17mg (IU) per day.

Recent studies have demonstrated that gamma-tocopherol may be superior to alpha-tocopherol, the type of vitamin E generally found in supplements, in the prevention of both prostate cancer and heart disease. A 1999 study from the University of Michigan showed that gamma-tocopherol was superior to alpha-tocopherol in inhibiting the growth of prostate cancer cells in the lab.

Gamma-tocopherol, but not alpha-tocopherol, reduces inflammation by inhibiting cyclooxygenase (COX-2) activity. Inhibition of COX-2 is not only thought to reduce the risk of prostate cancer but to reduce the chances of heart disease too.

Blood plasma levels of gamma-tocopherol (and lycopene) are strongly correlated with the amount of gamma-tocopherol in the prostate itself. A Johns Hopkins study reported in the December 2000 issue of the *Journal of the National Cancer Institute* found that increasing plasma amounts of alpha-tocopherol tended to reduce the risk of prostate cancer, but this trend did not reach statistical significance in a prospective study of 10,456 men. Gamma-tocopherol plasma levels, on the other hand, made a highly significant difference in the risk of getting prostate cancer. Men in the top 20% of gamma-tocopherol blood levels had 1/5 the risk of developing prostate cancer, when compared with men in the bottom 20%. Moreover, statistically significant protective associations for high levels of selenium and alpha-tocopherol were only seen when gamma-tocopherol levels were also high. For selenium and alpha-tocopherol to work effectively, they appear to require high levels of gamma-tocopherol.

Of particular importance is this fact: High doses of alpha-tocopherol *reduce* plasma levels of gamma-tocopherol. So men taking large doses of vitamin E in the form of alpha-tocopherol supplements are actually depleting themselves of the seemingly more beneficial,

---

HELPFUL HINT

Recent evidence indicates that gamma-tocopherol supplements may be more effective in reducing the risk of prostate cancer and heart disease than the widely-used alpha-tocopherol.

Alpha-tocopherol supplements deplete the body of gamma-tocopherol. Gamma-tocopherol supplements increase plasma levels of both gamma- and alpha-tocopherols.

and prostate cancer protective, gamma-tocopherol. Gamma-tocopherol supplements, however, increase plasma levels of both gamma and alpha-tocopherol. This new information strongly indicates that alpha-tocopherol supplements may be counter-productive. I take 400 IU of mixed tocopherols and related compounds that provide seven of the eight components of vitamin E, but are highly weighted toward gamma-tocopherol (Life Extension gamma-tocopherol; see "Sources of Supply" in the Appendix IV).

All vitamin E components are fat-soluble. They're better absorbed when combined with a small amount of oil or fat and are stored in the fatty tissues of the body. Unlike the easily excreted water-soluble vitamin C, which should be taken in divided doses, vitamin E can be taken only once a day. Since it's stored in fat, it's removed from the body more slowly.

Substantial evidence indicates that vitamin E protects against cancer. Vitamin E gained prominence in the prevention of prostate cancer based on two medical studies reported in the 1990s. The first, a Swiss study, examined 2,974 male smokers. Low vitamin E levels (alpha-tocopherol) were associated with a significantly higher risk of getting prostate cancer. But this study is small compared to the joint study done by the National Cancer Institute (NCI) and the National Public Health Institute of Finland. The study group comprised 29,133 male smokers. Men were randomly given 50 IU alpha-tocopherol, 20 mg beta-carotene, both, or neither. Surprisingly, it turned out that alpha-tocopherol did not influence the incidence of lung cancer that developed in these men over a five- to eight-year time framework. Although not the original object of this study, the group that received 50 IU of alpha-tocopherol daily had 32% fewer cases of prostate cancer than the supplement-free control group. There were 41% fewer deaths from prostate cancer over this 5-8 year follow-up period. Fifty IU of alpha-tocopherol is considerably lower than the 200-800 IU that is commonly recommended.

More is not necessarily better. Since vitamin E tocopherols and tocotrienols are fat soluble, they can't be quickly excreted from the body. Cases of bleeding disorders have been reported from large doses of vitamin E taken over a protracted time period. As you know, high doses of alpha-tocopherol also deplete gamma-tocopherol. Although doses up to 800 IU of gamma-tocopherol are considered safe, higher doses aren't recommended.

Going back to the Finnish study, a look at the effects of beta-carotene (a vitamin A pre-cursor), when taken as a sole supplement, helps illustrate the point that supplements are not always safe. In this group of men, the incidence of lung cancer *increased* by 16% and deaths from lung cancer increased by 14%, when compared with the control group that took no supplements. In fact, the investigators terminated the "beta-carotene-alone" group early, because the supplement was obviously harmful. This result was highly significant.

What happened to the men in the beta-carotene group as far as prostate cancer is concerned? This group had 35% more clinically overt prostate cancer than did the controls! Further analysis showed a high correlation of these cases of prostate cancer in men who drank alcohol. Moreover, it was dose dependent, meaning that the more alcohol these men consumed, the higher their risk of prostate cancer when taking beta-carotene. The investigators also found that men who drank large amounts of alcohol and took beta-carotene had a higher risk of developing lung cancer, too. In the subgroup of men who took beta-carotene and did not drink, the incidence of prostate cancer *decreased* by 33%. Obviously, something about alcohol and beta-carotene doesn't mix. This came as a total surprise to the researchers.

Vitamin E (alpha-tocopherol), when combined with beta-carotene, reduced the risk of prostate cancer as compared to the controls, but not to the same extent as alpha-tocopherol alone. Apparently, subgroups of drinkers and non-drinkers in the combined group were not broken out in this study. Too bad. I'd like to know the effects of alcohol on the men in these two groups. My guess is that the men who drank large amounts of alcohol fared more poorly in both, but this is mere conjecture.

How long did it take for vitamin E to start exerting its protective effects? Two years. This finding led Dr. Philip Taylor, M.D., Sc.D., and chief of the NCI's Cancer Prevention Branch, to speculate that vitamin E may delay the development of slow-growing prostate cancer to an active tumor. Dr. Taylor believes that factors that might otherwise convert a more benign tumor into a clinically significant more aggressive form are blocked by alpha-tocopherol. We now know that this protective effect is likely to be more pronounced in men with high plasma levels of gamma-tocopherol.

Key References

Jiang Q et al. Gamma-tocopherol, the major form of vitamin E in the US diet, deserves more attention. *Am J Clin Nutr* 2001; 74: 714-722.

Giovannucci E. Gamma-tocopherol: a new player in prostate cancer prevention? *J Natl Cancer Inst* 2000; 92: 1966-1967.

Helzlsouer K et al. Association between alpha-tocopherol, gamma tocopherol, selenium and subsequent prostate cancer. *J Natl Cancer Inst* 2000; 92: 2018-2023.

Moyad M et al. Vitamin E, alpha-and gamma-tocopherol, and prostate cancer. *Semin Urology Oncol* 1999; 17: 85-90.

Freeman V et al. Prostatic levels of tocopherols, carotenoids, and retinol in relation to plasma levels and self-reported usual dietary intake. *Am J Epidemiol* 2000; 151: 124-127.

Heinonen O et al. Prostate cancer and supplementation with alpha-tocopherol and beta carotene: incidence and mortality in a controlled trial. *J Natl Cancer Inst* 1998; 90: 440-446.

Vitamin D

This is another fat-soluble antioxidant that seems to be lacking in many people. Researchers from Harvard Medical School found low blood levels in more than 40% of a group of 290 consecutive patients admitted to the hospital for any reason.

Unlike vitamin E, our bodies have the ability to make vitamin D. But we need a little sunlight to do it. I know we've been taught that sun exposure is a bad thing. And so it is, if it's excessive. You need only about 15 minutes of sun exposure at least three times a week for your body to produce sufficient vitamin D. A brief walk in a short-sleeved shirt will do it. Sunscreens inhibit vitamin D production, so you need direct sun exposure. Walking in the early morning or late afternoon will keep you from being sunburned. This amount of sun exposure will not significantly increase your risk of getting skin cancer.

To be sure you're getting enough vitamin D, experts recommend vitamin D supplements. This is especially necessary for men with prostate cancer. Some clinicians recommend calcitriol (Rocaltrol), the active form of vitamin D, for men with prostate cancer, especially if their vitamin D levels are low or low-normal. This is available by prescription only and should be taken only under a doctor's care. Vitamin D3 supplements are available in health-food stores and don't require a prescription. The optimal dose of vitamin D3 supplements is 300-700 IU per day. The usual calcitriol does is 0.5 micrograms per day, but may be adjusted periodically by your doctor.

In the lab, vitamin D analogs successfully converted malignant white blood cells back to normal ones. Vitamin D has also been shown to be a factor in apoptosis, or programmed cell death. Vitamin D analogs may play a regulatory role in reprogramming malignant cells, once again making them mortal.

Dr. David Feldman of Stanford University, author of a book called *Vitamin D*, has shown that this vitamin slows the growth of both normal and malignant prostate cells. There appears to be a specific receptor in these cells for vitamin D. When the vitamin latches on to the receptor, prostate cell growth, both normal and malignant, is inhibited.

Vitamin D takes on added importance in men with prostate cancer who are taking androgen-blocking hormones. You might recall that use of these hormones can reduce bone density in the large bones by 4% or more in only nine months. For this reason many experts put their patients taking hormones on bisphosphonates, such as Fosamax or Aredia. These compounds are known to increase bone density. Some medical oncologists also add Rocaltrol, the active form of vitamin D, to this regimen. The combination of Rocaltrol with a bisphosphonate may help drive calcium back into bone. Rocaltrol also increases the absorption of calcium from the gastro-intestinal tract, and seems to have the ability to slow the rise in PSA by direct effects. For more on this, refer to the section on bone density in the chapter on hormone therapy.

Promising research is currently under way using vitamin D analogs to treat prostate cancer (see "New and Future Developments"). Some experts think this avenue of investigation is one of the most likely to be rewarding.

Selenium

Selenium is another antioxidant that has been associated with a reduced risk of prostate cancer. Numerous studies have shown the protective value of selenium supplementation in animals given a variety of cancer-causing chemicals. Selenium also protects animals that have had tumor cells implanted into them.

In humans, epidemiologic studies reveal that people who live in areas where the soil has low levels of selenium have a higher risk of cancer. In another study, blood levels of selenium were significantly lower in a group of cancer patients when compared with controls who did not have cancer.

Perhaps the most significant study of the anti-cancer effects of selenium came serendipitously. A large study involving several institutions was started in 1983 by Dr. Clark and his group at the University of Arizona. More than 1,300 patients were evaluated in terms of the effects of selenium supplements in preventing skin cancer. Although selenium was not found to be associated with a reduced risk of skin cancer, subsequent evaluation of these patients revealed that men who received selenium supplements had only a little more than a third as many incidences of prostate cancer as those men receiving placebos. That's a risk reduction of more than 60%! The average time for follow-up examination of these men was more than six years. Serum-selenium levels increased by about two-thirds in the men who took selenium supplements. The dose of selenium was 200 micrograms per day and there was no evidence of selenium toxicity in the men who took these supplements.

This study is especially significant because it was randomized and controlled. The odds of this reduction in prostate cancer happening purely by chance is 999 to 1 (p=.001). Selenium reduced the risk of all cancers by about 50%. The result for all cancers was also highly significant (p=.001). The two cancers that selenium seemed to reduce the most were prostate and esophageal.

This study was confirmed by a prospective controlled investigation out of Stanford University. Reported in the *Journal of Urology*, researchers found that plasma selenium levels measured on average nearly 4 years prior to diagnosis predicted the likelihood of developing prostate cancer. Men with low selenium blood levels were 4-5 times more likely to develop prostate cancer than men with normal levels.

Plasma selenium levels decrease with aging and, as you know, the risks of prostate cancer increase with age. Evidence now exists that part of the age-related risk of prostate cancer development may be low selenium levels.

How does selenium work its cancer-protection magic? No one knows for certain. Because it's an antioxidant, it helps prevent DNA damage from marauding free radicals. It's estimated that each cell in the body receives 10,000 potentially cancer-causing damages to its DNA daily! Selenomethionine, the most common form of selenium, induces DNA repair along with other reparatory systems in the body to repair these daily DNA insults before they become problems. This is one way that selenium seems to protect against prostate cancer.

But it seems to do more. In the lab it protects cells against a variety of chemicals known to cause cells to mutate (mutagens). It may kill cancer cells directly by having toxic effects on them, or it may induce programmed cell death in cancer cells that, by mutating, have overcome this normal cell death process.

In the laboratory, selenium inhibits the growth and proliferation of prostate cancer cells. The growth of androgen-sensitive LNCaP cells was reduced by 80% in one recent study. There is new evidence that one way selenium works in androgen-responsive prostate cancer cells is by reducing the number of androgen receptors—the sites where androgens dock on the cancer cells. Dr. Brooks at Stanford University has documented reduced androgen receptor activity in prostate cancer cells treated with methyselenic acid and noted reduced gene expression in 73 other androgen-responsive genes. The strong anti-proliferation effects of selenium may also be due, at least in part, to upregulation of the p21 and p27 cancer-suppressor genes. A number of nutrients, including silymarin and quercetin, increase the expression of one, or both, of these important cancer-suppressor genes. Although I know of no study that proves it, these nutrients may well work synergistically in helping to suppress cancer by this genetic up-regulation of cancer-controlling genes.

At this point, it seems likely that selenium works by several different and distinct mechanisms in exerting its anti-cancer activity. Besides those already discussed, selenium inhibits prostate cancer cell proliferation, increases apoptosis, increases detoxification, and interferes with the formation of new blood vessels (anti-angiogenesis) in prostate cancer.

I'm intrigued by a possible connection between the effects of a diet lacking the amino acid methionine in animal studies and the effects of selenium. The major form of selenium in food is in the form of selenomethionine. Ninety percent of selenomethionine is absorbed and when proteins are made in the body from amino acids, selenomethionine randomly substitutes for methionine. Here's the interesting part: Studies show that restricting methionine in animals that had received grafts of prostate cancer cells causes the tumor to shrink, according to researchers at Baylor College of Medicine in Houston, Texas. Restricting methionine inhibited the growth of both androgen-dependent and androgen-independent prostate cancer cells. Lack of methionine increased apoptosis and increased the expression of the p21 and p27 cancer-suppressor genes.

Selenium also inhibits prostate cancer cell growth, increases apoptosis, and up-regulates p21 and p27. Given that we know that by far the most common form of dietary selenium is selenomethionine and this compound randomly substitutes for methionine in the formation of proteins in the body, could it be that part of the way in which selenium works revolves around this substitution? Since the effects of selenium and of methionine restriction seem to mirror each other, it seems to me that this might be a fruitful area for further research. Bear in mind that all this is purely hypothetical and may turn out to be no more than ruminations of my overly imaginative mind, but the relationship is intriguing.

Dr. Moshe Shike, Head of Cancer Prevention and Nutrition at Sloan Kettering Memorial Hospital in New York City, is convinced that selenium supplementation is only beneficial in areas where the selenium level in the soil is low. He says that in most of North America the selenium level is adequate. It seems to be low in the southeastern part of the United States, parts of the Eastern seaboard, the Pacific Northwest, and in a number of foreign countries. He told me that, since I live in New Zealand, I should take it. New Zealand is known to have selenium-poor soil.

A report issued as we go to press supports Dr. Shike's contention. Researchers at the Arizona Cancer Center in Tucson, Arizona, Dr. Clark's institution, have gone back and looked at blood levels of selenium in all the men in the Nutritional Prevention of Cancer Trial, as Dr. Clark's original trial is called. They found that selenium supplementation significantly reduced the overall cancer risk (all cancers) only in men in the lower ⅔ of selenium blood levels. Selenium supplementation actually seemed to slightly increase the risk of cancer in men in the highest third of selenium blood levels. Additionally, they found that men who formerly smoked benefited the most from selenium supplementation.

Plants absorb selenium from the soil, so if the vegetables you eat come from selenium-rich soil, you'll absorb some. The question is how much. Researchers disagree on the need for supplemental selenium if people come from an area with selenium-rich soil and eat locally grown produce. The best approach would be to have your plasma selenium levels checked and to take selenium supplements if your level is less than 122 ng/mg.

Recently, researchers from Dr. Clark's lab in Arizona have been studying the effects of higher selenium doses on men with prostate cancer. It appears to be safe to take up to 800 mcg or more per day. Ironically, and tragically, Dr. Clark recently succumbed to prostate cancer. His studies are being continued, however, by his colleagues. Four new studies are currently under way at the Arizona Cancer Center. They include randomly testing selenium supplementation versus a placebo in each of the following groups:

• Men suspected of having prostate cancer, but who have a negative biopsy (to test the ability of selenium to prevent the development of prostate cancer).

• Men with high-grade PIN (again to see if cancer development can be prevented).

• Men with known prostate cancer scheduled for surgery (to test the effects of selenium supplementation on the tumor removed at surgery).

• Men with prostate cancer who have decided against definitive treatment (watchful waiting)—to test the ability of selenium supplementation to inhibit the progression of prostate cancer.

So what's the bottom line on the use of selenium to help prevent prostate cancer and for men that already have the disease? I suggest you have your plasma (blood) selenium level tested. If it's low, selenium supplementation is definitely warranted. Based on current evidence, it seems likely that selenium supplementation for men with low levels will reduce the risk of getting prostate cancer. It may well reduce the chances of the cancer spreading in men that already have cancer. Although it's possible to raise blood selenium levels by consuming selenium-rich foods like Brazil nuts, it's easier and more regulated to take a selenium supplement. Two hundred micrograms daily is sufficient for prevention and 200-400 micrograms daily is sufficient for men who already have cancer.

The National Cancer Institute has launched an enormous study to determine whether selenium and/or vitamin E (alpha-tocopherol) decreases the incidence of prostate cancer. Over the next 12 years, 32,000 men will be studied to determine the effects of these two nutrients. Hopefully, they will adjust the study protocol to take into account the new information about the apparent need for high levels of gamma-tocopherol for selenium and alpha-tocopherol to be effective.

Key References

Brooks JD et al. Plasma selenium levels before diagnosis and the risk of prostate cancer development. *J Urology* 2001; 166: 2034-2038.

Seo Y et al. Selenomethionine induction of DNA repair response in human fibroblasts. *Oncogene* 2002; 21: 3663-3669.

Venkateswaran V et al. Selenium modulation of cell cycle proliferation and cell cycle bio-markers in human prostate cancer cell lines. *Cancer Research* 2002; 62: 2540-2545.

Junxuan Lu and Cheng Jiang. Antiangiogenic activity of selenium in cancer chemoprevention: metabolite-specific effects. *Nutr and Cancer* 2001; 40: 64-73.

Grieger, J. Selenium: what's new? *Nutr Today* 2001; 36: 97-99.

Shan L and Epner D. Molecular mechanisms of cell cycle block by methionine restriction in human prostate cancer cells. *Nutr and Cancer* 2000; 38: 123-130.

Brooks JD. Mechanisms of action of the chemopreventive agent methyseleninic acid. Poster presentation number 7. Ninth Annual Prostate Cancer Foundation Scientific Retreat, September 20-22, 2002.

Waters D. Dietary selenium supplementation decreases DNA damage and upregulates apoptosis within the aging prostate. Poster presentation number 99. Ninth Annual Prostate Cancer Foundation Scientific Retreat, September 20-22, 2002.

Clark L et al. Decreased incidence of prostate cancer with selenium supplementation: results of a double-blind cancer prevention trial. *Brit J Urology* 1998; 81: 730-734.

Duffield-Lillico A et al. Baseline characteristics and the effect of selenium supplementation on cancer incidence in a randomized clinical trial: a summary report of the Nutritional Prevention of Cancer Trial. *Cancer Epidemiol Biomark Prev* 2002; 11: 630-639.

Clark L and Marshall J. Randomized controlled chemo-prevention trials in populations at very high risk for prostate cancer: elevated prostate-specific-antigen and high-grade prostatic intraepithelial neoplasia. *Urology* 2001; 14: 153-159.

Marshall J. Larry Clark's legacy: randomized controlled, selenium-based prostate cancer chemoprevention trials. *Nutr and Cancer* 2001; 40: 74-77.

Lycopene

Lycopene, a potent fat-soluble antioxidant found predominately in tomato products, has received much attention in the popular press lately. It's a "carotenoid," like beta-carotene, but is a more potent antioxidant. The hoopla is based on several dramatic studies that indicate powerful protective effects of lycopene on the prostate.

It started with a landmark study by Dr. Edward Giovannucci and his associates at Harvard Medical School, published in the *Journal of the National Cancer Institute* in 1995. The study evaluated the effects of eating 46 different fruits, vegetables, and related products on the risk of getting prostate cancer. It was a prospective study; none of the 50,000 participants was known to have prostate cancer at the start of the study. Between 1986 and 1992 there were 812 new cases of prostate cancer in the entire group. The intake of various fruits and vegetables of the men in whom prostate cancer appeared was compared to the consumption of the men who were still free of prostate cancer. The only foods that were significantly associated with a reduction in the risk of contracting prostate cancer were tomato sauce, tomatoes, pizza, and strawberries. The three tomato-based products are rich sources of lycopene. In fact, 82% of total lycopene consumption comes from these three foods. Other sources of lycopene include tomato juice, tomato soup, catsup, barbecue sauce, pink grapefruit, watermelon, apricots, and guavas. But tomato products are far and away the richest source of lycopene.

How much protection do tomato-based foods provide? Considerable. According to Dr. Giovannucci, men who ate as little as one to three servings a month decreased their risk of getting prostate cancer by 15%. The more tomato products they ate, the lower their risk. Men who ate 10 or more servings a week decreased their risk by 35%. Even more impressively, cases of metastatic prostate cancer were reduced by a whopping 47% in the tomato-guzzling group.

Although tomato juice did not show a significant association with a reduction in prostate cancer in the Giovannucci study, it was found to be an excellent source of bio-available lycopene in a subsequent study done at the University of Toronto. It appears as though lycopene from tomato juice is readily absorbed. Lycopene supplements were also easily absorbed in the Toronto study. It is absorbed most effectively when combined with oil. Olive oil would be an excellent choice. Without a little oil, lycopene is very poorly absorbed.

Because lycopene is fat-soluble, there's a carryover effect from day to day. It takes two or three days for half of the plasma level of lycopene to be removed. Eating tomato-based products with regularity will gradually build up the levels of lycopene in the blood and in the prostate. In fact, lycopene makes up about 50% of the total carotenoids in human serum, far greater than beta-carotene. Lycopene is also heavily concentrated in the prostate, adrenal glands, and testes.

Men with prostate cancer tend to have low lycopene intake, thus low levels of serum lycopene. Unlike beta-carotene and other carotenoids, lycopene levels are not reduced by tobacco or alcohol consumption. However, they are reduced by advancing age. This can be readily corrected by ingesting more tomato products.

Lycopene supplements show remarkable effects on existing prostate tumors in a very short period of time. Proof of this comes from a nifty study by Omer Kucuk, M.D. and his colleagues. Dr. Kucuk randomly assigned 30 men with prostate cancer, who were scheduled to undergo a radical prostatectomy three weeks later, into two groups. One group got 15 mg of a lycopene supplement twice a day; the other received a placebo twice daily. Dr. Kucuk then compared the removed prostate glands from the 2 groups. Significant shrinkage in the size of tumor was noted in the men who got the lycopene supplement. At surgery the tumors of these men were more likely to be confined to the prostate, as compared with those who did not take the lycopene supplement. In fact, 73% of the men receiving lycopene had clear surgical margins compared with just 18% in the group that did not receive lycopene. Additionally, there was a significant reduction in high-grade PIN in the lycopene-treated group. PSA levels also dropped by an average of 20% in the treated group, although this trend did not reach statistical significance, perhaps due to the small sample size of only 30 men. IGF-1 levels, the previously discussed growth factor related to insulin that has been implicated with increased risk of both the intiation and spread of prostate cancer, were significantly reduced in the lycopene group.

The fact that the time span for taking the supplement was only three weeks prior to surgery seems to indicate that lycopene has a fast-acting effect on prostate tumor cells. I want to point out that some researchers question these results. They point out that this study was small and underpowered. Larger studies need to be done to verify these effects and to show more conclusively the drop in PSA associated with lycopene intake. Also, longer time periods need to be evaluated to see if the tumors continue to shrink. Large randomized clinical trials are now under way.

How does lycopene work? Lycopene is the most effective antioxidant of the major carotenoids, including beta-carotene. Again, lycopene seems to indicate a clear connection between oxidation and the development of prostate cancer. Lycopene may also kill prostate cancer cells directly. This hypothesis is supported by the reduced tumor volume in Dr.

Kucuk's study. Whether this is a direct effect of lycopene or a secondary effect of lycopene's influence on other substances like IGF-1 remains to be determined. Lycopene intake has also been associated with a decreased risk of cancers, most notably lung and stomach, and has been associated with a reduced risk of heart disease.

Key References

Giovannucci E et al. A prospective study of tomato products, lycopene, and prostate cancer risk. *J Natl Cancer Inst* 2002; 391-398.

Giovannucci E et al. Intake of carotenoids and retinol in relation to risk of prostate cancer. *J Natl Cancer Inst* 1995; 87: 1767-1776.

Miller E et al. Tomato products, lycopene, and prostate cancer risk. *Urology Clin North Am* 2002; 83-93.

Kucuk O et al. Phase II randomized trial of lycopene supplementation before radical prostatectomy. *Cancer Epidemiol Biomark Prev* 2001; 10: 861-868.

Herber D and Lu Q. Overview of mechanisms of action of lycopene. *Exp Biol Med* 2002; (Nov.) 227: 920-923.

Giovannucci E. A review of epidemiologic studies of tomatoes, lycopene, and prostate cancer. *Exp Biol Med* 2002; (Nov.) 227: 852-859.

Rao A and Agarwal S. Bioavailability and in vivo antioxidant properties of lycopene from tomato products and their possible role in the prevention of cancer. *Nutr and Cancer* 1998; 31: 199-203.

The Forgotten Strawberry

Lycopene has received substantial popular press coverage since Dr. Giovannucci's landmark article. Of the four foods found to be significantly associated with a reduction in prostate cancer, three were tomato-based, in which lycopene was thought to be the most active anti-cancer component. Yet a close reading of the Giovannucci paper shows that strawberries appear to be quite active against prostate cancer too.

Strawberries are not high in lycopene. An entirely dif-

HELPFUL HINTS

• Freeze strawberries in early summer, when they are abundant and inexpensive, for use later.

• Strawberries are often heavily sprayed with pesticides. Look for organically grown berries or soak them in water for 20-30 minutes before eating them.

ferent substance seems to account for their bio-activity against prostate cancer—ellagic acid. Since a different chemical is at work, strawberries are likely to be additive in their effect to lycopene-rich foods. I have added strawberries in all forms to my diet: fresh, dried, jam, and stewed (especially with rhubarb). Other berries, such as raspberries and blueberries, are also rich in antioxidants. Not only are they healthy, they're delicious. It's time for the forgotten strawberry to share equal billing with lycopene. Act accordingly.

Milk: Friend or Foe

Through the years we've been indoctrinated with the benefits of milk: strong bones, healthy teeth, etc. People of all ages have proudly sported a "milk mustache" as an enduring emblem of good health.

It may surprise you to learn that when it comes to prostate cancer, recent evidence indicates that milk and milk products are not protective. In fact, they may be harmful.

Some of the most compelling work in this regard comes out of Dr. Ed Giovannucci's study of 50,000 men at Harvard Medical School and Harvard School of Public Health. This Health Professionals Study is the same one that catapulted lycopene and tomatoes onto the national health stage as protectors against the proliferation of prostate cancer. While the popular press lapped up the protective effect of tomatoes, an even more striking result of this study received virtually no attention.

Dr. Giovannucci found that men with high calcium intake (2,000 mg/day or more), whether from diet or supplements, had 4.5 times the risk of developing metastatic prostate cancer when compared to men with low calcium consumption (500 mg/day or less). Interestingly, it did not seem to make a difference whether the men drank skim milk, whole milk, ate lots of yogurt, or took calcium supplements. The association was with calcium, regardless of the vehicle. Milk fats, previously implicated with metastatic prostate cancer in some studies, did not seem to be a key variable. Somehow, calcium itself seemed to be stimulating the growth and spread of prostate cancer in a dose-dependent manner.

At a recent meeting, I asked Dr. Giovannucci why this striking observation had not received more attention in the popular press. "I really don't know," he said. "It certainly should have. Calcium intake is clearly associated with a dramatically increased risk of advanced prostate cancer."

Supporting data for Dr. Giovannucci's findings were published in 1999 in the journal *Alternative Medicine Review*. Using a multi-country statistical approach, Dr. William Grant found that, in combined data from 41 countries, the highest dietary risk associated with death from prostate cancer was the non-fat portion of milk. That's right. His study showed that, ounce for ounce, skim-milk consumption posed a greater risk of death from prostate cancer than whole milk, and this risk was higher than any other dietary component!

How can this be? The working hypothesis among experts in nutrition and prostate cancer, such as Drs. Giovannucci, Ornish, and Myers, is that calcium's role in prostate cancer involves its effect on vitamin D.

High calcium consumption reduces the conversion of one form of vitamin D, 25-hydroxy-vitamin D, to another form, 1,25-hydroxy-2 vitamin D. This latter form is an active suppresser of prostate cancer. It's produced when 25-hydroxy vitamin D is altered in the liver and kidney to this more active form. High calcium levels interfere with the production of this active form of vitamin D (calcitriol). Low calcitriol levels are commonly found in men with prostate cancer. Since calcium reduces this key substance, this provides a potential mechanism to support the work of Drs. Giovannucci, Grant, and others.

Additional support for the vitamin D hypothesis comes from the fact that prostate cancer mortality is higher in the northern states, where men get less sunshine, than in the southern states. This trend is virtually linear as you progress from south to north. As Dr. Grant points out, "Surface UV-B radiation is predicted to decrease from 34-43 in the Southwest to

10-18 in the Northeast." Put another way, men living in the Southwest are exposed to nearly three times the amount of sunshine, which, as we know, is converted into vitamin D.

In his multi-country statistical analysis, Dr. Grant found an interesting relationship between milk intake (especially skim milk) and tomatoes. As we've discussed, tomatoes are a rich source of lycopene. Dr. Grant confirmed Dr. Giovannucci's findings that tomatoes, presumably due to their lycopene content, significantly reduce the risk of prostate cancer from milk intake.

A ratio can be established between increased risk from milk consumption as the numerator and decreased risk from tomato ingestion as the denominator. According to Dr. Grant's analysis, it takes about one calorie from tomato products to counteract three calories from skim milk. A cup of skim milk has 86 calories and 300 mg of calcium. Five ounces of fresh tomatoes, a half a can of canned tomatoes, a half-glass of tomato juice, or an ounce and a quarter of tomato paste would be enough to offset this amount of skim milk, using Dr. Grant's formula.

His statistical analysis showed the more skim-milk calories consumed, the greater the risk of dying from prostate cancer; the more calories from tomatoes, the lower the risk of prostate cancer mortality. This relationship is linear. The conclusions I draw from this study are these:

• It's best not to consume milk products.

• If you do drink milk or eat yogurt and other milk products, eat enough tomatoes daily to offset the potential risk.

As you can see, the effect of the equivalent of a glass or less of skim milk per day is relatively easy to neutralize by the lycopene in a bowl of spaghetti with tomato sauce or a

---

HELPFUL HINT

It's probably best not to drink milk at all, but if you do, eat lots of tomato products to counteract any stimulatory effects milk may have on prostate cancer growth. Based on Dr. Grant's research, drinking skim milk won't protect you from milk's ill-effects.

small glass of tomato juice. But if you consume two or more glasses of milk per day or their equivalent, it may become difficult to eat enough tomato products to keep the proper balance, according to Grant's formula.

This conclusion is supported by a study reported in the journal *Oncology* in 1991. Researchers found that men who drink two or more glasses of milk daily had five times the risk of dying from prostate cancer compared with men who didn't drink milk. An earlier study showed nearly twice the risk of succumbing to prostate cancer in men who drank one to two glasses of milk per day compared to less than one glass daily. This increased to about $2\frac{1}{2}$ times the risk when three or more glasses were drunk daily.

A 1999 Athens Medical School study also showed an increased risk of prostate cancer associated with milk, dairy products, and seed oils; olive oil was neutral. Cooked tomato products, and to a lesser extent raw tomatoes, were associated with decreased risk.

Population studies give further support to the milk/tomato relationship. The country where people eat the most tomatoes is Greece: an average of 73 calories of tomatoes per day. Greeks also consume 122 calories from milk. Note that the ratio of 122/73 is less than 2/1. According to Grant, in 1986 there were 50 cases of death from prostate cancer in Greece per 100,000 men aged 65-74. Compare this with Hungary. In the same year 117 men per 100,000 aged 65-74 died of prostate cancer. Hungarian men consume 102 calories from skim milk each day and only 16 calories from tomatoes: 102/16 is nearly a 6/1 ratio. Grant's work shows a consistent correlation between high ratios and countries with high rates of prostate cancer mortality. Death from prostate cancer is almost twice as high per capita in Hungary than in Greece.

Also of interest is the fact that milk-product consumption is practically non-existent in most adult Asian cultures, where the incidence of fatal prostate cancer is low. True, this may also be due to their high intake of soy, green tea, fewer calories, and meager meat consumption. But the fact that their dietary supply of milk is next to nil cannot be overlooked as a risk-reduction factor.

As stressed before, studies like these are not proof that milk is hazardous to the health of your prostate, or tomatoes are protective. There may be other factors involved. If you stop drinking milk and start guzzling tomato juice, there is no certainty that you won't die from prostate cancer. But to my way of thinking, there is enough evidence here for me to eliminate milk and milk products from my diet, while greatly expanding my intake of tomato-based foods. There is a high probability, I believe, that this will reduce my risk.

Using the same logic, I don't take supplemental calcium. Many doctors recommend calcium, especially for patients on hormones. Although this may be okay for men who also take Rocaltrol (calcitriol), the active form of vitamin D, I think the available evidence supports a fair degree of risk from calcium supplements, especially without added calcitriol. You needn't worry about becoming calcium deficient. You'll get enough if you eat sufficient broccoli and green leafy vegetables, or small amounts of sea vegetables (seaweed); kelp has more than 1,000 mg of calcium per serving. Japanese people are not deficient in calcium despite their lack of dairy products. In fact, elderly Japanese have a lower incidence of osteoporosis than Western people of a comparable age. Although part of the reason for this may be attributed to their high soy intake, they obviously have sufficient amounts of calcium to maintain healthy bones. Based on Dr. Giovannucci's findings, optimal calcium intake might be in the range of 300-500 mg per day.

So, in relation to prostate cancer, milk may not be as healthy as we have been led to believe. Other studies have shown an association between milk consumption and coronary heart disease, colon cancer, Alzheimer's disease, and diabetes. And, as Dr. Grant points out, tomatoes do not seem to be nearly as protective against the development of these conditions as they appear to be against metastatic prostate cancer. Overall, it seems to me that, for adults, the downside to milk and dairy products far exceeds the upside.

> ### Caveat
> Not all experts believe that calcium increases cancer risks. This has not been *proven*. They correctly point out that associations are not proof.

Key References
Chan J M et al. Dairy products, calcium, and prostate cancer risk in the Physician's Health Study. *Am J Clin Nutr* 2001; 74: 549-554.

Giovannucci E. et al. Calcium and fructose intake in relation to risk of prostate cancer. *Cancer Research* 1998; 58: 442-447.

Chan JM, Giovannucci E, et al. Dairy products, calcium, phosphorus, vitamin D, and risk of prostate cancer. *Cancer Causes Control* 1998; 9: 559-566.

Grant WB. An ecologic study of dietary links to prostate cancer. *Alternative Medicine Review* 1999; 4: 162-169.

La Vecchia C et al. Dairy products and the risk of prostate cancer. *Oncology* 1991; 48: 406-410.

Tzonou A et al. Diet and cancer of the prostate: a case-control study in Greece. *International Journal of Cancer* 1999; 80: 704-708.

Giovannucci E. Dietary influences of 1,25 (OH) vitamin D in relation to prostate cancer: a hypothesis. Cancer Causes Control 1998; 9: 567-582.

Snowdon D et al. Diet, obesity, and risk of fatal prostate cancer. *Am J Epidemiol* 1984; 120: 244-250.

Conjugated Linoleic Acid (CLA)

As you've probably become aware from reading this book, all fats are not created equal. There are good ones and bad ones. Harmful ones include saturated fats, polyunsaturated oils, and alpha-linolenic acid. Beneficial fats include the two prevalent fatty acids found in fish, DHA and EPA, and monounsaturated fats like olive oil. Conjugated linoleic acid (CLA) is also a helpful fat. It has been shown to have anti-inflammatory and anti-cancer effects. It seems particularly beneficial for people with prostate or breast cancer.

CLA is an isomer of linoleic acid (LA). An isomer is a chemical with the same molecular structure as another, but with the atoms arranged differently. This altered arrangement gives the two compounds different properties. CLA is a strong antioxidant.

CLA has been scarcely studied in humans. The one human study I know of is a small, randomized, double-blind, placebo-controlled study that shows that 4.2 grams of CLA daily significantly reduced the abdominal fat in obese men. Apparently, it does this by reducing the size of the fat-containing cells known as adipocytes. I have it on good authority that study protocols for CLA for men with prostate cancer are now being prepared. By the time you read this, human studies may well be under way.

In the laboratory, CLA affects prostate cancer cells very differently from linoleic acid (LA). LA stimulates prostate cancer cell growth; CLA inhibits it. Animal studies confirm this beneficial effect. Mice with implanted prostate cancer cells that were fed a CLA-supplemented diet had smaller local tumors than mice fed a normal laboratory diet. They also had dramatically fewer lung metastases. In distinct contrast, mice fed an LA-enriched diet had increased local tumor volume when compared with controls.

Even more impressive results were reported in another study with implanted breast cancer cells. Interestingly, the effects of CLA on cancer cell growth and proliferation appear to be independent of the level of fat in the diet.

How does CLA work? Although this hasn't been definitively determined, recent research indicates that CLA interferes with the metabolism of LA. The June 1999 issue of *Carcinogenesis* reports a study by Dr. Banni and colleagues. These investigators found that LA metabolites were consistently depressed in mice fed a diet comprised of 1% CLA.

One of the LA metabolites that was significantly reduced was arachidonic acid. As previously mentioned, arachidonic acid is now being extensively investigated as a strong promoter of prostate cancer cell growth and spread. CLA reduces the formation of arachidonic acid from LA, and consequently has anti-inflammatory properties. Another just-released study shows that CLA up-regulates genes in prostate cancer and breast cancer cells involved with apoptosis.

We have three key prongs that point to the likely efficacy of CLA for preventing the development of prostate and breast cancer: laboratory evidence; animal evidence; and a cogent mechanism for its action. What's still missing are more human studies, and these should be under way soon.

Ironically, CLA is naturally found in grilled meats, cheese, and other whole-fat dairy products. In fact, some food manufacturers are now experimenting with the idea of commercially producing CLA-enriched butter. Cows, when fed certain plant oils and fresh greens, can produce milk with up to five times the normal amount of CLA by a process called biohydrogenation. This was reported in the December 1999 issue of the *Journal of Nutrition*. CLA is also readily available as a supplement.

Should you take CLA supplements now or wait for the results of the human studies? Tough question. It depends a lot on your outlook. Since it has yet to be proven to be an effective anti-cancer agent in humans and there could possibly be some undesirable effects from consuming it, you may choose to wait. On the other hand, you may be sufficiently impressed with the laboratory data, animal studies, and mechanism for achieving benefits that you think it's worth taking now. There are no known harmful effects. It appears to be safe. But as you know, beta-carotene used to be considered safe too, but not when it's combined with cigarettes and alcohol. Until CLA is studied further, all we can say is that it's probably safe.

What do I think? If you have not been diagnosed with prostate cancer, I don't think it's necessary to add CLA supplements to your diet. If you do have prostate cancer, then it depends on your thinking as outlined in the preceding paragraph. Personally, I find the evidence compelling in favor of taking CLA. The predominate fatty acid in my vegan diet is LA. One of the main reasons I chose this diet was to reduce the amount of arachidonic acid. Vegans have only about 20% as much arachidonic acid as their carnivorous companions. Since LA can be converted in the body to arachdonic acid and since I eat plenty of soy products that contain LA, taking CLA seems like a reasonably safe way to keep my arachidonic acid levels to a minimum. It also seems to help keep me trim around the middle. In short, for me the potential rewards of taking CLA significantly outweigh the risks.

Key References

Wahle K and Heys S. Cell signal mechanisms, conjugated linoleic acids (CLAs) and anti-tumorigenesis. *Prostaglandins Leukot Essent Fatty Acids* 2002; 67:183.

Banni S et al. Decrease in linoleic acid metabolites as a potential mechanism in cancer risk reduction by conjugated linoleic acid. *Carcinogenesis* 1999; 20: 1019-1024.

Cesano A et al. Opposite effects of linoleic acid and conjugated linoleic acid on human prostatic cancer in SCID mice. *Anticancer Research* 1998; 18: 1429-34.

Ip C. Review of the effects of trans fatty acids, oleic acid, n-3 polyunsaturated fatty acids, and conjugated linoleic acid on mammary carcinogenesis in animals. *Am J Clinical Nutrition* 1997; 66 (supp.): 1523s-1529s.

Riserus U et al. Conjugated linoleic acid (CLA) reduced abdominal adipose tissue in obese middle-aged men with signs of the metabolic syndrome: a randomized controlled trial. *Int J Obes Relat Metab Disord* 2001; 25: 1129-1135.

Curcumin

Curcumin is a constituent of tumeric, a popular East Indian spice used in curries. Tumeric is a rhizome (a creeping stem that grows just beneath the surface) in the ginger family. It looks like a small version of yellow-orange-colored ginger. It's readily available in Asian markets as a whole root and is found as a yellow powder in many supermarkets and health food stores. Curcumin has recently come to the attention of Western researchers.

What has attracted modern scientists to this spice is its anti-inflammatory properties. Additionally, it seems to have anti-cancer effects. Besides the cancer protection that its anti-inflammatory action may have, curcumin also induces self-destruction (apoptosis) in a number of cancer cell lines. These effects would not surprise traditional Indian-medicine practitioners. They have used curcumin to combat cancer and arthritis for more than a millennium. Parts of India where tumeric is widely used have very low cancer rates.

Curcumin is a potent antioxidant. It also seems to affect

several enzymes involved in cancer cell growth. One such enzyme, COX-2, is involved in the inflammatory process. Curcumin supresses COX-2.

What, if any, effect curcumin has on prostate cancer in men is unknown. Since some prominent researchers, such as Don Coffey at Johns Hopkins, currently believe that inflammation is an important promoter of cell changes that can lead to prostate cancer, it's conceivable that the anti-inflammatory properties of curcumin may provide some protection.

In colon cancer this appears to be the case, at least in male rats. A report published in the February 1999 issue of *Cancer Research* showed that daily intake of curcumin significantly suppressed the development of colon cancer over a year's time. Like aspirin and other non-steroidal anti-inflammatory drugs (NSAIDS), curcumin may interfere with the production of inflammatory prostaglandins. The equivalent human dosage in this study was 2,000-6,000 mg per day.

Curcumin is available in capsules generally ranging from 500 to 900 mg each. As with CLA, human studies have yet to be performed. Until prospective, randomized, double-blind studies are conducted, we can't be sure that any of these products are helpful. It remains to be seen if curcumin is absorbed and carried to the prostate where it might inhibit cancer cell

> **HELPFUL HINTS**
>
> • Add tumeric powder to soups, stews, and curries to get the benefit of curcumin.
> • Consider using curcumin supplements if you don't like food made with curcumin or tumeric or if you travel frequently.
> • Men with untreated prostate cancer or rising PSAs after definitive therapy should avoid curcumin supplements.

development. Even so, I do think there are sound reasons to include lots of tumeric in your diet. If this is inconvenient, or incompatible with your tastes, I see nothing wrong with taking the supplement, although men with newly diagnosed cancer or a rising PSA after treatment, should be cautious. Men with existing active prostate cancer should probably not take curcumin supplements, according to Dr. Myers, since it seems to interfere with one of the apoptotic pathways of prostate cancer cells. If you decide to take curcumin supplements, limit the amount consumed to 1,000 mg per day. Curcumin at this dose is a potent antioxidant. At higher doses, it has an undesirable pro-oxidant effect. Of course, as always, it's preferable to get it from dietary sources.

HELPFUL HINT

It's best to get antioxidants and phytoestrogens from food. Supplement what you can't eat naturally.

Key References

Rao C et al. Chemoprevention of colon carcinogenesis by dietary curcumin, a naturally occurring plant phenolic compound. *Cancer Research* 1995; 55: 259-266.

Kawamori T et al. Chemopreventive effect of curcumin, a naturally occurring anti-inflammatory agent, during the promotion/progression stages of colon cancer. *Cancer Research* 1999; 59: 597-601.

Rao C, Kawamori T et al. Chemoprevention of colonic aberrant crypt foci by an inducible nitric oxide synthase-selective inhibitor. *Carcinogenesis* 1999; 20: 641-644.

Huang M et al. Inhibitory effects of curcumin on tumorigenesis in mice. *J Cell Biochem Suppl* 1997; 27: 26-34.

Phytoestrogens: Soy and More

Phytoestrogens are plant-derived nutrients with weak estrogenic effects. Some, including isoflavones, lignans, and coumestans, show promise as anti-cancer nutritional agents. Isoflavones, from a practical standpoint, are found in significant quantities only in soy-based foods. Lignans are found in beans (including soybeans), lentils, grains, nuts, seeds, and berries. Coumesterol is found in beans, peas, and bean sprouts.

Soy

The isoflavones genistein and daidzein are found mostly in soy products. Epidemiologic, laboratory, and animal studies predominately show these isoflavones to be active against prostate cancer. A number of experts believe that soy plays a big part in the success of Japanese men in avoiding clinical prostate cancer. Ninety percent of these isoflavones come from only three foods prevalent in the diet of these men: tofu, miso, and natto. Miso (soybean paste) and natto (fermented soybeans) have higher levels of isoflavones than tofu. Fermentation releases them from the fiber in the bean, making them more available for absorption by the body. Soy sauce has practically no isoflavones. The average Japanese man consumes about 20 times as much genistein as his American or British counterpart. Not surprisingly, blood levels of isoflavones in Japanese men also exceed those of Western men by 20-fold.

Epidemiologic studies have shown that eating lots of soy products is associated with a decreased risk of not only prostate cancer, but stomach, lung, rectal, and breast cancer as well.

These studies involve not only the Japanese, but Caucasians too. A Norwegian group at the University of Tronso prospectively studied more than 12,000 Seventh-day Adventist men. The study began in 1976 and was reported in 1998. Over time, 225 men developed clinical prostate cancer. Nutritional studies revealed that men who drank soy milk more than once a day had 70% less risk of prostate cancer than men who drank a glass a day or less. This study suggests that high soy milk consumption may reduce prostate cancer risk in a Caucasian population. This is interesting because soy milk has less genistein than the three soy products that comprise most of the soy in the Japanese diet.

Another large international study involved 59 countries. Data were obtained from United Nations sources. It was reported in the November 1998 issue of the *Journal of the National Cancer Institute*. In this study Hebert and colleagues found that for all foods, calorie for calorie, soy had by far the greatest effect on reducing prostate cancer *mortality*. In fact, it was *four times* more effective than any other dietary factor.

Other food sources that showed a significant reduction in deaths from prostate cancer include cereals, grains, seeds, nuts, and fish. Consumption of nuts and seeds should be limited, in my opinion, due to their high caloric and fat content. Since eating soy is better than any other food as a cancer fighter by several levels of magnitude, it seems sound to use soy products as the major source of dietary protein. When combined with grains or cereal, the result is complete protein.

Fish consumption adds DHA and EPA to the diet and is far preferable to meat. Whether it's more beneficial than an exclusively plant-based high-soy diet is debated by experts in nutrition. I think current evidence favors eating fish as part of a high-soy predominately plant-based diet.

Whole Soy Versus Genistein

In the laboratory, genistein inhibits a variety of cancer cells, including prostate, by a number of different mechanisms (see Table 1, later in this section).

What puzzles researchers, however, is that the concentration of genistein required for prostate cancer cells to stop growing or self-destruct is way more than what can be reached by eating soy foods. Ten to twenty times as much soy would have to be consumed by Japanese men to achieve blood concentrations comparable to those that affect prostate cancer cells in the lab. So how does soy provide protection for men? The answer isn't known. One way that soy might work is by reducing inflammation (see page 319). Studies in rats show that soy reduces prostatitis. Imflammation increases DNA damage to prostate epithelial cells and increases cell turnover. Slowing this down may reduce the risk of prostate cancer.

Soy, like other foods, may be more potent in men than genistein in laboratory experiments, due to the complexities of interactions of its composite chemicals. There may also be an additive effect when these elements combine. And, as always, there may be as yet unidentified factors in soy that play a role in cancer cell inhibition.

It's possible to achieve significant blood elevations of genistein by using supplements. These concentrations are similar to those in the lab that destroy prostate cancer cells. There has not been a well-designed, prospective, randomized, medical study that proves that soy inhibits or helps kill prostate cancer cells in man. Until such a study is done, and its results are replicated, all conclusions about the efficacy of soy are inferential. Dr. Heber, head of Nutrition at UCLA Medical Center, believes that soy supplements should be avoided. He recommends soy protein isolate, available in most health food stores as an easy to take source of soy isoflavones.

But as I've said, if you have prostate cancer, especially an aggressive form, you may need to make judgment calls before all the evidence is in. I eat lots of soy in all forms, about 50-75 grams of soy protein per day. Michael Milken, emulating the long-lived Okinawans, consumes about 100 grams daily. When I travel, I bring soy protein isolate packets with me. If you travel a lot, it's sometimes difficult to get soy products, especially in foreign countries. On a recent visit to Vienna, I could find neither soy milk nor tofu in any conveniently located market. I was glad I'd brought my soy protein.

If I had cancer cells in my lymph nodes or bone, I would definitely step up my soy protein intake to at least 100 grams daily. Whether I'd use soy supplements to provide enough genistein to raise my blood levels to those seen to be effective in the lab is a tougher call. There is currently no evidence in humans that this would be effective in helping to control the cancer. There is also no current evidence that this would be harmful. Hopefully, studies will help resolve these issues. At the moment the jury is still out.

If you do decide to take soy supplements for advanced prostate cancer, the dose to bring blood levels up to those comparable to laboratory studies would be about 1,000 mg of genistein per day. Taking soy-protein supplements may be more acceptable to your doctor than genistein supplements.

Remember, the final decision about your health and treatment is yours. But it's imperative to keep your medical team informed. Supplements may interfere with or augment prescription medicines. Your doctors must know what you are taking. Hopefully, you can establish an open dialogue with your physicians about your complementary health program, but regardless, you must keep your medical team informed about what you're taking if you want an optimal result.

How Soy Works

Soy isoflavones and lignans are converted by bacteria in the intestines to hormone-like chemicals. These compounds are weakly estrogenic and can modulate sex-hormone output. There is also substantial evidence that they affect prostate cancer cell growth and proliferation in a number of important ways independent of their estrogen effects (see table 1). Activating cancer cells to self-destruct has already been discussed. Other important influences of soy isoflavones include anti-angiogenesis, interfering with cancer-cell DNA synthesis, inhibiting enzymes in cancer cells required for growth, and making cancer cells more normal in both appearance and function. In addition, soy isoflavones, vitamin D, selenium, and silymarin all share an anti-cancer property—they stimulate the production of a protein produced by the p21 cancer-suppressor gene. This protein has a direct effect in slowing prostate cancer cell growth and is knocked out early in the cancer-forming process.

Of these various actions, anti-angiogenesis may be the most promising. Cancer cells need oxygen and nutrients to grow. Small colonies clump together and release chemicals that stimulate the growth of new blood vessels (called "angiogenesis"). Anti-angiogenesis is the process of stopping the formation of these new blood vessels. Anti-angiogenetic agents, if effective, will help stop metastasis. Interestingly, in the lab, much lower levels of isoflavones are needed to stop new blood vessels from forming than to stimulate apoptosis (cell suicide).

A 1999 article in the *Journal of Nutrition*, a combined effort between Harvard and Ohio State medical schools and a Japanese hospital, showed that mice innoculated with prostate cancer cells and fed a diet of 20% soy protein plus 1% soy isoflavone concentrate had 40% lower tumor volume than control mice fed 20% casein (a milk protein) and no soy. This result was highly significant ($P=<0.005$). Even when the amount of soy isoflavones was reduced to 0.2% of the diet, a 20% soy protein diet reduced tumor volume by 28%, still statistically significant ($p=<0.05$).

When the researchers examined the tumors from the soy-fed mice and the casein-fed mice, they found that the soy-fed mice had a significant reduction in their tumor microvessel density, i.e., less angiogenesis. They also found that insulin-like growth factor (IGF-1), a protein known to increase angiogenesis, was reduced in the blood of the soy-fed mice. Whether soy reduces angiogenesis by reducing IGF-1 levels, by direct anti-angiogenic effects on prostate cancer cells, or by a combination of mechanisms remains to be determined.

One factor to consider in this study is the use of casein as a control. Since this is milk-based, it may have a stimulating effect on tumor growth. If so, this would not be a good control diet. What can be safely concluded from this study, however, is that the effects of a soy-based diet were considerably more beneficial than those of a casein- (milk-) based diet.

Needed now are clinical studies on soy diets in men without any sign of prostate cancer to determine its protective influence. Additionally, soy and soy isoflavone supplements need to be tested in well-designed trials on men with untreated low-grade prostate cancer, men with treated prostate cancer but a rising PSA, and in men with advanced prostate cancer.

My opinion is that soy should be eaten in large quantities by most men. I drink a soy protein isolate shake made with 1% fat vanilla soy milk, 2 scoops of soy protein powder, and blueberries daily. This has more than 35 grams of soy protein. I also eat lots of tofu, miso soup, natto, and soy yogurt.

Recently, soy products have been approved for labeling as effective against heart disease when used as part of a healthy diet. Although the jury is still out on whether soy will be definitively proven to protect men from prostate and other cancers, its beneficial effects on the heart have now been recognized. If you needed another reason to increase your soy intake, this is it.

> **HELPFUL HINT**
>
> Look for soy products with the lowest fat content to optimize the beneficial effects, while reducing calories and linoleic acid consumption. Low-fat (1%) or non-fat soy milk and "lite" tofu will help reduce fat.

Table 1

Reported mechanisms of soy isoflavone action on prostate cancer cells from laboratory and animal studies:

1. Antioxidant action—May reduce alterations in DNA in normal cells, reducing cancer cell numbers.

2. Inhibits angiogenesis—Helps prevent spread of existing tumors; decreases microvessel density.

3. Inhibits tyrosine kinase—Inhibits cancers cell growth.

4. Induces apoptosis—Increases programmed cell death of cancer cells.

5. Up-regulates p21—Increases the protein production of a prostate cancer cell growth suppressor gene.

6. Stimulates sex hormone binding globulin synthesis (SHBG)—May decrease the effects of male sex hormones.

7. Induces differentiation—Makes malignant cells more normal in appearance and function.

8. Decreases IGF-1—Decreases the amount of this angiogenic protein in the circulation.

9. Inhibits DNA topo-isomerases I & II—Suppresses DNA synthesis inhibiting prostate cancer cell growth.

10. Decreases the release of PSA from hormone dependent prostate cancer cells—A compound in soy, biochanin, changes testosterone metabolism.

Key References

Adlercreutz H and Mazur W. Phyto-oestrogens and Western diseases. *Annals of Medicine* 1997; 29:95-120.

Sun X et al. Increased UDP- glucuronosyltranserase activity and decreased prostate specific antigen production by biochanin A in prostate cancer cells. *Cancer Research* 1998; 58: 2379-2384.

Zhou J et al. Soybean phytochemicals inhibit the growth of transplantable human prostate carcinoma and tumor angiogenesis in mice. *Journal of Nutrition* 1999; 129: 1628-1635.

Wakai K et al. Dietary intake and sources of isoflavones among Japanese. *Nutrition and Cancer* 1999; 33: 139-145.

Strom S et al. Phytoestrogen intake and prostate cancer: A case-control study using a new database. *Nutrition and Cancer* 1999; 33: 20-25.

Hebert J et al. Nutritional and socioeconomic factors in relation to prostate cancer mortality: a cross-national study. *J Natl Cancer Institute* 1998; 90: 1637-47.

Jacobsen B et al. Does high soy milk intake reduce prostate cancer incidence? The Adventist health study. *Cancer Causes Control* 1998; 9: 553-557.

Davis J et al. Genistein-induced upregulation of p21WAF1, downregulation of cyclin B, and induction of apoptosis in prostate cancer cells. *Nutr Cancer* 1998; 32: 123-131.

DeMarzo A et al. New concepts in tissue specificity for prostate cancer and benign prostatic hyperplasia. *Urology* 1999; 53 (Supp 3A): 29-40.

Soy and Inflammation of the Prostate

At the 1999 Prostate Cancer Foundation conference, Professor Donald Coffey from Johns Hopkins University, a brilliant scientist, presented a fascinating theory. He postulated that prostate cancer starts with inflammation. This may come from an earlier infection. Circulating hormones, specifically the combination of estrogen and DHT, increase the amount of inflammation. They also stimulate prostate cells to grow.

You may be surprised to learn that men have circulating estrogen. Although not nearly as much as women, men do have significant amounts. DHT is formed by the action of the enzyme 5-alpha reductase on testosterone. DHT is 5-10 times as potent a stimulator of prostate cell growth as testosterone. Estrogen combined with testosterone results in normal prostate cell growth. But estrogen combined with DHT causes highly abnormal prostate cell development. Besides increasing cell growth and inflammation, these changes include atrophy (shrinking of cells) and DNA damage.

Diet also appears to be a key factor in both cellular pro-liferation (dividing to form new cells) and inflammation. Mice fed a Western diet for 12 weeks had a significant increase in the number and size of their prostate cells. Regarding in-flammation, soy intake makes a huge difference. Without soy, 80% of the prostate shows signs of inflammation. With moderate soy consumption, only 20% of the gland is affected. And with high soy diets, almost no inflammation can be found.

Under the microscope the combination of hyper-cellular growth and inflammation have a characteristic pattern. In multiple locations in the prostate, this proliferation sur-rounded by inflammation can be identified. This may even-tually become cancer. A high-calorie, high-fat, low-soy diet may accelerate this process.

Dr. Coffey's intriguing theory for the development of pros-tate cancer goes something like this:

• Hit-and-run infections lead to multiple locations of inflammation in the prostate.

• Estrogen in combination with DHT increases this in-flammation and stimulates prostate cell growth and DNA damage.

• Dietary soy reduces inflammation. A high-fat diet may increase inflammatory changes. Curcumin, an extract from tumeric, also decreases inflammation (see pages 307-308).

Dr. Coffey conjectures that non-steroidal anti-inflamma-tory agents (NSAIDS), such as Motrin, Celebrex, or Vioxx, may ultimately play a role in prostate cancer prevention. A NSAID a day might reduce inflammation in the prostate suf-ficiently to decrease the incidence of clinically significant prostate cancer. (For more information, see "New and Fu-ture Developments.")

Thus far, there's no medical study showing that inflam-mation causes prostate cancer. At this point, it's only a theory, though based on factual medical evidence. In the near fu-ture, studies will undoubtedly be designed to test its merits.

This research should prove to be most interesting.

Five years from now, men over 40 may be taking a Motrin a day to deter the development of prostate cancer, just as millions currently take a baby aspirin daily to help prevent heart disease.

Green Tea

Green tea is one of the most promising dietary sources for anti-cancer agents. In 1997 there were about 560,000 cancer deaths in the United States. Researchers estimate that 33% of these could have been prevented by only a change in diet. Green tea may prove to be a key part in this change.

Green, Black, and Oolong Teas

Surprisingly, all the tea in the world comes from only one plant species—*Camellia sinensis*. With the exception of water, tea is drunk by more people than any other beverage. Tea-drinking is believed to have begun 5,000 years ago. Green tea is made from the freshly picked leaves of the tea plant, which are then steamed and dried. Black tea comes from the same leaves, which are fermented and allowed to oxidize, changing color from green to black. This fermentation process also changes the taste of the tea leaves. Oolong tea is partially fermented, giving it its unique taste. The taste of tea may be further modified by adding flowers or fruits. Jasmine tea, for example, is green tea with added jasmine flowers. The quality, price, and flavor of the tea depend on the area where it's grown and the care with which it's picked and processed. Soil conditions, humidity, and age of the leaves can affect the taste.

All tea contains potent antioxidant substances called polyphenols. Green tea, consumed primarily in Asian nations, has the highest concentration of these polyphenolic compounds. These beneficial chemicals are partially lost by fermentation. Oolong tea, consumed in Okinawa and parts of China, has less polyphenols than green tea. Black tea, popular mainly in Western countries, has the least. Green tea has less than half the caffeine content of black tea or coffee.

Green-Tea Polyphenols—EGCG

Green tea is brimming with polyphenols. Up to 50% of the weight of the dry solid extract is composed of these strong antioxidants. The most copious and active of these is epigallocatechin-3-gallate, or EGCG for short. About 40% of the polyphenols (20% of dry solids) is composed of EGCG. Both laboratory and animal studies have confirmed this to be the most potent ingredient in green tea, although it does have other beneficial catechins and flavonoids.

One cup of green tea has about 350 mg of polyphenols. Various studies have shown that cancer cells are affected by green tea in a dose-dependent manner. At least four cups per day are required for a significant anti-cancer effect. Green tea, even in large amounts, appears perfectly safe. Four cups supply about 1,400 mg of polyphenols, but if you drink twice this amount, you may kill more cancer cells.

Men who are sensitive to caffeine, however, may have difficulty handling large amounts of tea. Decaffeinated green tea, or decaffeinated green tea extract capsules, are an option. You should be aware, however, that the studies on green tea have been done using the caffeinated form. Some observers think that caffeine may accentuate the effects of green tea, as discussed later.

For this reason I think it's best, if you can tolerate the caffeine, to drink the real thing, or take the lightly caffeinated extracts. I'm aware of the thinking that caffeine adversely affects calcium absorption (perhaps not such a bad thing— see the milk section). A recent study, however, shows that when adjustments are made for confounding factors like smoking and body weight, no association could be found between caffeine and bone loss.

Caffeine has also been thought by some to increase the

risk of heart disease, but this has been repudiated by recent studies. Some studies have shown caffeine to be protective against colon cancer. There may be an argument that caffeine negatively impacts certain neuro-hormones, leading to feelings of agitation, irritability, or loss of concentration in some people. But a large number of people who consume caffeine regularly report increased mental alertness, better mood, better memory, and improved reasoning ability.

If caffeine affects you adversely, you may wish to limit your green-tea consumption. Or you may wish to drink decaffeinated brands. There's no proof that they won't work; they just haven't been studied. Green tea has been used for centuries, however, at Buddhist temples in Asia where adepts have been able to meditate and reach deep levels of serenity, if not enlightenment. Personally, I find the caffeine in green tea not to be a problem, and I am not convinced that it poses a health concern.

How Green Tea Works

Although the exact way that it works on prostate cancer cells is still being researched, green tea, or extracted EGCG, triggers the suicide program in these cancer cells (apoptosis). The higher the concentration of polyphenols, the greater the effect.

Laboratory and animal studies have been done with crude green tea extracts, purified polyphenols, or EGCG. All of these appear to be active against prostate cancer cells. In the lab these effects are seen on both androgen-dependent and androgen-independent cell lines. Green tea also inhibits hormone-sensitive prostate cancer cells from growing when exposed to testosterone in the lab. Reduction in prostate cancer cell growth has also been observed in mice, even when the animals are given testosterone.

When it comes to humans, studies are inferential. Epidemiologic evidence indicates that men who consume green tea regularly (four or more cups per day) have less chance of dying from prostate cancer. In China and Japan, where large quantities of green tea are regularly consumed, death from prostate cancer is low, although other factors (soy, low calories, etc.) may also be involved. As discussed with soy, prospective human studies are warranted to better determine just how valuable green tea is in preventing the development or spread of prostate cancer.

Other important questions also need to be answered. Are green tea polyphenols concentrated in the prostate? If so, what effect does drinking tea more frequently, or at higher concentrations, have on the intraprostatic levels of these polyphenols? Are green tea extracts or purified EGCG as effective as drinking tea? More effective? What is the optimal daily intake for men who have prostate cancer? For men who don't have prostate cancer, how much green tea is required for prevention? Studies are now under way to answer some of these important questions. One recent study shows that many of the components of green tea extract are beneficial, not just EGCG, and advocates green tea or green tea extract as opposed to EGCG alone.

Recent evidence has led to several theories as to how green tea might help men fight prostate cancer:

An enzyme called ornithine decarboxylase (ODC) is produced in greater than normal quantities in men with prostate cancer. This enzyme helps regulate the rate of growth of prostate cancer cells. The gene that produces this enzyme responds to stimulation from androgens (testosterone and DHT).

Several studies by investigators at Case Western Reserve University in Cleveland, Ohio, led by Dr. Hasan Mukhtar, show that extracts of green tea significantly decrease ODC production in prostate cancer cells in both the lab and in animals. ODC levels in response to testosterone were reduced by 20%-50% in mice that had 0.2% green tea polyphenols added to their drinking water for a week before receiving testosterone. The researchers propose that lowering ODC levels may be one way that green-tea polyphenols work.

Another way has been proposed by Dorothy and James

Morre, professors at Purdue University. They noticed that an enzyme called quinol oxidase, or NOX, is required for both normal and cancerous prostate cell growth. It operates at the cell surface, a location that has been linked to the action of EGCG. NOX is required for cell division. In fact, in normal prostate cells the only time this enzyme is found is when cells are dividing. But prostate cancer cells have the ability to produce this enzyme all the time, facilitating their growth. In tumor cells this enzyme is referred to as tNOX (t for tumor). EGCG inhibits this enzyme. When this happens, the cancer cells stop growing and commit suicide.

To accomplish this effect, concentrations of EGCG equivalent to about four cups of green tea a day are required. As you'll recall, this is the same amount that has been associated with a reduction in prostate cancer mortality in population studies, which adds credence to the four-cups-a-day theory. Inhibition of tNOX was also observed by these scientists in breast and colon cancer cells. Population studies have found that people who drink equivalent amounts of green tea (four or more cups/day) tend to have less of these two cancers. Learning more about the action and properties of tNOX in prostate cancer could possibly lead to new drugs for controlling its production. For now, EGCG, or green tea consumption, seems a safe seemingly effective method.

A third possible effect of green tea may be on sex hormone-binding globulin (SHBG). SHBG binds to testosterone in the blood, theoretically providing less free testosterone to the prostate. You might recall that free testosterone is converted to DHT in the prostate, which strongly stimulates prostate cancer cell growth. So far, the only study of green tea and SHBG has been done in Japan on a group of 50 premenopausal women. Here, the research scientists found that green tea significantly raised SHBG levels and decreased the amount of circulating estrogens. Like testosterone in men, SHBG binds estrogens in women. If studies in men show the same magnitude of increase in SHBG levels as this study in women, and there is every reason to believe that they will, this will provide yet another cogent mechanism for the protective effect of green tea.

Of interest is the fact that in the above study, caffeine also independently raised SHBG levels. Green tea and caffeine may work synergistically in increasing SHBG—a case for caffeinated green tea.

There's also some additional evidence that male hormones may be affected by catechins in green tea. Work done at the University of Chicago showed EGCG to be a potent inhibitor of one type of 5 alpha-reductase, the enzyme that converts testosterone to DHT. As you know, DHT is about five to ten times more potent in its stimulation of prostate cell growth than testosterone.

As you can see, although there is as yet no conclusive proof as to the benefits of green tea in preventing the development of clinical prostate cancer, there are many reasons to believe that its ingestion will ultimately prove to be effective. More than 100 studies have been done linking green tea to anti-cancer effects for a variety of cancers. Additionally, there are hundreds of studies on other beneficial health effects of green tea (see the table below). I'm confident this list, although extensive, is not exhaustive.

Is there any known downside to drinking green tea? There is. A number of studies have reported that if green tea is drunk while it's very hot, it increases the risk of stomach and esophageal (but not prostate) cancers. Drinking warm (or cold) tea has the opposite effect. One Chinese study found that drinking very hot tea or soup increased the risk of cancer of the esophagus five fold! Obviously, this leads to the conclusion that green tea itself protects against stomach and esophageal cancers, but hot beverages increase risk. Whether you drink tea, coffee, or soup, you should allow it to cool a bit first. The same is true for hot (temperature) food. An Italian study showed that this also increases the risk of stomach cancer.

Reported Beneficial Effects of Green-Tea Polyphenols

- Decreases risk of cancer of the stomach, esophagus, colon, breast, bladder, and prostate
  - Lowers LDL cholesterol and triglycerides
  - Lowers blood pressure
  - Protects against DNA damage by free radicals
  - Inhibits bad breath odors
  - Reduces heart disease
  - Reduces strokes
  - Has anti-bacterial and anti-viral effects
  - Regulates blood sugar and insulin levels
  - Protects skin against U-V radiation
  - Helps neutralize cancer-causing agents in the diet
  - Inhibits angiogenesis
  - Reduces inflammatory cytokines
  - Increases detoxifying enzymes

Undoubtedly, some of these claims will ultimately be refuted; others will be supported. Meanwhile, green tea is being hyped as a panacea. It's not. But it seems likely that it will prove to be a useful nutrient as part of an overall diet for better health. Whether it turns out to specifically slow the spread of prostate cancer remains to be seen.

I drink about 6 cups of green tea per day and take 3 green-tea-extract capsules daily. The capsules provide a total of 375 mg EGCG per day. I take both the supplement and the food. Why? Because I don't know which may turn out to be more effective. With no known risk factors other than temperature, green tea in either form appears safe.

The green tea at your grocery store or health-food shop may taste bland or bitter. You needn't suffer. There are many tasty forms of green tea. Personally, I prefer Japanese *genmai cha*, green tea with toasted-rice kernels. I mix this in equal amount with another Japanese emerald-green tea called *kona cha*. This makes a delicious nutty-earthy blend, sweet enough

to eat the leaves after brew-
ing. You can find these two
teas at most Japanese markets. The Chinese-flavored
green teas, such as jasmine or
lychee, are another good option. Visit a Chinese tea shop
and take in the luscious teas
available. Tell the proprietress
you're interested in good-tast-

> **HELPFUL HINT**
>
> Brew green tea freshly each time
> you drink it for optimum effect.
> When it sits around, it oxidizes
> and loses potency. Brew it
> strongly (more tea). A major study
> reported strong tea to be more
> protective than weak tea. Enjoy
> different varieties and flavors.

ing green teas. She'll likely overload your palate with choices.
Health and pleasure need not be mutually exclusive.

Key References

Bushman J. Green tea and cancer in humans: a review of the literature. *Nutrition and Cancer* 1998; 3: 151-159.

Gopta S, Ahmad N, and Mukhtar H. Prostate cancer chemoprevention by green tea. *Semin Urology Oncol* 1999; 17: 70-76.

Paschka A, Butler R, and Young C. Induction of apoptosis in prostate cancer cell lines by the green tea component epigallocatechin-3-gallate. *Cancer Letter* 1998; 130: 1-7.

Gupta S et al. Prostate cancer chemoprevention by green tea: in vitro and in vivo inhibition of testosterone-mediated induction of ornithine decarboxylase. *Cancer Research* 1999; 59: 2115-2120.

Nagata C, Kabuto M, and Shimizu H. Association of coffee, green tea, and caffeine intakes with serum concentrations of estradiol and sex hormone-binding globulin in premenopausal Japanese women. *Nutrition and Cancer* 1998; 30: 21-24.

Hiipakka R et al. Structure-activity relationships for inhibition of human 5 alpha-reductases by polyphenols. *Biochem Pharmacol* 2002; 63: 1165-1176.

Bachrach U and Wang YC. Cancer therapy and prevention by green tea: role of ornithine decarboxylase. *Amino Acids* 2002; 22: 1-13.

Steele V et al. Comparative chemopreventive mechanisms of green tea, black tea and selected polyphenol extracts measured by in vitro bioassays. *Carcinogenesis* 2000; 21: 63-67.

Hogan E et al. Communicating the message: Clarifying the controversies about caffeine. *Nutrition Today* 2002; 37: 28-35.

A Lesson in Japanese Green Tea

Kyoto is considered by many to be the center for Japanese green tea; the ritualistic tea ceremony can still be expe-

rienced here. While in Kyoto, I visited the Horaido Tea Shop, which has been in the same location since 1803, and met with the proprietor, Nagahiro Yasumori. He's a direct seventh-generation descendant from the original owner and, naturally, is a tea expert. It was his family that invented *genmai cha,* Japanese green tea with toasted rice kernels, more than 75 years ago. Uji, a short 20 minutes by train from Kyoto, is renowned as the premier tea-growing area in Japan. The tea in this shop comes from Uji.

All Japanese tea is steamed immediately after the leaves are picked. Steaming stops fermentation and locks in the polyphenols. Even though all Japanese tea comes from the same genetic source, *Camellia sinensis,* growing conditions and processing can significantly alter taste. Also, the part of the plant used makes a difference in taste. Below is a brief description of the main categories of Japanese teas (*cha*):

Sencha—This is the standard Japanese green tea that most of us are familiar with. It's grown in full sun. It's usually bitter, especially the low-quality leaves often found in green tea bags in the United States. There are various grades. The better grades have a rich taste that's actually rather sweet. Only a hint of bitterness remains. Tea of this quality costs $15-$30 for three ounces.

Gyokuro cha—Tea plants are grown under reed blind coverings for the first 10 days. This provides them with reduced light (about 50%). They're then covered with straw, blocking out 95%-99% of the light. This results in a sweeter-tasting leaf. *Gyokuro cha* is sweet tasting without any bitterness at all. It's quite mild. It costs $15-$60 for three ounces. A less expensive version is grown under black shade cloth.

Matcha—*Matcha* is grown the same way as *gyokuro cha*: under reed blinds, then straw. The broad thin leaves are steamed, dried, and ground into powder. Japanese tea experts believe that *matcha* and *gyokuro cha* have the highest concentrations of both polyphenols and caffeine of all Japanese teas. However, I found nothing in the English literature to support this contention. *Matcha* is best drunk after being stirred with a bamboo tea whisk. When ready to drink, it makes a bright emerald green frothy brew. This is the form of tea often used by Zen monks, and in the traditional Japanese tea ceremony (*cha-no-yu*).

Genmai cha—This is *sencha* with roasted rice mixed in giving it a light toasty taste and an aroma similar to popcorn. It's easy to drink and inexpensive. Most Westerners are fond of its taste.

Hoji cha—This tea is roasted. Roasting changes the leaf color and brewed tea from green to brown. The roasting process removes nearly all the tannin and caffeine from the tea leaf. It may also remove much of the polyphenols. I could not find any studies comparing the polyphenolic content of the various forms of Japanese tea. Best to stick with other varieties if you're seeking maximum concentrations of polyphenols. *Hoji cha* is a lovely tasting tea and can be enjoyed even late at night without fear of caffeine-induced insomnia. (Studies on green-tea polyphenols are imprecise. They don't distinguish between the types of green tea consumed. Quantity is measured in "cups per day," obviously a crude measure. More precise work needs to be done on the polyphenolic content of specific amounts of particular green teas).

For further information on Japanese green tea, including how to order it, Horaido's web site is http://www.kyoto-teramachi.or.jp/horaido.

Other Beneficial Foods

Capsaicin

Capsaicin is a pungent component of hot chili peppers. It helps protect against genetic mutations induced in laboratory experiments. It also has direct apoptotic effects on a variety of cancer cell lines. Its role, if any, in prostate cancer has not been determined, but if you like spicy food, go for it.

Sesame Seeds

A new study shows that eating sesame seeds significantly raises blood levels of gamma-tocopherol. In a study done at the University of Hawaii and reported in 2001 in *Nutrition and Cancer*, Dr. Robert Cooney and colleagues found that as little as 5 mg of sesame seeds daily raised gamma-tocopherol in blood serum by an average (mean) of 19.1%. Interestingly, consuming walnuts containing an equivalent amount of gamma-tocopherol to the sesame-seed portions in this study did not show a rise in gamma-tocopherol levels. The researchers conclude that the dietary source of gamma-tocopherol makes a difference in blood levels achieved after consumption and that sesame seeds are highly effective in this regard. This study in humans confirms similar findings in animal studies. Sesame seeds contain a lignan called sesamolin. All subjects in the University of Hawaii study had detectable blood levels of this unique lignan. The investigators postulate that this lignan may account for the high retention of gamma-tocopherol in people who regularly consume sesame seeds.

Sesame seeds appear to be more effective and less caloric than nuts. Less than 11 grams of seeds have the equivalent gamma-tocopherol content as 17 grams of walnuts. I have added sesame seeds as a regular part of my diet.

Key Reference

Cooney R et al. Effects of dietary sesame seeds on plasma tocopherol levels. *Nutr and Cancer* 2001; 39: 66-71.

Allium Vegetables

Allium vegetables, such as garlic, scallions, onions, chives, and leeks, contain varying amounts of organic sulfur compounds. Although a number of population studies show an association of allium vegetable consumption and a reduced risk of a variety of cancers, little appeared in the medical literature about this class of vegetables and prostate cancer until November 2002, when a study on this subject was published in the *Journal of the National Cancer Institute*. This study, done in Shanghai, China, in coordination with the National Cancer Institute, compared the intake of allium vegetables in 238 men with confirmed prostate cancer with 471 normal men. They divided the men into four equal groups based on consumption. They discovered that men in the highest three categories of intake (more than 10 grams/day) had a significantly lower risk of prostate cancer than men with the lowest 25% of consumption (less than 2.2 grams/day). The risk reduction was independent of caloric intake, body weight, or intake of other foods.

The two foods with the greatest effect were garlic and scallions. Consumption of onions and chives, also allium vegetables, did not show a significant reduction in risk. Of note is the fact that in this study, 46% of the control men who didn't have prostate cancer consumed at least 6 grams of garlic (approximately 2 cloves) weekly. This compares to only 15% of British males who consume at least 6 grams per week and 20% of United States women who consume half this much (3 grams/week) or more. In other words, considerably higher amounts of garlic and scallions are consumed in Shanghai than in Britain or the United States. This study indicates that this consumption helps protect against prostate cancer.

Some studies seem to indicate that heating garlic may decrease its cancer-fighting properties. For this reason I make a salad dressing out of extra virgin olive oil, soft tofu, finely chopped raw garlic, half a teaspoon of honey, and a little hot mustard. It's delicious and provides raw garlic regularly. Throw a few scallions in the salad and you're set.

How do garlic and scallions work? One way may be by reducing inflammation. They may also protect against environmental carcinogens and reduce the proliferation of cancer cells.

Key References

Hsing A et al. Allium vegetables and risk of prostate cancer: a population-based study. *J Natl Cancer Instit* 2002; 94: 1648-1651.

Fleischauer A and Arab L. Garlic and cancer: a critical review of the epidemio-logic literature. *J Nutr* 2001; 131: 1032S-1040S.

Milner J. A historical perspective on garlic and cancer. *J Nutr* 2001; 131: 1027S-1031S.

Song K and Milner J. Heating garlic inhibits its ability to suppress 7, 12-dim-ethyl benz (a) anthracene-induced DNA adduct formation in rat mammary tissue. *J Nutr* 1999; 129: 657-661.

Ali M et al. Garlic and onions: their effect on eicosanoid metabolism and its clinical relevance. *Prostaglandins Leukot Essent Fatty Acids* 2000; 62: 55-73.

Red Wine

A number of recent medical studies have shown that regular moderate consumption of red wine may reduce the risk of heart disease and cancer. A study of 34,000 middle-aged French men reported that 2-3 glasses of red wine daily was associated with a reduction in cancer deaths by 22% and lowered deaths from all causes by 33%.

Red wine contains high concentrations of phenolic compounds, the best known and most widely studied being resveratrol. This has been shown to have the following properties in fighting cancer:

- Decreases DNA oxidation
- Inhibits the activation of environmental cancer-causing agents in the body
- Reduces inflammation by inhibiting both COX-1 and COX-2

Of these effects, reducing inflammation may be the most important in protecting against cancer and heart disease. In the lab, resveratrol inhibits the growth of both hormone-dependent and hormone-independent prostate cancer cell lines. It also helps induce apoptosis.

Although red wine has gotten considerable press as a heart-friendly cancer-fighting food, red and purple grapes or grape juice are also beneficial. There is some evidence, however, that the fermentation of wine makes resveratrol and other grape polyphenols more bio-available. So if you prefer wine to grape juice, you've got all the excuse you'll need, so long as you keep the intake moderate (2 glasses per day). What if you drink more? Alcohol consumption (wine, beer, or liquor) beyond 2 glasses daily has been associated with an increased risk of bleeding into the brain and stroke. How much each drink beyond 2 adds to the risk of stroke is debatable, but one study showed that 6 glasses of any kind of alcohol nearly doubles the risk; another study showed a 3-fold increase in the risk of stroke with 7 or more glasses per day. It should be noted that small amounts of alcohol from any source seem to afford some protection against coronary artery disease, but red wine is best.

Grape polyphenols are also available as supplements made from grape skins and seeds. For most of us, taking this supplement is not as pleasant as a glass or two of a fine red wine. But if you find the effects of even small quantities of alcohol to be unpleasant and don't like grapes or grape juice, these supplements will provide the beneficial polyphenols. Some men I know who travel frequently prefer the supplements for their convenience and regularity. I see no harm in this approach, but personally go for the natural sources.

Key References

Hsieh TC and Wu JM. Differential effects on growth, cell cycle arrest and induction of apoptosis by resveratrol in human prostate cancer cell lines. *Exp Cell Res* 1999; 249: 109-115.

Waffo-Teguo P et al. Potential cancer-chemopreventive activities of wine stilbenoids and flavans extracted from grape (Vitis vinifera) cell cultures. *Nutr and Cancer* 2001; 40: 173-179.

Luceri C et al. Red wine and black tea polyphenols modulate the expression of cycloxygenase-2, inducible nitric oxide, and glutathione-related enzymes in azomethane-induced F344 rat colon cancers. *Nutr and Cancer* 2002; 132: 1376-1379.

Kampa M et al. Wine antioxidant polyphenols inhibit the proliferation of human prostate cancer cell lines. *Nutr and Cancer* 2000; 37: 223-229.

Klatsky A et al. Alcohol drinking and risk of hemorrhagic stroke. *Neuroepidemiology* 2002; 21: 115-122.

Stampfer M et al. A prospective study of moderate alcohol consumption and risk of coronary disease and stroke in women. *New Engl J Med* 1998; 319: 267-273.

Burns J et al. Alcohol consumption and mortality: is wine different from other alcoholic beverages? *Nutr Metab Cardiovasc Dis* 2001; 11: 249-258.

Modified Citrus Pectin

Citrus pectin is the soluble fiber from citrus fruit. It's been modified so that it's more readily absorbed. Modified citrus pectin has been found to reduce prostate cancer cell growth in a hormone-independent line of prostate cancer cells. These studies created a flurry of interest in its use by men who have prostate cancer. Animal studies done by Dr. Ken Pienta and his group at the University of Michigan support the idea that modified citrus pectin may help prevent the spread of prostate cancer. Dr. Pienta's group observed a significant reduction in the number of lung metastases in rats fed modified citrus pectin compared with control animals.

Several mechanisms for its action have been proposed. One is that it may suppress the production of the protein produced by the nm23 gene. Studies have shown over-production of this protein in metastatic disease. Reducing its production could reduce metastases.

Key References

Pienta K et al. Inhibition of spontaneous metastasis in a rat prostate cancer model by oral administration of modified citrus pectin. *J Natl Cancer Instit* 1995 87: 348-353.

Hsieh T and Wu J. Changes in cell growth, cyclin/kinase, endogenous phosphoproteins and nm23 gene expression in human prostatic JCA-1 cells treated with modified citrus pectin. *Biochem Mol Biol Int* 1995; 37: 833-841.

Chocolate

For those of you who may be feeling deprived with a vegan diet, here's a tidbit you'll probably like: Chocolate may be helpful in reducing the risk of prostate cancer.

In the Physicians Health Study at Harvard, one of Dr. Giovannucci's observations was that men with high blood levels of a fatty acid called stearic acid had reduced chances of getting prostate cancer. Doctors with the highest levels of stearic acid reduced their risk of getting metastatic prostate cancer by 70%! By far the richest source of stearic acid is chocolate—not milk chocolate, but dark chocolate, the darker the better.

European chocolate quantifies the percentage of cocoa, the ingredient in chocolate that contains the stearic acid. The highest I've found is 88% in a Belgian chocolate manufactured by Dolfin. Parisian chocolatier Michel Cluizel makes an 85% cocoa chocolate. Seventy percent cocoa is more common. This is made by Nestlé, Lindt, and Jacques (72%). Look for at least 70% cocoa content. Check the Appendix for addresses of European chocolatiers if you're unable to find suitable chocolate in your local area.

I limit my chocolate intake to a square or two a day. More than this provides too many calories for me to be able to control my weight. But if you can spare the calories, up to three ounces per day may have beneficial antioxidant effects. I let it melt in my mouth and savor the flavor. A real treat!

Limonene

I also use lots of citrus peel in everything from rice pudding to spaghetti sauce. Citrus peel contains limonene, another compound that has received attention for its anti-cancer properties.

Silymarin

Silymarin is an extract from the milk-thistle plant. It's a potent polyphenolic antioxidant. Its main active ingredient is called silibinin. The only food with significant amounts of silibinin is the artichoke, in the milk thistle family of plants. The recent work of two academicians, Drs. Zi and Agarwal, has focused attention on this milky-white flavonoid as a potentially useful agent in the fight against prostate cancer.

In the laboratory, these researchers showed that "silymarin possesses exceptionally high to complete protective effects against experimentally induced tumorigenesis." They found that it works on several key pathways in prostate cancer cell growth, causing the cells to stop growing. Of particular interest is the finding that silymarin seems to stop the growth of both hormone-dependent and hormone-independent prostate cancer cell lines. It seems to up-regulate the p21 cancer-suppressor gene. Cells also became more differentiated (normal).

It's still too early to know how important silymarin will become in the treatment of prostate and other cancers (silymarin is strongly active against skin cancer). Human studies have not yet been done. Dosages have not been determined. Studies in mice show that orally administered silymarin does produce increased levels of silibinin in the prostate and other tissues.

This is another supplement where you pay your money and you take your chances. It seems safe. It works in the lab and has several known mechanisms for inhibiting prostate cancer cell growth. New evidence shows that silibinin may raise insulin-like growth-factor binding protein 3 (IGFBP-3) blood levels, while reducing insulin-like growth hormone 1 (IGF-1) levels. IGF-1 has been associated with an increased risk of prostate cancer onset and progression, while IGFBP-3 has been shown to reduce IGF-1 levels and seems to kill prostate cancer cells directly. For a full discussion, see pages 418-423). Silymarin supplements might also be considered as part of a prostate cancer prevention regimen for men with elevated IGF-1 levels.

Key References

Zi X and Agarwal R. Silibinin decreases prostate-specific antigen with cell growth inhibition via G1 arrest, leading to differentiation of prostate carcinoma cells: implications for prostate cancer intervention. *Proc Natl Acad Sci USA* 1999; 96: 7490-7495.

Zhao J, and Agarwal R. Tissue distribution of silibinin, the major active constituent of silymarin, in mice and its association with enhancement of phase II enzymes: implications in cancer chemoprevention. *Carcinogenesis* 1999; 20: 2101-2108.

Zi X, Agarwal R, et al. A flavonoid antioxidant, silymarin, inhibits activation of erbB1 signaling and induces cyclin-dependent kinase inhibitors, G1 arrest, and anticarcinogenic effects in human prostate carcinoma DU-145 cells. *Cancer Research* 1998; 58: 1920-1929.

Functional Foods—A New Working Paradigm In Food Selection

Okinawans, the longest-lived people on Earth, think of food as medicine. Doctors Aliza Stark and Zecharia Mador use the term "functional food" when referring to olive oil. I think the paradigm of functional food has merit. A functional food is one that serves a constructive purpose in maintaining optimal health. They come in many forms that span the globe. Although there is an enormous difference in the foods eaten by the Greeks and the traditional Japanese, both diets are predominately comprised of functional foods. And despite the diversity, there are some striking similarities between the Mediterranean and East Asian cuisines. Both are rich in vegetables, fruits, legumes, grains, and fish. Red meat is consumed in relatively small amounts.

Interestingly, the traditional Japanese diet is low in tomatoes, especially cooked tomatoes, with their protective lycopene. This is compensated for by a low dairy intake. By contrast, the Mediterranean diets are relatively high in dairy intake (yogurt and low-fat cheese like feta), but this is offset by an exceptionally high consumption of cooked tomatoes. Remember, studies indicate that the ratio of tomato intake to dairy intake seems to have the greatest impact on health. Cholesterol-lowering olive oil and antioxidant-rich red wine, both functional foods, seem to compensate for the lack of soy and green tea in the Mediterranean diet.

Functional foods are diverse. This provides a wide range of choices. In fact, constantly varying the selection of functional food probably provides optimal health benefits, as this diversity is likely to provide the body with proper amounts of micro-nutrients, antioxidants, and anti-inflammatories. Dr. Heber recommends selecting a variety of the brightest colored fruits and vegetables to optimize their nutrient content.

Eating functionally does not mean eating boringly. The

choice of dishes and cuisines is enormous. Even dishes that are unhealthy can be modified by substituting some key healthy ingredients in the recipe for unhealthy ones. Substituting applesauce for oil in cakes, for example, makes a constructive difference.

Michael Milken and Beth Greenberg have published two superb cookbooks that detail the concept of substituting functional food for dysfunctional food in a variety of recipes from around the world (see Appendix IV).

Nutrients not available in sufficient quantities in the diet, like silymarin, can be provided through supplements. Supplements are also a useful source of nutrients for men who travel frequently and have their normal eating routine disrupted.

Charts listing functional foods and what they provide can be found in Appendix III.

Supplements Summary

I think it's prudent to get most vitamins, minerals, and micro-nutrients from your diet. A vegan diet, or a vegan diet with added fish, will provide you with almost all your nutritional needs. There are a few exceptions.

• Vitamin E (mixed tocopherols with high gamma-tocopherol levels)—You cannot get adequate amounts from your diet. I recommend 400 IU/day (range 200-800 IU). Your daily dose should not exceed 800 IU. Doses above this may have a pro-oxidant effect instead of working as an antioxidant. High doses can also result in bleeding problems. If taken with gingko biloba, it may cause gums to bleed.

• Selenium—200 micrograms/day is recommended, especially in areas with low selenium levels in the soil, such as the Pacific Northwest or the Eastern seaboard, and some countries (New Zealand and Scandinavia). Higher doses are currently being tested.

• Vitamin C—Since it's water soluble, 500 mg 2-3 times a day is recommended. Although if may be possible to get enough from dietary sources, intake is often sporadic, so supplements make sense for cancer-prevention purposes. Some medical experts caution men with existing prostate cancer against vitamin C supplements. They point out that it nourishes the cancer cells, as well as the normal cells, in the body.

• Green-tea capsules—Since the effects of the polyphenols in green tea are dose dependent, it pays to be sure you're getting enough. Few of us regularly consume the required 4-10 cups a day. The supplements insure that you're getting enough. I recommend four to six capsules per day in divided doses. Since the studies use caffeinated green tea, I take lightly caffeinated capsules except at bedtime. I don't know if the process of decaffeination alters the beneficial effects; it hasn't, to my knowledge, been investigated. If you're sensitive to caffeine, decaffeinated capsules are readily available. Green-tea extract capsules are preferable to EGCG capsules.

• Sulforaphane—One of the active anti-carcinogen ingredients in cruciferous vegetables like broccoli. Researchers at Johns Hopkins University found it to be highly concentrated in broccoli sprouts (now available in selected stores as "BroccoSprouts®"). You can also either grow your own sprouts from seed or purchase a standardized extract as a dietary supplement. Probably not necessary if you eat four to six ounces or more of crucifers daily. One tablet per day is sufficient for a prevention regimen. Three tablets/day for men who have prostate cancer.

• Vitamin B-12—This one is for vegans: 300 micrograms/day. It's difficult to get enough naturally.

• Silymarin—Not available from diet unless you eat a lot of artichokes. Recommended dose two to three 100-mg capsules/day in divided doses. May be especially important for men with elevated IGF-1 levels. Silibinin, the most active component of silymarin, is also available in capsule form.

• Lycopene—Best to get from diet through tomato products. But if you hate tomatoes, it's best to take a lycopene supplement. 20-30 mg/day. These are also handy when traveling. Men with existing prostate cancer might consider taking 30 mg lycopene in supplement form and eat lots of tomato products.

Additional Supplements for Men Who Have Prostate Cancer

• Modified Citrus Pectin—Five grams two to three times daily. Can be mixed into soy protein shake.

• Genistein—Best to get this one from soy products like tofu, miso, and soy protein isolate. But if your palate rebels or if these products are not available when you travel, genistein supplements can be substituted.

• Conjugated Linoleic Acid (CLA)—Not studied yet in humans, but strong lab and animal evidence of inhibition of prostate cancer proliferation and metastases. Dose is three 1,000-mg softgel caps/day (optional).

• Silibinin—Although not yet proven, there's evidence that silibinin raises beneficial cancer-killing and IGF-1-lowering IGFBP-3 levels. Silibinin (and silymarin) supplements appear to be safe at high doses. I currently take 6 silibinin capsules (from Life Extension) daily in divided doses. Each capsule provides 266 mg of silibinin and 60 mg of silymarin. My IGFBP-3 level is in the 98th percentile for men my age and my IGF-1 levels have been reduced by 40%.

• Chinese Herbs/Mushrooms—Widely studied in China and Japan, but not in the United States. Immune-system stimulants include ganoderma lucidum (*reishi*), astragalus (*huang chi*), and maitake extract (extract from edible mushroom). These supplements are all optional. Some brands of astragalus may have high levels of selenium. Men taking high doses of astragulus should be aware of this, especially if they are also taking selenium supplements. If you take these, the recommended amount is one to two caps of each three times a day. The Chinese herbs scuttelaria (scute) and licorice root have been shown to have anti-prostate cancer effects. They (and *reishi*) are part of the PC-SPES formula. A balanced formula including these two herbs can be prepared by a doctor trained in traditional Chinese medicine.

Remember, whenever possible look for food sources for nutrients. If you can find and regularly eat fresh immune-system-enhancing mushrooms, for example, you probably don't need to also add supplements. Supplements should provide vitamins and nutrients not available through food. Food provides numerous micro-nutrients, many of which have not been studied. When you take only one isolated active ingredient, you may lose some of the beneficial effects that you would get from eating the whole food.

Supplements to Avoid

Beta-carotene—May increase the risk of prostate cancer growth. Especially true for smokers.

Chromium Picolinate—Can react with vitamin C and other antioxidants to produce a form of chromium capable of damaging DNA in the cells of the body. Avoid.

Coenzyme Q-10—Widely publicized for its beneficial effects on the heart. Several labs have shown that this compound stimulates the growth of prostate cancer cell lines in the test tube. Avoid if you have prostate cancer.

Curcumin—Although excellent as a prevention agent for prostate cancer, men with existing prostate cancer should avoid this supplement, as it seems to interfere with one of the apoptosis pathways of prostate cancer cells.

Factors Associated with Increased Prostate Cancer Risk

1. Obesity
2. High caloric intake
3. High fat diet (40%, or more, of total calories from fat)
4. High intake of red meat
5. Milk and dairy products
6. High IGF-1 levels
7. Inactivity

8. Low serum selenium levels
9. Low blood vitamin D levels

Factors Associated with Reduced Prostate Cancer Risk

1. Low fat diet (20%, or less, of calories from fat)
2. Eat about 2000-2200 calories/day
3. High fiber intake (25-35 grams, or more, per day)
4. High intake of vegetables, especially crucifers.
5. Consuming soy products and green tea
6. High SHBG levels
7. Regular exercise
8. High IGFBP-3 levels
9. High blood lycopene levels
10. High blood lutein levels

Foods to Avoid

1. Red meats (beef, veal, pork, lamb)
2. Cheese and cream
3. Whole & reduced fat milk and yogurt
4. Mayonnaise
5. Butter
6. Nuts (due to high fat content), but are okay in moderation.
7. Polyunsaturated oils (salad oils). Olive oil is fine, but watch the calories
8. Margarine
9. Egg yolks
10. Farm-bred (low DHA and EPA) fish, farm-bred salmon, trout, and yellowtail (*hamachi*) tuna; wild varieties are okay.
11. Fried foods
12. Chips cooked with oil
13. Packaged foods with "partially hydrogenated" oils.
14. Coconut & coconut milk
15. Alcohol. More than two ounces of spirits per day, or more than two glasses of wine daily. One or two glasses a day

seem to be beneficial, especially red wine.

16. Charbroiled foods (produce carcinogenic heterocyclic amines). Chicken cooked under high heat seems to have the highest concentration of heterocyclic amines.

Foods to Increase

1. Fruits of all kinds, except coconuts

2. Tomato products of all kinds—tomato sauce, pastes, juice, ketchup, non-fat barbecue sauce, tomato relish, pizza (cheese-less). Cooked tomato products are best, but fresh tomatoes are still nutritious.

3. Soy products: tofu, miso, tempeh, soy milk, soy protein isolate, natto, boiled green soybeans (edamame), soybean sprouts, low-fat soy cheese, dried soy beans, non-fat soy protein bars.

4. Use olive oil spray for cooking.

5. Vegetables of all kinds: raw and lightly steamed or baked. Fresh vegetable soups. Crucifers are especially good.

6. Beans and lentils (but watch the calories).

7. Healthy snacks: air-popped popcorn, rice cakes, dried fruit, fat-free soy protein bars, rye wafers, fat-free unsalted pretzels (watch the calories), and roasted chestnuts. Fresh fruit's always a good snack alternative.

8. Low-oil-content breads, such as flat dark breads, sprouted grain breads, pita. Add pure fruit jams, if you wish.

9. Egg whites or egg-beaters.

10. Cereals and grains of all kinds: brown rice, white rice (but not as good as brown rice due to fewer nutrients and a higher glycemic index), basmati rice (low glycemic index), bulgar wheat, millet, etc; All Bran, Grape Nuts, Raisin Bran, Shredded Wheat; whole-grain hot cereals.

11. Green tea, black tea, oolong tea, non-fat cocoa. Coffee in moderation is okay unless you're sensitive to caffeine.

12. Spaghetti (with lots of tomato sauce).

13. Mushrooms and fungi of all kinds: shiitake, maitake, enoki, shimeji, portobello, oyster, Chinese black fungus, Chinese white fungus.

14. Organically grown produce.

15. Fruit juices of all kinds (watch calories).

16. A glass or two of red wine, or red grape juice, daily.

17. Most fish, including shellfish (crabs, shrimp, lobster, clams, mussels), sashimi, sushi. Raw, steamed, or grilled with olive-oil spray.

18. Garlic, scallions, ginger, and tumeric.

For those with prostate cancer, a low-fat vegan diet may be preferable, provided that DHA supplements are included in the diet.

Twenty Steps to a Healthier Lifestyle

• Eat more fruits and vegetables—at least 5 servings/day.

• Eliminate or reduce consumption of meat. Substitute fish whenever possible. Continue to move toward a vegan diet. If you eat chicken or turkey, stick with breasts and remove the skin prior to cooking.

• Use olive oil (sparingly) as your only oil. Use olive-oil spray for cooking. Remember, although probably not directly harmful, olive oil is high in calories. Do not use polyunsaturated oils (corn, safflower, soybean, etc.). Macadamia nut, walnut, and avocado oils can be substituted for olive oil as a matter of taste.

• Eliminate butter, egg yolks, margarine, mayonnaise, and creamy salad dressings from your diet.

• Reduce your overall caloric intake; reduce calories from fat to 20% of total calories, or less.

• Eat whole grains and cereals for their fiber content.

• Eat lots of soy.

• Drink four or more cups of green tea daily.

• Add garlic, curcumin, and chilis to your cooking whenever possible.

• Eat your crucifers. Consider broccoli-sprout supplements; look for "BroccoSprouts®."

- Eat strawberries, raspberries, and blueberries. Use frozen berries when fresh ones are not available. Try to have a daily serving (½ cup per day). Organic strawberries are highly preferable due to heavy spraying.
- Reduce or eliminate milk and milk products.
- Eat lots of tomato products—Seven to ten times/week, if possible. A daily 8-ounce glass of low-sodium tomato or V-8 juice is an easy routine to guarantee sufficient lycopene, but a little oil (½ teaspoon of olive oil) is required for optimal lycopene absorption.
- Use citrus rind in sauces and desserts.
- Drink a glass or two or red wine or grape juice regularly.
- Take selected supplements, including vitamin C, vitamin E, and selenium. If you have prostate cancer, consider adding silibinin (silymarin), or Rocaltrol if prescribed by your doctor, green-tea extract, and modified citrus pectin. Some may want to add immune-system-stimulating mushroom extracts and other Chinese herbs.
- Get 15-20 minutes of unprotected sunshine every two to three days.
- Exercise regularly (see "Exercise").
- Reduce stress (see "Stress Reduction").
- Laugh a lot.

19

EXERCISE AND PROSTATE CANCER

Men Who Exercise Live Longer

Is exercise important for health? Studies consistently show that it is. Probably the best way to test the benefits of exercise is to see if men who exercise regularly live longer. Just such a study was done in Holland by Dr. Bijnen and reported in 1999 in the *American Journal of Epidemiology*. The researchers asked a group of 472 elderly Dutch men to complete a questionnaire that quantified physical activity. Then they followed the men for five years, during which time 25% died.

The study found that the risk of dying from all causes was highest in men with the lowest level of physical activity. Similarly, the risk was lowest in the men with the greatest amount of activity: 2½ or more hours a day of walking or cycling. The intensity of physical activity did not seem to matter in this study. Casual walking proved as good as strenuous walking. Men who were recently physically active lived longer than men who were active within the past five years, but had recently stopped exercising. After adjusting their results to account for chronic illnesses that might cause men to become sedentary, the research team concluded that 23% of the risk of dying from any cause was due to lack of physical activity. In short, physical activity extended life expectancy.

Another large study of nearly 10,000 men was reported in *JAMA* in 1995. Steven Blair and colleagues at the Cooper

Institute in Dallas, Texas, found that men 60 years of age and older decreased their risk of dying by 50% by being fit. This was true for both healthy and unhealthy men. While this is an impressive statistic, exercise had an even more profound effect on unfit men who improved their fitness. This group reduced their death risk by an amazing 64%!

These investigators found that a *change* in fitness level, either up or down, made a difference in survival expectations. A reduction in fitness increased mortality risk; an increase in fitness reduced the chance of dying. Also, the effect of exercise was incremental. Men who were fit, then became more fit, continued to reduce their mortality risk by an additional 15%.

This was a prospective study that tested fitness levels of each man twice, separated by about five years. Men determined fit at both examinations had the lowest death rates.

It's important to note that this study not only demonstrates the benefits of fitness, but more significantly, demonstrates that changes in fitness levels alter life expectancy. The investigators quantified this effect: "For each minute increase in maximal treadmill time between the first examination and the second (mean interval 4.9 years), there was a 7.9% decrease in the risk of mortality." As previously mentioned, reducing physical activity reduces life expectancy proportionately.

The researchers conclude: "Men who maintained or improved adequate physical fitness were less likely to die from all causes and from cardiovascular disease during follow-up than persistently unfit men. Physicians can have confidence that their patients will reduce risk of mortality by increasing physical activity and improving fitness."

Why Do Men Who Exercise Live Longer?

The cardiovascular benefits of exercise have been widely publicized. There is little question that exercise helps prevent heart disease. It also reduces the chances of developing diabetes. How? Primarily by keeping down your weight. There is a clear correlation between obesity and heart disease and diabetes. Fat men produce more insulin, a characteristic of the early stages of adult-onset diabetes. Exercise lowers blood insulin levels.

Recently, researchers at the Harvard School of Public Health found that exercise decreases levels of a "fat hormone," called leptin, in the blood. Men who exercised most had the lowest levels of leptin; men who exercised the least had the highest leptin levels. Surprisingly, it did not seem to matter whether the men who exercised were fat or not. If they were fat and in the group that exercised the most, they had low leptin levels. Although there is little doubt that losing weight protects against heart disease, stroke, diabetes, and perhaps cancer, it hasn't yet been conclusively determined how much protection is provided by lowering leptin levels without losing weight. The main point is to exercise and receive the benefits, while scientists continue to work out the mechanics of why exercise works.

For elderly men, exercise becomes more important as muscle mass shrinks and the risk of osteoporosis increases. Men 75 years of age or older can increase their muscle mass by as much as 20% with just three months of weight training. They can also improve their lung capacity by comparable amounts with about six months of exercise.

Regularity of exercise is more important than the type of exercise. Regular moderately strenuous exercise has repeatedly been shown to increase strength, endurance, and balance—keys to maintaining health and vigor with aging. This kind of exercise, besides the protection against heart disease and stroke previously discussed, also reduces the risks of high blood pressure, osteoporosis, and hip fractures. A study just out as we got to press shows increased exercise also reduces the risk of Alzheimer's disease.

Exercising for Prostate Health

When it comes to prostate cancer, exercise works in several important and helpful ways. A massive combined prospective study of 13,000 men who responded to long-term questionnaires was launched by the Strang Cancer Prevention Center, the Harvard School of Public Health, and the Cooper Institute. Reported in 1996 in the journal *Medicine and Science in Sports Medicine*, the researchers monitored the development of prostate cancer in men whose fitness had been tested at the Cooper Institute over an 18-year period. On follow-up the scientists found that men in the top 50% for fitness had significantly less chance of developing clinical prostate cancer than men in the lowest 25% for fitness. When adjusted for age, this correlation between fitness and reduced risk of prostate cancer was limited to men under age 60. The researchers point out that there were very few men over 60 in this study (average age 44) and this may account for the lack of statistical significance of exercise in reducing the incidence of prostate cancer in the older group.

A second supportive study on the positive effects of exercise on prostate cancer came from a group of researchers at the National Cancer Institute (NCI). This NCI group reviewed the records of 29,000 men in a large study from Finland. Although the original objective was to determine the effects of vitamin E and beta-carotene on the risks of prostate cancer, exercise data were also collected. The NCI investigators found that over a nine-year period, men they characterized as "occupational walkers" had 40% less risk of developing prostate cancer than inactive men. Men who combined walking with weight lifting had 20% less risk than sedentary men. The NCI group concluded: "These results are consistent with a protective effect of physical activity on prostate cancer." More prospective studies need to be done to better determine the effects of exercise on the development of prostate cancer in older men. For men under 60, cardiovascular fitness is associated with a decreased risk of prostate cancer.

The authors postulate that the reason for the reduction in cancer may be due to a reduction in testosterone levels. Athletes, they point out, have lower blood-testosterone levels than non-athletes. Also, when men exercise, their testosterone level is reduced immediately after working out, although only temporarily. What effects, if any, this has on prostate cancer remains unclear, although as we've seen, some investigators have found a correlation between high testosterone levels and prostate cancer. Of course, there is no conclusive proof that this causes prostate cancer to develop—only an association. Some other studies show no effect from higher testosterone levels.

Other possible influences of exercise on hormone levels include a decrease in blood insulin and IGF-1 levels and an increase in SHBG levels. It makes good sense that a decrease in testosterone and IGF-1 levels, combined with an increase in SHBG levels, protects against prostate cancer, although proof is not yet in hand. It's well known, however, that Chinese and Japanese men, who have much less clinically significant prostate cancer, have far higher concentrations of SHBG and lower levels of testosterone than Western men. Since regular exercise has no downside and unequivocal upside as far as heart disease, stroke, obesity, etc. are concerned, it makes good sense to establish a regular exercise program. Beside diet, exercise is one of the activities within your control. Men who exercise feel stronger, are more mentally alert, have reduced levels of stress, and have more energy than sedentary men. Overall, exercise improves health and attitude. Go for it!

Exercise and Androgen-Ablating Hormones

As we know, hormones are becoming increasingly important in the treatment of prostate cancer. In the near future, I predict there will be substantially more combination therapy, integrating androgen-ablating hormones with either surgery or radiation. Because hormones have a systemic effect (throughout the body), they can cause some undesirable side effects. With prolonged hormone use, men have a tendency to gain weight (fat), while losing muscle. In addition, hormones virtually eliminate testosterone and other androgen production, which can lead to bone loss. Men on complete androgen blockade lose more bone density every year than post-menopausal women.

Exercise helps reverse these unwanted events. It reduces weight, increases muscle mass, and reduces bone loss. When combined with bisphosphonates, exercise is especially effective in combating osteoporosis. Michael Milken actually *increased* his bone density by 4% in one year by combining exercise with bisphosphonates and diet. Before I started hormones I weighed 182 pounds, of which 22% was fat. Sixteen months after starting hormonal therapy, I weighed 179 pounds with 18% fat. I'd increased my muscle mass, while reducing my weight and body fat despite complete androgen blockade. So, with the help of exercise and diet, it's possible to keep fat levels down without sacrificing muscle. The trick is to conscientiously stick to your diet and exercise programs. It works!

I also took bisphosphonates (Fosamax) during and after hormonal therapy. My bone density is the same today (age-adjusted) as it was when I started hormones.

What Kind Of Exercise To Do

The best exercise for men with prostate cancer is moderately strenuous activity that combines the following elements: strength, endurance, balance, flexibility, and breathing. Here are the ones I like best.

Walking

The simplest and most convenient exercise is walking. You can walk at home, at work, on the road, anywhere. It requires no special equipment; a good pair of walking shoes is all you'll need. Walking regularly improves strength, endurance, and balance. If you increase your pace and move your arms vigorously, you'll get the aerobic benefits you need too. Start slowly (10-20 minutes every other day) and increase to 30-40 minutes at least three times per week. If you walk in the early morning or late afternoon without sunscreen, you'll get the sun required to generate critical vitamin D needed to help fight your cancer.

Several studies have shown that regular walking increases life expectancy. The chance of dying early from all combined causes is reduced by up to 55% if you walk only 30 minutes a day. This has been confirmed by recent studies reported in the *New England Journal of Medicine* and *JAMA*. The latter paper related significant benefits from as little as one 30-minute walk per week.

Other studies indicate that men who walk at least a mile a day tend to have less prostate enlargement than inactive men. Walking also reduces stress and improves the sense of well-being. One research group documented improved scores on memory tests by men who walked a mile a day.

Overall, walking is probably the easiest and one of the most beneficial of all exercises.

Hatha Yoga

Hatha yoga is the yoga most people are familiar with. It's another ideal exercise for men with prostate cancer. In fact, yoga might be *the* ideal exercise for anyone. It has all the key elements, and then some. Besides being superb for balance, strength, and endurance, yoga incorporates controlled breathing. This reduces stress. Like walking, yoga can be done anywhere and requires no equipment, not even shoes. It can be done indoors or out, rain or shine.

Yoga is also a good way to increase *chi*. *Chi* is a Chinese term that, roughly translated, means "life force." In the West, it's sometimes called "bio-energetic current." Like trying to describe the taste of an orange to someone who has never tasted one, *chi* is difficult to characterize. Every living human has *chi* and it's "there" all the time. The closest description I can come up with is this: an ever-present rhythmic pulsation throughout the body best perceived with a quiet mind (free from thought). The Chinese believe that keeping this current strong is crucial to optimal health.

Yoga generates *chi*. At the end of a one-hour yoga session, lie on your back. Relax completely. Concentrate on your breathing. Take a few deep breaths, filling your chest first, then your abdomen, then exhale. Repeat this three times, then lie quietly. Move your focus to two inches below your navel. Relax completely. By doing this, you have a good chance of observing the flow of *chi*. The more yoga you do the more you'll become aware of *chi*. *Chi* will also get stronger with regular yoga practice. Shiatsu or ayurvedic massage and a variety of breathing techniques also help generate *chi*.

Other forms of yoga are centered more on breathing than on movement and postures. For some practitioners, these forms, such as kundalini yoga, generate and strengthen *chi* more powerfully than hatha yoga. I do not recommend starting with kundalini yoga. Hatha yoga is much more practical for men with prostate cancer. But if you get into yoga and enjoy it, or want to rev up your *chi*, you might want to give kundalini a try.

Yoga combines mind and body: stretching the body while relaxing the mind. Don't push yourself too hard. Stretch as far as you can comfortably stretch, then relax into each pose. Allow your mind to gently focus on your body sensations. Continue to relax. Gradually you'll become more aware of what's happening in your body and be more free from thought. Stretch, relax, and enjoy it.

High-Resistance Weight Training

High-resistance weight training uses machines that provide resistance while minimizing the chances of injury. It builds muscle mass and reduces osteoporosis (bone loss). This type of exercise is particularly useful for men taking hormones. The side effects from hormones are reduced with proper weight training. For best results, weight training should be combined with aerobic exercise, such as walking, swimming, or yoga.

Some men get "addicted" to weight training. This is probably due to release of endorphins. These "natural opiates," as they've been called, induce a sense of euphoria in many men. After a while, they may come to "crave" the training. This is one addiction you can well afford.

Swimming

Swimming combines stretching, aerobics, strength, and endurance. The risk of injury is probably the lowest of any exercise, even walking. Swimming is an excellent way to maintain fitness. The only problem is that it requires a body of water, and these are not always readily available. If you're lucky enough to have a swimming pool or if you have access to a lake or ocean, swimming can be an enjoyable exercise choice. As with walking, swimming will help maintain your levels of vitamin D.

Tai Chi

Walk into the large parks in Beijing, China, any morning and you'll see hundreds of men and women, mostly elderly, practicing tai chi. It's a daily ritual. Tai chi is considered a form of martial art, but is performed in slow motion. It looks more like a dance. It enhances strength, endurance, and flexibility. Superb balance training, it's also excellent for amplification of *chi*. Tai chi classes are offered in most major cities. Start slowly, especially if you have knee problems. As your body adjusts to the unfamiliar moves, you'll become more graceful and fluid. If you stick with it, you're likely to be happy with the results.

Qi Gong

Another popular exercise in China, qi gong (pronounced "chi goong") combines rhythmic motions with breathing and walking meditation. It's not commonly practiced in the United

States, but is great for stress reduction and chi generation. The Chinese believe that qi gong is especially good for cancer patients, where low levels of *chi* is common. Qi gong and acupressure massage are part of routine patient care in many Chinese hospitals. You may have difficulty finding a good qi gong teacher. If you're lucky enough to find one, you might give it a try. It's especially good for men whose exercise capability is limited due to physical limitations.

For Couch Potatoes

For a variety of reasons, regardless of its virtues, some of you will chose not to exercise. You may be too busy, too lazy, or too bored. Even if you don't work some sort of regular exercise into your day, remember this principle: Be as active as possible. Take the stairs instead of the escalator; walk through airports instead of standing on the moving walkways; walk a few blocks to the market instead of taking the car. Each day you'll have similar choices to make. If you pick the "exercise way," you'll improve your fitness and help control your weight.

An article published in the December 30, 1999, issue of the *New England Journal of Medicine* determined that if you did nothing more than chew gum during all your waking hours, you would lose 11 pounds a year! Although it's a bit absurd to contemplate chewing gum incessantly, you get the point. Increase your activity level. Move around. Get active. All signs indicate this will help your heart, weight, and bones. It may also help your cancer.

My Exercise Routine

Men with whom I consult often ask me what I choose to do for exercise. This was my routine while on hormonal therapy:

- Walking: 30 minutes (about two miles) six days a week.
- Hatha yoga: one-hour session three days a week.
- High-resistance weight training: three days a week for one hour each time.
- I walked to the gym for either yoga or weight training six days a week. It was just over a mile in each direction. On the seventh day, I had no planned activity, except for a shiatsu massage. Sometimes I'd take a walk along a beach or in the mountains; more often I'd just hang out and let my body rest. A day of rest is constructive. Don't feel obliged to exercise every day. After I finished my androgen-blocking hormones and the effects were eliminated from my system, I reduced my weight training to one to two times per week. Walking and yoga, however, I continued without reduction in frequency. Simply put, I feel better when I'm active and limber.

Key References

Blair SN et al. Changes in physical fitness and all-cause mortality. *JAMA* 1995; 273: 1093-98.

Oliveria S, Blair SN, et al. The association between cardiorespiratory fitness and prostate cancer. *Medicine and Science in Sports and Exercise* 1996; 28: 97-104.

Hartman TJ et al. Physical activity and prostate cancer in the alpha-tocopherol, beta-carotene (ATBC) cancer prevention study (Finland). *Cancer Causes Control* 1998; 9: 11-18.

Levine J. The energy expended in chewing gum. *The New England Journal of Medicine* 1999; 341: 2100.

Lindsay J et al. Risk factors for Alzheimer's disease: a prospective analysis from the Canadian Study of Health and Aging. *Am J Epidemiol* 2002; 156: 445-453.

20

ATTITUDE

Does attitude really make a difference if you have cancer? I posed this question to each clinician I interviewed for this book. Virtually all believe it helps. Frequent responses included, "Men with a positive constructive outlook seem to do better," or, "That's my impression, though I can't prove it." As Dr. Snuffy Myers puts it, "In my clinical practice, I've been impressed that the men who seem to do best are those who fully confront the implications of their disease and take an active part in developing the treatment plan." He referred to a 1999 study on women with breast cancer that characterized this attitude as "realistic optimism." In the words of Dr. Spiegel, the author of this study, "Optimistic women appear to accept more readily the reality of the challenge they face, whereas pessimistic women try to push this reality away."

I first became aware of a possible influence of mental factors in medicine while still a medical student (too many years ago to mention). Part of our training in the final year included clinical experience. While on the surgery wards, a respected surgeon was talking with a patient scheduled for surgery the next day. The surgeon asked the patient, "Are you ready? How do you feel about your operation?"

She responded, "Doctor, I'm really scared. I don't think I'll make it through the surgery. I think I'm going to die," and she burst into tears.

I've never forgotten the surgeon's response: "Well, in that case, I'm canceling your surgery." Additionally, the doctor withdrew from the case!

I was spellbound. Why? I sought out the surgeon and asked him. He said, "This has happened to me several times before and in each case the patient died. I won't operate on patients who are convinced they won't survive."

Wow! I was thunderstruck. Although the surgeon's opinion was clearly based on what researchers refer to as "anecdotal evidence," from then on I began paying close attention to how patients approached their disease and observed their outcome.

Just what is the relationship between mental factors and disease? Is there a mind-body connection? If so, how does it work? It probably won't surprise you that we have only a rough guideline to the interaction between the brain and nervous system and the immune system. How emotions influence this interaction is fuzzier still. But there have been some fascinating observations that have practical implications.

What Is the Immune System?

The immune system is comprised of white blood cells, lymph nodes, the spleen, thymus, and bone marrow. The job of the immune system is to protect the body from "foreign invaders," such as bacteria, viruses, and the body's own damaged cells (cancer).

The "soldiers" of the immune system are the lymphocytes, specialized white blood cells. These circulating cells are armed with receptors on their surface that recognize alien molecules (antigens). When lymphocytes recognize antigens, it triggers the "immune response." Part of this response is the production of an increased number of special lymphocytes, called "natural killer" (NK) cells. These and other specialized lymphocytes defend the body from everything that they recognize as "other than self." In other words, they're constantly poised to identify and destroy any molecule determined to be foreign to the functioning organism. They behave as if they can "think," constantly re-evaluating an ever-changing interior chemical environment and participating in its response to a multitude of external influences.

Medicine and Information

How does the immune system distinguish "self" from "other?" How does it "think?" The answer to this question is redefining the entire medical paradigm: information.

The DNA sequence that makes a gene is information. Like Morse code, which uses combinations of dots and dashes to form words, the genetic code uses sequences of DNA to form genes. Each gene has the code to produce a single protein. Proteins then become the "biological information superhighway." They form information pathways that interconnect with other streams of information. In this way the nervous, immune, and endocrine systems are perpetually interacting. Chemical signals (messages) are constantly being sent and received, which produces responses.

Chemical signals from proteins are received at sites on the cell surface. Until recently, these were thought to exist only in the brain. We now know that receptors are present on circulating immune-system cells and are capable of responding to messages from hormones produced by the central nervous system. These hormones, called "neuropeptides," affect our mood.

Not only can hormones from the brain affect the immune and endocrine systems, but immune and endocrine hormones can also affect the brain. Communication is not one way. An all-powerful brain is not solely sending out commands to ever-obedient body systems, like a puppeteer pulling the strings of a marionette. Rather, information flows in multiple directions. Each body system is interdependent on other body systems. As Dr. Candace Pert recounts in her excellent book *Molecules of Emotion*, immune-system cells not only have surface receptors to receive neuropeptides from the brain, they also make their own neuropeptides that act on the brain and affect our mood. This has opened up a whole new way of looking at the interaction between mind and body. Called by Dr. Pert "psychoimmunoendocrinology," this big word encompasses the effects of thinking and emotions on the immune and endocrine systems.

Geneticist Dr. LeRoy Hood of the University of Washington sums it up, "Medicine is informational science."

Not only are messages generated internally by the body's systems, but external environmental messages also affect the on-going interchange of the body's signals and responses. Laurence Foss, author of *Healing Biological Medicine* and co-author of *The Second Medical Revolution: From Biomedicine to Infomedicine*, points out that the environment includes not only the physical and ecological environments, but the psychological, social, and cultural environments as well. Thoughts and feelings form an integral part of the environment and, as Foss points out, can produce physical responses. Conversely, physical responses can generate thoughts and emotions. This differs from the traditional biomedical model that doesn't account for intercommunication between the body and mind in any significant way. In Foss' words, "In the infomedical but not in the biomedical picture, a thought or emotion can manifest itself bodily; and, conversely, a body process can translate itself into a thought or emotion."

Examples of the two-way communication between the mind and body include:

• An embarrassing thought and feeling (mind) can lead to blushing, a dilation of blood vessels in the face triggered by neuropeptides acting on receptors on these blood vessels (body).

• Turning "white with fear" or "red with anger." Intense fear can cause uncontrollable shaking (quivering with fear). This is a physical response to an emotion.

• Recalling past noxious events can provoke a physical

response. Someone with a fear of snakes may shudder upon hearing a conversation about an encounter with one. A cancer patient may feel nauseous while sitting in the waiting room prior to chemotherapy.

This kind of "conditioned response" has potential therapeutic ramifications. Just as a negative association can lead to an undesired physical response, so too can a positive association produce a desirable physical change. Dr. Spector and associates at the University of Alabama in Birmingham, working together with Italian colleagues, demonstrated a three- to 39-fold increase in natural killer (NK) cells in response to conditioned activity in mice. Typically, this increase is seen in response to an antigen. But when these researchers combined a "conditioner," such as a certain taste, with the introduction of an antigen, they found that mice could be "trained" to dramatically increase their NK cells by experiencing the taste without the antigen. NK cells are one of the key lymphocytes in the fight against cancer. As you'll see, their production can be influenced by thinking and emotions.

All these are physical responses to thoughts and feelings.

Other emotions—joy, depression, and amusement—are also expressed both mentally and physically. Biochemically, it appears that neuropeptides produced by the brain are then received by receptors in the body, resulting in a variety of physical responses. Emotions can, therefore, be the catalysts for physical responses, which, in turn, can evoke emotions. In other words, the body processes are constantly changing in response to the mind's interpretation of external events. This change is reflected in alterations of pulse rate, respiration rate, blood pressure.

When it comes to coping with cancer, perception of events is a critical variable. How we think about events is perhaps more consequential than the events themselves. Cancer itself can be interpreted by one person as punishment for a body-abusive lifestyle, creating feelings of guilt and helplessness, while another regards it as the sternest warning for the necessity of a drastic change in lifestyle. Framing events in a consistently constructive way not only makes dealing with cancer easier, it also improves the quality of life. The emotions evoked by constructive interpretations of events are also likely to bolster your immune system.

Key References

Foss L. The necessary subjectivity of bodymind medicine: Candace Pert's *Molecules of Emotions—Advances in Mind-Body Medicine* 1999 15: 122-134.

Pert C. *Molecules of Emotions* 1997 Scribner Press, New York.

Spector N. Neuroimmunomodulation: a brief review: can conditioning of natural killer cell activity reverse cancer and/or aging? *Regul Toxicol Pharmacol* 1996; 24:S32-S38.

Block K. The role of the self in healthy cancer survivorship: A view from the front lines of treating cancer. *Advances: The Journal of Mind-Body Health* 1997; 13: 6-26.

How Moods Affect the Immune System

What are the effects of neuropeptides produced by our various moods on the immune system? One measure of immune function is immunoglobulin A, or IgA. It's the primary immunoglobulin in tears and saliva. Because saliva IgA is so readily accessible, it's frequently used as a measure of immune strength.

It has been shown in a series of studies by Dr. Arthur Stone, professor of psychiatry at State University of New York at Stony Brook and his associates, that salivary IgA levels are influenced by moods. Debilitating emotions, like anger, depression, anxiety, and despair, lower salivary IgA levels. So do stressful events in daily life. On the other hand, positive emotional states like joy, happiness, and serenity, raise salivary IgA levels. Supportive social interactions, humor, and meditation also raise IgA levels.

Emotions and Natural Killer (NK) Cell Levels

Emotional states have also been correlated with the number of NK cells in the circulation. Stress, anxiety, and depression have been associated with a decrease in the number of NK cells. Positive moods correlate with an increase in NK cells. Activities like meditation and massage have also been associated with increases in NK cells. There are even suggestions in the literature that intensive meditation and religious or spiritual epiphanies may lead to a spontaneous remission of cancer in some people. While this is conjecture, there is some logic in the premise that if positive moods strengthen the immune system, then extremely positive experiences could conceivably trigger a disease-altering immune response. No studies have been done to verify this hypothesis. The combination of a peak experience and spontaneous remission of cancer occurs so rarely that reports must be anecdotal. Still, the possibility is extremely intriguing.

Emotions and Disease

If the hypothesis that emotions can affect disease is true, then we should be able to identify an association between negative emotions and illness. A number of studies have demonstrated such a connection.

The May 2, 2000, issue of the journal *Circulation* reports that in people with normal blood pressure, anger is associated with heart attacks. The investigators from the University of North Carolina found that people who were most prone to anger had three times the chance of a heart attack, or sudden death due to heart failure, as those least prone to anger.

One of the most interesting and poignant recent studies comes from Dr. Stone at Stony Brook. It's germane for men who have prostate cancer, as well as those trying to prevent it. Dr. Stone found that stressed-out men, or men lacking social support, were two to three times more likely to have an elevated PSA. Men with high stress levels were three times as likely to have a high PSA; men with a poor social-support network were twice as likely to have an elevated PSA as those with good social support. Not surprisingly, the stressed-out men reported frequent feelings of anger and nervousness.

One possible explanation is that stress reduces immune

function, which may make a man more susceptible to prostate cancer. Stress consistently reduces NK cells. Another possibility is that the hormonal response to stress stimulates prostate cancer cell growth. According to Dr. Snuffy Myers, researchers at his former institution, the University of Virginia, led by Dr. Michael Weber have shown that epinephrine (adrenalin) stimulates the growth of prostate cancer cells. It's possible that chronic stress with its associated increased levels of "stress hormones," like epinephrine, stimulates the proliferation of prostate cancer cells and increases PSA levels. Dr. Myers, in his private clinical practice, has observed a frequent correlation between periods of particularly intense stress and the onset of clinically relevant prostate cancer. Yet another possibility is that high stress promotes an unhealthy lifestyle. Anxious men are likely to have poor eating and exercise habits.

As for social support, a good support network may increase immune function by generating positive emotions that come with a sense of belonging and helping others. Men lacking social interconnections might not receive this immune benefit.

These studies do not prove that stress or lack of social support cause prostate cancer. As with diet there is an association, but an association is not a cause. However, as Dr. Stone points out, it's "not likely" that the cause of the high stress levels was the elevated PSA. The men in the study filled out questionnaires that were used to determine their level of stress. At the time they answered the questions they had no knowledge of their PSA results.

Key References

Williams J et al. Anger proneness predicts coronary heart disease risk: prospective analysis from the atherosclerosis risk in communities (ARIC) study. *Circulation* 2000; 101: 2034-2039.

Stone A et al. Psychosocial stress and social support are associated with prostate-specific antigen levels in men: results from a community screening program. *Health Psychol* 1999; 18: 482-486.

Myers CE. *Prostate Forum* 2000; volume 5, number 6, page 4.

Can Attitude Influence Outcome

Is there any evidence that attitude makes a difference in the prognosis of cancer patients? Dr. Steven Greer addressed this issue by interviewing women three months after radical mastectomy (breast removal) for breast cancer. He divided the women into four categories.

Group 1

Fighting Spirit—Accepted diagnosis and optimistically approached the disease by learning about it and getting involved in the decision-making process.

Group 2

Positive Avoiders—Denied or diminished the seriousness of their condition.

Group 3

Stoics—Accepted the diagnosis, but did not try to learn more. Accepted their fate submissively.

Group 4

Helpless and Hopeless—Convinced that they were going to die and that there was nothing they could do about it.

Survival Data for Each Group Five Years Later

Group 1	80% survival
Group 2	70% survival
Group 3	32% survival
Group 4	20% survival

After 10 years, "Fighting Spirit" still led in survival benefits. If these data are to be believed, it appears as though attitude may play a role in survival.

Two things particularly stand out in the above study. I found it interesting that denial was nearly as effective as fighting spirit in five-year survival outcome. Other studies have included denial in their list of positive attitudes. This seems to me to be counterintuitive. Second, women with attitudes characterized as "pessimistic" (helpless, hopeless, fatalistic) were two to four times as likely to die in the first five years, when compared to optimistic women. Denial would have to be classified as optimistic. If you don't have cancer, or believe it's not serious, it certainly can't do you much harm—a strong reason for optimism.

Researchers at Ohio State University conducted a study and found that pessimism may have a stronger negative influence on disease than the positive impact of optimistic thinking. They discovered that pessimistic adults were more likely to report higher levels of stress and anxiety than optimistic people. When they looked at the two groups a year later, the pessimistic group reported poorer overall health.

It seems to me that one role for physicians should be helping patients to maintain hope and optimism. This doesn't mean becoming a Pollyanna. I don't think, however, that physicians should make pronouncements like "You've got three months to live." This can become a curse. Look at it this way. The patient has a great deal of respect and confidence in his doctor. He has developed a deep trust in his doctor, much like the relationship between a religious devotee and his spiritual leader. The doctor's opinion has great importance in this context. A statement like the one above may be tantamount to a death sentence in this setting. If not one before, the patient immediately becomes a member of the "helpless and hopeless" set. This can lead to depression and lassitude. As we've seen, such suppression of emotional response has been linked with a decline in natural killer cell activity. Logically, this may accelerate the tumor's growth, resulting in a downward spiral. The prophecy is fulfilled.

Not only is this unfortunate, it's also inaccurate. The physician has no way of knowing that this particular individual will survive three months. It may be accurate that the median survival for men with comparable disease is three months, but as we've discussed, statistics don't apply to individual cases. Median survival means that half the men will live longer than three months, some much longer. The truth is that the doctor is extrapolating from a group statistic to an individual case and, in the process, stripping the man of hope. To me, this is not good medicine.

What's a better approach? I'd respond this way, "Survival depends on a complex set of factors and is difficult to predict. I could give you a statistic that would apply to a large group of men with similar levels of disease, but this almost certainly does not apply to your situation. Some studies show that people who keep battling live longer. Let's discuss the available options and determine together the best course for you to take from now on."

A statement like this supports the patient in his battle and reinforces the thinking that's most likely to be helpful in extending survival. Pronouncements, such as the first example, seem to me to have the opposite effect.

In the words of Dr. Keith Block, director of the Block Medical Center in Evanston, Illinois, "Initial coping responses, such as despair and helplessness, may trigger a cascade of neuroendocrine processes that compromise the very immune mechanisms the individual needs to keep malignant tumors and micrometastases in check. Conversely, positive coping behaviors appear to help keep the immune system actively engaged in neoplastic surveillance and cytotoxic activities, thereby discouraging the progression of cancer." One role of a care-giver, according to Dr. Block, is to provide "an unrelenting life-affirming attitude," allowing patients to experience "the optimism of possibility." This way "people feel more whole, more alive, more engaged with life, and inspired to go on living."

Excellent clinicians are careful not to strip patients of hope. Quoting earlier investigators Dufault and Martocchio, Dr. Block provides this excellent definition of hope, "A multidimensional life force characterized by a confident yet uncertain expectation of achieving a good future that, to the hoping person, is realistically possible and personally significant."

Good doctors provide the tools for positive coping. Although this hasn't been conclusively proven to improve outcome, it will certainly provide a better quality of life. As Dr. Block points out, "Quality of life is inseparable from the biological, psychological, and psychosocial context for maintaining sound health." It may also improve immune function.

Bottom line: The patient feels better and may be better equipped to fight the cancer.

Key Reference

Block K. The role of the self in healthy cancer survivorship: A view from the front lines of treating cancer. *Advances: The Journal of Mind-Body Health* 1997; 13: 6-26.

Will Power

I have read about many cases where people with terminal diseases survive far longer than "expectation" when they have a specific target or time goal. This goal is often an important event: a child's wedding, a college graduation, or an anniversary.

Although I found this interesting, I didn't pay much attention to it. Then, one day, events emblazened this phenomenon in my memory.

When my mother was dying of lung cancer, she vowed that she would "make it" to her 79th birthday. Several months prior to her birthday her cancer progressed dramatically. She became totally bedridden, was jaundiced (yellow skin and eyes), and had a large mass of cancer in her abdomen. She was on supportive care only.

She said, "It doesn't look good, but I will make it to my birthday." I lived a great distance from her and she told me to "make travel plans to be here on my birthday."

"I wouldn't miss it for the world," I replied.

She continued to slowly decline until a week before her birthday, when her condition started to rapidly deteriorate. She had trouble breathing and required continuous oxygen. She flitted in and out of consciousness. In response to an urgent summons, I arrived two days before her birthday. My mother was unconscious. She did not open her eyes and did not acknowledge my presence. Her breathing was heavy and labored. She was severely jaundiced.

The next day, one day before her birthday, she was still alive. It seemed to me that she was struggling to stay alive. Each breath seemed a tremendous effort. Knowing her vow to survive until her birthday and thinking she might still be able to hear me, I decided to ease her burden. I said softly, "Mom, it's your birthday. You can let go now."

To my utter amazement, her eyes opened suddenly and she said, "Not till tomorrow." These were the only three words she had uttered in two days! How she could keep track of the time she needed to fulfill her goal is beyond me. At 4 a.m. the day of her birthday, a scant four hours into the day, her fight ended.

Had I, and others, not witnessed this, I might have been incredulous. The power of will can be marvelous. Just how this works physiologically is a mystery to which I'd love to know the answer.

Helpful Mental Factors

- Learn all you can about prostate cancer.
- Be actively involved in the decision-making process. Take control of your disease.
- Determination to defeat the cancer and maintain an active engaging existence may help improve outcome.
- Adherence is important if you make the decision to change your lifestyle.
- Seek out physicians with whom you can establish a close working rapport. A physician-patient partnership is likely to be more effective than a dominant-submissive doctor-patient relationship.

21

STRESS REDUCTION

What Is Stress?

The human body is equipped with hormones that get "switched on" in potentially dangerous situations. These stress hormones provide added strength for fighting or improve the ability to run away from a threat. These "fight-or-flight" hormones are produced primarily by the adrenal glands. Epinephrine (adrenalin) and norepinephrine (noradrenalin) are the main stress hormones.

When we respond to an acute situation, such as rescuing a drowning child from a swimming pool, we get a burst of stress hormones. This temporarily raises our heart rate, respiration rate, and blood pressure, pumping more oxygenated blood into our muscles where it's needed. Soon after the emergency has passed, hormone levels subside and body functions return to normal.

Modern society has introduced new sources of stress (stressors) into daily life. Psychological stress, prevalent for many individuals attempting to cope with the ever-increasing rate of change, also causes release of stress hormones. Unlike physical stressors that are acute but intermittent, psychological stressors occur far more frequently. For some they become almost constant. In situations such as this, stress hormones have little or no opportunity to return to baseline levels. They may remain continually elevated. This can lead to persistently elevated blood pressure, rapid pulse, and rapid shallow respiration. Experientially, the individual feels a sense of anxiety or nervousness, responses that are characterized as "chronic stress."

Does Stress Impact Life Expectancy?

This is difficult to measure in a prospective randomized study, so it cannot be said conclusively that chronic stress reduces life expectancy. However, a plethora of evidence indicates that high stress levels and long life don't go together.

The association of stress with a variety of chronic diseases is well-established. High stress levels are associated with increased incidence of heart attacks and high blood pressure. Reports in the literature associate stress with increases in everything from colds to cancer.

Stress is caused by environmental changes. Even so called "positive" environmental changes, such as taking a trip, moving to a new house, or getting married, can be stressful. Individual adaptation to stress varies. Some people cope well with change, while other get stressed-out.

Dr. Thomas Perls at Harvard Medical School studied 150 centenarians in an attempt to discover traits associated with long life. Here's what he reported.

"*Every person* [italics mine] we studied tested low for levels of neuroticism—unhealthy feelings of extreme anger, fear, anxiety, or sadness. These feelings can disturb heartbeats, reduce immune functioning, and even accelerate the aging process. The people in our group all had the ability to easily shed emotional stress, tended to be calm and collected during crises, and easily adapted to changes in their environment."

Dr. Perls suggests, "Stress-reduction techniques, such as daily meditation and deep-breathing exercises, can be helpful. Learning to adapt to changing situations is another common characteristic among our winning 100-year olds. But adaptability entails more than responding to outside forces. Equally important is the ability to take charge of life situations."

Ways To Reduce Stress

Change your environment—To some extent stress can be reduced by eliminating stressful environmental influences. Avoiding toxic people (ATP) is a good start. I shy away from people who anger easily, exhibit high levels of anxiety, are depressed, or tend to chronically complain. If you hang out with people like this and are empathetic, you can't help but raise your own stress level in the process. ATP is a good start in removing environmental stress.

Change your thinking—How you think about things that happen can also make a difference in stress levels. Case in point: prostate cancer. For some it's viewed as a death sentence; for others it's a wake-up call. This latter group uses cancer as a catalyst for constructive lifestyle changes. Their nutrition and exercise programs improve and they interlace stress-reduction techniques into their lives while treating their disease. They come out the other side as better rounded, more adaptive, and in better physical and mental condition than ever before. For others, prostate cancer can be a downward spiral of despondency, neglect, helplessness, and depression from which they never recover.

Stress-Reduction Techniques

Stress-reduction techniques include meditation, breathing, yoga, tai chi, qi gong, progressive relaxation training, biofeedback, guided imagery, massage, and aromatherapy. Many books have been written on these subjects, and it's beyond the scope of this book to examine these in detail. It might be helpful, though, to tell you about a few methods that have worked for me.

Meditation—Many years ago when I started meditating, I found it to be difficult to do even for 20 minutes. My mind kept ticking over. Every minute or two I'd open my eyes and check my watch. Rarely, if ever, did I experience a "relaxation response," a state of complete relaxation accompanied by a slowing of pulse and respiration and a drop in blood pressure (the opposite of a stress response).

Then I discovered "high-tech" meditation. Although purists may shudder, high-tech meditation "meditates you," entraining your brain waves into patterns associated with deep meditation states. Using a Walkman, earphones, and brain-entrainment cassette tapes, I was soon able to meditate for 30 minutes at a sitting. I did this twice a day. Gradually, I was able to extend the sessions to an hour.

Brain-entrainment tapes provide pleasant listening. The functional program that entrains the brain into progressively slower brainwave patterns is masked by a music overlay. As I sat in my chair listening to the pleasant drone of East Indian musical instruments, I could feel the relaxation response being triggered as thoughts melted away. Brain-entrainment tapes or CDs can be obtained from Synchronicity at 800/962-2033.

Yoga—Yoga is discussed in the section on exercise. It provides strength, endurance, flexibility, balance, and stress-reduction benefits. I go to an hour-long yoga class three times a week. Tai chi and qi gong are useful alternatives to yoga. All these Eastern disciplines have one thing in common: deep abdominal breathing. Some experts believe this is why they reduce stress (see below).

Massage—Massage, especially one of the Eastern techniques, if received regularly will help reduce stress and may stimulate the immune system. Studies show that natural killer cells may increase after massage. I prefer shiatsu, ayurvedic, or Thai massage to the more common Swedish massage. Practitioners of one or more of these Eastern disciplines are available in most big cities (see Appendix IV).

Breathing techniques—Techniques involving breathing are generally underutilized. In my opinion, breathing exercises are one of the most important adjuncts to stress reduction, chi generation, and the ability to fight disease.

Why is breathing so important for stress reduction? We've already touched on the fact that stress is linked with shallow rapid breathing. This has physical consequences. It can cause blood vessels to constrict, reducing the amount of oxygen that's delivered to the brain and muscles. This can result in tense muscles and headaches that add to feelings of anxiety.

It's important to break this debilitating cycle. Breathing should be deep, flowing, and slow. It's a learned behavior, like learning how to ride a bike. Once learned, it's easy to do. Often, it becomes a new salubrious pattern of behavior. I find the best time to practice stress-reducing breathing techniques is while driving my car or sitting at my desk. At stoplights or in heavy stop-and-go traffic, or while working at the computer, I practice breathing. I breathe in deeply through my nose, filling my abdomen, then out, forcefully, through my mouth. As I repeat this pattern over and over, my breaths start to come more regularly. After a while they become rhythmic, smooth, and flowing. Together with this rhythmic slow pattern of deep abdominal breathing comes a diminution of tension and headaches. I begin to feel calm and relaxed. Over time, this has become my new breathing habit, an essential change for the better.

To complement this breathing exercise, I use a similar technique at home. Why not give it a try? Lie on your back on a bed or the floor with bent knees and the soles of your feet flat on the floor. Breathe deeply through your nose, filling your abdomen first, then your chest. Exhale forcefully through your mouth. Inhale again in the same fashion as soon as you feel the urge. Exhale forcefully. Don't force the inhalations and don't hold your breath by conscious effort. In other words, just allow a flow to be established. Start by doing this breathing exercise for just a few minutes per session. Two sessions daily, one upon awakening and one just before sleeping, are recommended. Gradually increase the time to about 10-15 minutes.

As you increase the duration of this breathing exercise, you may feel a tingling in your fingertips or around the corners of your mouth. Don't be alarmed. This is due to a change in blood gases induced by the breathing. Should your hands start to cramp, breathe normally for a minute or two until the cramp subsides, then continue the exercise. Don't push yourself to the point where you feel uncomfortable. As you gain experience, you'll be able to breathe deeply for longer periods of time.

The goal here is gradually to re-train your habit of shallow breathing to a more healthy pattern. By combining this home exercise with your driving and office exercise, you'll eventually change your breathing pattern from a stress-related pattern to one associated with relaxation. Establishing salubrious breathing habits complement the balance established by better eating, drinking, and exercise habits.

Changing your breathing pattern reduces stress. When you feel tense or anxious, pay attention to your breathing. If you notice it's rapid and shallow and limited to your chest, override it and start breathing more deeply and slowly into your abdomen. It works!

Guided Imagery

Guided imagery uses imaginary visuals to help evoke a relaxation response. Cassette tapes or CDs are the most common sources of imagery, although live sessions are also provided in the office by some adjunctive cancer therapists. In a typical session, you may be asked to visualize yourself in a place that you associate with peace and calm. It may be stretched out at a beach with gently breaking waves, lying in tall fragrant grass beside a bubbling brook, or perched on a mountain watching a magnificent sunset. You'll be encouraged to relax more deeply, to breathe more slowly and deeply, to imagine wafting fragrances or the salt air.

Sometimes you may be asked to focus on a blue-purple ball in your mind's eye or travel to a golden waterfall. "The closer you get the more relaxed you'll feel," drones the soothing voice of the facilitator.

Guided imagery can also be used more actively. You may be asked to visualize your immune cells as colored Pac-men roaming through your blood stream and gobbling up any cancer cells they may encounter.

Chemical Changes Associated with the Relaxation Response

A variety of neuroimmunologic chemical changes have been associated with a regularly induced relaxation response. Here they are.

• An increase in endorphins—hormones released by the brain with a chemical structure similar to Valium. These not only facilitate relaxation, but also increase feelings of well-being or euphoria.

• An increase in the number of natural killer cells and other cytotoxic lymphocytes. The stress hormones epinephrine (adrenalin) and norepinephrine (noradrenalin) have been shown to stimulate prostate cancer cell proliferation in the laboratory. Interestingly, recent autopsy studies of men who died of prostate cancer reveal that the fifth most common site of prostate cancer metastases is the adrenal glands. It appears as though an affinity exists between prostate cancer cells and stress hormones. Deep relaxation reduces stress, lowers stress hormones and, presumably, decelerates the rate of growth of prostate cancer.

The Importance of Good Social Support

Can social support influence survival? A number of studies indicate that it can. One study prospectively followed a group of more than 300 cancer patients (154 men) for 17 years. The researchers found that men with the fewest social contacts survived a significantly shorter time. Similarly, in a group of women with breast cancer, Dr. Maunsell and colleagues found a positive association between social support and survival.

Married men with prostate cancer tend to fare better than men who live without a partner. Men with closely knit families also seem to benefit. Why? Perhaps these social connections are "de-stressors." Perhaps the comfort of close relationships strengthens the immune system by defusing debilitating emotions and helping men better deal with stress.

Man is a social animal. Social support reduces stress for

most of us. Besides close family ties, additional support can come from religious groups and prostate cancer support groups.

Prostate Cancer Support Groups

Support groups for men with prostate cancer have been organized worldwide. Us Too and Man-to-Man are two of the largest organizations. Here men can share their cancer-related problems, including their emotions, with like-minded men. Besides providing valuable social support and comraderie, these groups also help disseminate valuable new innovations in the treatment of prostate cancer. I believe such support groups should be considered by most men with prostate cancer. (For contact information, see Appendix IV.)

Key References

Anderson J. The immune system and major depression. *Adv Neuroimmunol* 1996; 6: 119-129.

Leonard B and Song C. Stress and the immune system in the etiology of anxiety and depression. *Pharmacol Biochem Behav* 1996; 54: 299-303.

Newschaffer C et al. Causes of death in elderly prostate cancer patients and in a comparison non-prostate cancer cohort. *J Natl Can Inst* 2000; 92: 613-621.

Reynolds P and Kaplan G. Social connections and risk of cancer: prospective evidence from the Alameda County study. *Behav Med* 1990; 16: 101-110.

Maunsell E et al. Social support and survival among women with breast cancer. *Cancer* 1995; 76: 631-637.

Conclusion

Regardless of how you get there, a number of experts in prostate cancer, including myself, believe that regularly triggering a relaxation response and clearing your mind of cluttering thoughts is beneficial to overall health and quality of life. Reducing stress will probably also reduce your risk of heart attacks. Other undesirable symptoms (headaches, head and neck tension) are likely to be relieved. Blood pressure may drop a few points. You're also likely to feel better. Stress and anxiety are not pleasant. Getting rid of them is a great boon. If you're successful enough, perhaps you'll be one of the 100-plus-year-old men in Dr. Perls next study.

Recent autopsy studies reveal that about 40% of men diagnosed with prostate cancer ultimately succumb to the disease, while about 23% die of heart disease and more than 11% die of other cancers. Learning how to reduce stress, improve nutrition, and exercise is known not only to reduce heart disease, but is associated with reduced risks of many cancers. Making appropriate lifestyle adjustments now may not only be remedial for your present cancer, but is likely to help prevent other debilitative conditions in the future. This is something totally within your control. All it requires is changing your habits. Once you make the switch, these changes will become habitual too. You'll be replacing debilitating habits with more salubrious ones. It's difficult for me to conceive of a situation that provides more incentive than this.

22

PUTTING IT ALL TOGETHER

Japanese Lifestyle and Prostate Cancer

I wrote this section in Japan. Although I've traveled to Japan on numerous occasions, I'd never before done so with prostate cancer as my focus. I wanted to get a first-hand peek at what might be protecting these people from developing clinical prostate cancer. Here's what I found.

Diet

Japanese men consume an average of 2,000 calories/day. In the three weeks I spent in Japan on this particular trip, green tea was served at every meal. It was provided in my room at every inn and hotel. It was also served at business meetings, as a welcome drink at the home of friends, and by some shops that I visited. Drinking 10 cups a day was easy. Some days I drank much more. Green tea in Japan is as common as water in America. It's rare to see water served in a restaurant in Japan, however. Green tea is the predominant national drink. It's available in most vending machines as iced green tea. It's even used in many desserts, such as green-tea ice cream, green-tea and bean muffins, and ice with green tea syrup. In short, it's ubiquitous.

Soy is another dietary staple. I ate soy several times a day without having to seek it out. Miso soup is served for breakfast and often for dinner too. Natto, fermented soybeans, is a popular breakfast food in the countryside. Tofu is prepared often and creatively. I had several meals in Buddhist temples made exclusively from soy and vegetables, yet with the flavors of duck, chicken, and fish. The variety of flavors and textures was unbelievable. The aesthetically sensitive presentation added to the experience.

Milk, cheese, cream, butter, and yogurt are uncommon. Ice cream is popular, but not often consumed in rural areas, especially at home.

As for fiber, besides soybeans, the Japanese consume large quantities of other beans. Japanese red (adzuke) beans are found in an amazing array of sweets available in numerous shops. They're eaten regularly. Rice, of course, is a staple, generally eaten 2-3 times a day. Soba (buckwheat noodles) and udon (thick rice noodles) are popular lunch items. Add to this a variety of vegetables (spinach is the most popular) and fruits, and you have a high fiber diet rich in antioxidants.

Fish is eaten often, but meat only occasionally and in small quantities. This pattern is changing in the big cities, but continues in agrarian areas.

The Japanese love edible mushrooms: shiitake, maitake, enoki, matsutake, shimeji, etc. Many of these mushrooms seem to have stimulating effects on the immune system, according to a number of Japanese studies. An anti-cancer preparation extracted from the shiitake mushroom has been approved by the Japanese equivalent of the FDA for use in Japan. Mushroom extracts have not been widely studied in the West. Eating these mushrooms in their natural food forms seems quite safe, and may help the immune system.

Exercise

The Japanese often ride bicycles, especially in rural areas. In the big cities they ride subways, which are economical and widely used. Now, you wouldn't think that riding a subway would be good exercise, would you? Well, it is. Subway stations are underground. They average about 40 steps to reach the platform. Escalators are rare. A Japanese man taking the subway to work and back daily must navigate 160 steps, 80 up and 80 down. If he has to change trains (which is usual), add another 160 steps. If he goes off to a business lunch, it's 160 more. Add an afternoon business meeting? You get the picture. Their daily routine includes a fair amount of walking and a lot of stairs. Just for kicks, I counted the stairs I climbed (including ups and downs) in a day of sightseeing. More than 800! Who needs a stair machine when you've got this kind of natural "subway exercise"!

Downsides

Are there any downsides to the Japanese lifestyle? Several. They work long hours and generally have high stress levels. Meditation is not nearly as common as it once was (no time). Japanese also smoke more than Americans. They eat large quantities of heavily salted preserved foods, such as pickled vegetables *(tsukemono)*. These are served at nearly every meal. Numerous stores sell only these salty pickled vegetables.

The Japanese also relish very hot temperatures for their tea, soups, and noodles. I saw Japanese people eating noodles that were too hot for me to even put in my mouth. The combination of high stress, heavy smoking, a lot of salty preserved foods, and scalding beverages is believed to be related to the high incidence of esophageal and stomach cancer in Japan. Lung cancer is also a problem. But as far as prostate (and breast) cancer is concerned, the Japanese lifestyle seems practically ideal.

The Michael Milken Saga

If you don't happen to be Japanese, you can still live a prostate-cancer-friendly lifestyle. Perhaps the best way to illustrate how to use the principles elucidated in this section is by reviewing an exemplary case history—that of Michael

Milken, international financier and philanthropist.

In 1993, Mike went to his internist for a routine physical exam. It was completely normal. According to the physician, Milken was in excellent health. A DRE was done. The doctor said Mike's prostate was "normal." Routine blood work was ordered. It did not include a PSA. The physician assured Mike that he was "too young" (46 years old) to get prostate cancer, so a PSA was unnecessary. But Milken had a premonition. One of his closest friends had just died of prostate cancer. He'd also lost seven relatives to cancer. He told the doctor, "I can afford the test. Humor me." When his PSA came back at 24, the doctor told him it had to be a lab error. It wasn't.

Mike went to see Dr. Stuart (Skip) Holden, an excellent urologist in private practice in Los Angeles. A repeat DRE, now by a more skilled finger, identified a mass on Milken's prostate. (Once again, this emphasizes the importance of having your annual prostate exam done by a urologist rather that by an internist or general practitioner.) From here, Mike was barraged with a spate of bad news. A repeat PSA confirmed a reading in the mid-20s. A prostate biopsy revealed a highly aggressive (Gleason score 9) adenocarcinoma of the prostate. An MRI was grossly abnormal, indicating the likelihood of pelvic lymph-node involvement. This was subsequently confirmed by biopsy; the cancer had already spread beyond the prostate to the pelvic nodes. Mike was devastated.

Milken now underwent more tests to see if the cancer had spread even further. A bone scan was negative. This was the first bit of good news that he had received since his nightmare began. So, although the disease had spread to the pelvic lymph nodes, there was no sign that it had spread to bone.

After the initial shock wore off, Mike approached his medical condition with the same cool logic and discipline that had served him so well in the investment community.

"The day after my diagnosis, I stopped eating," Mike

recalls. "I had lost seven relatives to cancer. They had tried many things, all of which had failed. But none had changed their diet. So that's the first thing I did—I changed my diet drastically. I cut way back on my food intake and stopped eating meat. I lived almost entirely on steamed vegetables and fruit."

Mike read everything he could get his hands on about prostate cancer. He traveled across the country talking with experts in the field. He concluded that his disease was too far along to consider surgery, so he started hormonal therapy: complete androgen blockade.

"I went to more than a dozen cancer centers," Mike recalls. Having received the best information that Western medicine had to offer, he turned to complementary medicine to strengthen his immune system and reduce stress. He visited with Dr. Deepak Chopra, the well-known and respected ayurvedic medicine physician. From him, Mike learned meditation and experienced immune-system-stimulating ayurvedic massage. To this day Milken meditates regularly and gets a weekly ayurvedic massage.

Next, he went to China to study *chi* with a *chi* master in the mountains outside of Beijing. As you'll remember from the section on incorporating Eastern medicine in your treatment plan, *chi* is the body's natural bio-electrical current. Accentuating the flow of this *chi* current, according to Chinese medicine, strengthens the immune system and creates balance and harmony in the body. This helps ward off disease; it primes your immune system to kill cancer cells. Mike learned *qi gong* and other *chi*-generating techniques.

Returning to the United States, he met with Tom Laughlin, author of *The Six Psychological Factors that May Lead to Cancer—And What You Can Do About Them: Plus Proof that the Mind Plays a Significant Role in Cancer and Other Diseases.* From Laughlin, Milken learned about the mind-body connection and the importance of mental attitude in combating disease.

Mike visited Dr. Dean Ornish in Sausalito, California.

He'd known Dr. Ornish since 1983, when he first funded his research. From Ornish, an expert in human nutrition, he learned more about diet. Dr. Ornish extolled the virtues of a low-fat, high-fiber, vegan diet. Dr. Ornish also emphasized exercise, yoga, and meditation as part an anti-cancer heart-friendly lifestyle.

Vowing to keep an open mind and explore all possibilities, Milken met with Dr. Tenagawa at M.I.T. Dr. Tenagawa is an expert at aromatherapy. Mike learned how various scents may strengthen the immune system, promote relaxation, and reduce stress.

Armed with all this information, Mike established a new lifestyle for himself. Religiously, he stuck to his new diet, consuming less than 10 grams of fat daily, mostly in the form of soy products. He ate sparingly, controlling his calories. He established a regular exercise, meditation, and massage routine.

"I visited gardens and rented a house by the beach," Mike recalls. "I went out there every other day. I meditated or just sat and listened to the ocean. I took walks along the sea and smelled the water. I still go regularly to smell the sea. There is something therapeutic about the smell of the ocean."

After four months of hormonal therapy combined with the complementary techniques he had assimilated, Milken's PSA dropped to undetectable levels and stayed down. Several months later he decided that his cancer had reached a point of minimal activity. Now, he reasoned, it was at its most vulnerable point. This was the optimal time to hit it with what would, hopefully, be a knockout punch. He opted for a course of high-intensity 3-D conformal external beam radiation.

Amazingly, he sailed through the course of radiation without any side effects. He's stayed on hormones since the day he started. He's avoided osteoporosis, a common side effect from long-term hormone therapy, by using bisphosphonates as part of a clinical trial. He also does high-resistance weight training. Last year he gained bone density by 4%. As you may recall, this is normally the annual loss of bone density for men taking hormones.

In 1993 Mike started the Prostate Cancer Foundation, a non-profit public charity dedicated to finding controls and cures for prostate cancer. Since then, the Prostate Cancer Foundation has funded some 1,100 research awards, mostly for clinical research on prostate cancer. The Prostate Cancer Foundation is the world's largest non-governmental source of funds for research on prostate cancer. Recently, CaP CURE has changed its name to the Prostate Cancer Foundation.

By providing funding for complementary therapy as well as traditional approaches, Milken has helped establish a role for prostate cancer treatments such as PC-SPES. Research such as this would have been very difficult to fund without the help of the Prostate Cancer Foundation. As Dr. William Catalona, Chairman of the Department of Urology at Washington University Medical School in St. Louis, put it, Milken "has done more to advance the cause of prostate cancer than anyone."

In 1995, Milken recruited Beth Ginsberg as his personal chef. With the help of nutritionalists like Dean Ornish and David Heber, combined with her own prodigious culinary talents, Beth started improvising. Her mission was to duplicate the taste of the things Mike liked to eat, but to change the ingredients. She substituted healthy foods, such as tofu, applesauce, and vegetables, for meat, oil, and fats. Beth is wonderfully creative and worked out ways to make healthy Reuben sandwiches, manicotti, French fries, brownies, and even—get this!—Hostess Twinkies. Beth believes that by substituting ingredients, the taste of any dish can be duplicated, converting it from a health hazard full of fat, to a heart-, prostate- and breast-friendly food. This is a revolutionary concept in health. As Milken puts it, "We must educate the kids, not to choose different foods, but on how to use and understand the need for healthy ingredients. It is important to start education on nutrition when children are young."

Milken and Ginsberg have produced two cookbooks, containing a cornucopia of delectable dishes from all over the world. The first book, *The Taste for Living Cookbook—Michael Milken's Favorite Recipes for Fighting Cancer,* is a best seller. The second cookbook, released in 1999, is called *The Taste for Living World Cookbook, More of Mike Milken's Favorite Recipes for Fighting Cancer and Heart Disease.* In these two books you will find all the recipes you'll need to provide you with great variety and flavor while improving your health. My wife easily learned how to make these dishes and now does her own improvisations. She tells me the recipes are easy to follow. I can attest to the great taste. The bottom line is that it's possible, in fact easy, to eat healthfully without sacrificing taste. Great stuff!

I asked Milken about supplements. He regards them as part of his diet. He makes a daily drink using soy protein isolate, brewed green tea, fruit, fruit juice, vitamin E, selenium, modified citrus pectin, and green-tea capsules. He says, "I don't know whether it's better to get these things from food or supplements, so I do both."

Well, there you have it. Has all the study, effort, and discipline paid off for Milken? It's now more than 10 years since he was diagnosed with aggressive metastatic prostate cancer. Today, his PSA is zero—undetectable! He feels great and is as active as ever.

Just lucky? I don't think so. He did his research and applied himself assiduously to the task of re-establishing wellness. He is a prime example of the rewards that can be reaped by taking control of your disease, getting the best medical care available, and implementing lifestyle changes designed to promote physical and mental well-being. You can do the same thing. All the tools are available to you.

Although prostate cancer is a great catalyst for significant lifestyle modifications, I urge those of you who are free of cancer to make these changes now. This way, you'll reduce the odds of getting cancer or heart disease. Why wait? The life you save may be your own.

SECTION III:

NEW AND FUTURE DEVELOPMENTS

23

WHAT'S ON
THE HORIZON

This chapter was both the most fascinating and the most difficult to write. I could literally write a whole book about new and experimental agents currently being investigated to treat or prevent prostate cancer.

The future for men with prostate cancer is brightening. These days, deaths from prostate cancer are down 10,000, or about 25%, from five years earlier. According to urologist and Medical Director of the Prostate Cancer Foundation, Dr. Stuart Holden, "Patients today unequivocally live longer at every stage of prostate cancer. Prostate cancer is becoming a chronic illness, not immediately life-threatening." For those of us with prostate cancer, this is of some comfort. It provides new hope that we can survive until remedies are developed that either provide a cure or hold the disease at bay long enough that it is no longer life-threatening.

Here are some reasons for hope:

• Spending on prostate cancer increased from $100 million in 1996 to $400 million in 2000.

• Many quality people are now involved at all levels of prostate cancer research. Brilliant minds are focused on finding new treatments and a cure.

• Biotech and pharmaceutical companies have become very interested in prostate cancer. At the seventh annual Prostate Cancer Foundation retreat in September 2000, thirty-one companies gave presentations.

New developments are exploding, in large part due to the genetic-medicine revolution. With the completion of the mapping of the human genome has come a scramble to identify genes involved in cancer. Already five hereditary genes involved in prostate cancer have been identified. Environmental factors that affect gene expression have also been identified. As Dr. Richard Klausner, Director of the National Cancer Institute, puts it, "Cancer is a disease of genomic instability leading to cellular change." The normal balance between cellular growth stimulation and suppression is lost in the cancer cell. They become immortal.

Clinical Trials

On the following pages, you'll see frequent mention of clinical trials. These occur in varying stages, designated Phase I, Phase II, and Phase III. Sometimes Phase I and Phase II trials are combined into a single trial designated Phase I/II.

Here's what these various trials mean:

Phase I—A trial used to determine the safety, dosage, and side effects of an experimental drug or therapy.

Phase II—A trial used to determine the preliminary activity and efficacy of a new drug or treatment.

Phase III—A large randomized study often involving multiple medical centers used to conclusively determine the efficacy of a new drug or treatment as compared to the standard treatment currently available. This is the final step in the long process of FDA approval for the clinical use of a new treatment.

It now appears that multiple mechanisms may be at work, resulting in these cellular abnormalities.

Thanks to the Human Genome Project, it will ultimately be possible to pinpoint the exact genetic defect(s) in each cancer patient. Knowing this will allow doctors to categorize patients into different prognostic categories and to recommend therapeutic programs tailored to individual genetic abnormalities.

By understanding the mechanisms by which cancer cells attain immortality and invade, migrate, and colonize in distant tissues, scientists can create specific therapies to intercede in this process. Genes will be manipulated either to shut off the production of undesirable proteins, or to increase the output of protective ones.

• Vaccines are being developed. Some are already in clinical trials. More vaccine-based therapies are under development in the field of prostate cancer than in any other disease.

• Advances are also being made in chemotherapy. Some regimens provide clear survival advantages for men with late-stage disease. Several protocols consistently provide more than a 50% reduction in PSA levels in more than 60% of men. This response rate is on a par with breast cancer. It may now be possible to alter the progress of prostate cancer by using chemo early in the disease when it has the potential to cure, especially when combined with radiation, surgery, or hormones. This is how it is currently used in women with breast cancer.

• Investigators are finding that combination therapies may be synergistic and additive. Two remedies, each individually active against prostate cancer, may be more than twice as effective when combined. Some approaches involve combining a drug that kills prostate cancer cells with one that strengthens the immune system or blocks the development of new blood vessel formation to the tumor.

In the following pages, I summarize some of the most promising advances in our understanding of prostate cancer. New information on nutrition, diagnosis, surgery, radiation, brachytherapy, and hormones is presented. I also cover vaccines, angiogenesis inhibitors, and a variety of innovative drugs and drug combinations. Due to the sheer volume of material, I've encapsulated the information as much as possible.

Much of this information comes from the Prostate Cancer Foundation retreats. I am deeply indebted to Dr. Howard Soule and the people at the Prostate Cancer Foundation for providing me with the opportunity to attend these retreats, allowing me to conclude this book with many of the exciting events currently under way. As one investigator at a retreat put it, "Prostate cancer has reached an inflection point from which developments will now grow exponentially."

Here goes.

Nutrition

Leafy Greens

Dr. David Heber, Director of the UCLA Center for Human Nutrition, is studying dietary differences between men in rural Shanghai who have very low rates of prostate cancer, men from rural Shanghai who migrated to the United States at least 15 years ago, and American Caucasians. He has discovered that the men in rural Shanghai eat much less polyunsaturated fat than men living in the U.S. Additionally, the men living in China eat much more green leafy vegetables than their American compatriots. The Chinese men in China have lutein levels that are four times higher and zeaxanthin levels that are twice as high as U.S.-based men.

Dr. Heber thinks that the high levels of lutein and zeaxanthin in the Shanghainese diet may play a role in protection against prostate cancer. Interestingly, men in Shanghai consume very few tomato products (lycopene), yet their rate of prostate cancer is still very low. The high consumption of leafy green vegetables may compensate for this. Other lifestyle factors, such as heavy manual labor, different bacteria in their digestive tracts (see "Equol" later in this chapter), soy consumption, calories, etc., may also play a role in limiting prostate cancer in China.

Dr. Heber recommends increasing the diversity of fruits and vegetables consumed, especially green leafy vegetables like spinach, kale, broccoli, and collard greens. If you like Chinese vegetables, try bok choi, choi som, and gailan (Chinese broccoli) available at most Chinese markets. Avocados are also high in lutein.

New Developments From Dr. Ed Giovannucci and the Harvard Health Professionals Study

Fish, if consumed four or more times weekly, is associated with a 50% reduction in the risk of prostate cancer. Whether this is due to the replacement of meat in the diet by fish or due to the nutrients in fish, such as omega-3 fatty acids or vitamin D, or both, is unknown. Dr. Giovannucci points out that fish is one of the best food sources of vitamin D. The omega-3 fatty acids in fish (DHA and EPA) may block arachidonic acid production. Arachadonic acid can be converted to harmful prostaglandins by the enzyme cyclooxygenase-2 (COX-2) and lipooxygenases (more on this later in this chapter).

Aspirin, when used long-term at least five times per week, is associated with greater than a 50% reduction in the risk of prostate cancer.

Calories and the amount of body mass (body mass index, or BMI) are associated with an increase in the risk of prostate cancer. The more calories you ingest and the more weight you put on, the greater the risk of prostate cancer. This may be related to the effect increased caloric intake and BMI have on hormonal factors like IGF-1, testosterone, and DHT. Men with the lowest caloric intake and the lowest body mass have the lowest incidence of prostate cancer.

Recommendations

- Replace red meat and chicken in your diet with fish.
- Take one baby aspirin daily to protect against both heart disease and prostate cancer.
- Eat fewer calories and exercise more to reduce your BMI. Stay lean and mean—and green!

Nutritional Factors That May Be Helpful in Avoiding Osteoporosis

The following may be especially useful for men on hormones:

• Green leafy vegetables are rich in vitamin K. High levels of vitamin K are associated with a reduced risk of hip fractures.

• An English study shows that women who drink tea have higher bone density that those who don't.

• High soy consumption has been associated with a reduced risk of osteoporosis.

The Latest on Lycopene

Dr. Gann from Northwestern University Medical School and Dr. Giovannucci from Harvard collaborated to study serum lycopene levels in men in the Physicians' Health study. They compared 578 men who developed prostate cancer within 13 years from the time the study started with 1,294 men who remained cancer free. The men were matched for age and smoking status. Lycopene levels were found to be significantly lower in the group of men who got prostate cancer. This was especially true for the men who developed aggressive cancers.

Higher blood levels of vitamin E were also associated with a reduced risk of aggressive prostate cancer, but this trend did not reach statistical significance.

These results confirm Dr. Giovannucci's earlier dietary studies, which showed a protective effect of tomato products against prostate cancer. The investigators conclude: "These data provide further evidence that increased consumption of tomato products and other lycopene-containing foods might reduce the occurrence or progression of prostate cancer."

Although smoking does not seem to be associated with an increased risk of getting prostate cancer, it is associated with a reduction in life expectancy for men who have it, according to Dr. Giovannucci.

Key Reference

Gann P, Ma J, Giovanucci E et al. Lower prostate cancer risk in men with elevated plasma lycopene levels: results of a prospective analysis. *Cancer Research* 1999; 59: 1225-1230.

Equol

At the September 2000 Prostate Cancer Foundation retreat, the now deceased Dr. Gary Miller, Professor of Pathology and Urology at the University of Colorado, presented some fascinating findings. Daidzein, one of the isoflavones in soy, can be converted in the body to a substance called "equol" (not to be confused with the artificial sweetener "Equal"). Equol is 100 times more potent than daidzein. It also decreases the proliferation of prostate cancer cells (which Daidzein doesn't).

Asians living in Asia have 100 times as much equol in their blood as Europeans. Two bacteria have been identified that convert daidzein to equol. These are found in Asians, but not in Europeans. There's a difference in the ability of Asian and Western men to convert daidzein to equol. This may be due to environmental factors, like food and water, or to a hereditary component.

If these bacterial differences can be isolated and put into a form that can be ingested and repopulate the digestive tract in Westerners, equol levels in Westerners can be raised to levels typically found in Asian men and prostate cancer may be able to be suppressed. Although this work is still in its early stages, it's pretty exciting stuff.

Exercise

Researchers from Duke University Medical Center tested exercise against the anti-depressant Zoloft, or a combination of the two, on a group of seriously depressed patients.

After four months, improvement was noted in 60% to 69% of the patients. But exercise was significantly better at keeping the depressive symptoms from returning than either Zoloft alone, or Zoloft combined with exercise.

Patients who exercised and were no longer clinically depressed after four months had only an 8% chance of a recurrence of their depression after 10 months; 38% of patients on Zoloft alone and 31% of patients on Zoloft combined with exercise had their depressive symptoms return. Why exercise alone seems to work better than exercise combined with Zoloft is not known.

Diagnosis and Screening

• In the past 10 years, the number of prostate cancer patients diagnosed with T1c disease (cancer detected by PSA, though not palpable by DRE) has increased from 11% to 64%. Average initial PSA readings have dropped from 11.0 to 6.6 during this same time period. Extracapsular extension has decreased from 80% of men to 40%. As discussed, the death rate has dropped 25% in the past five years. These results are due in large part to earlier detection of cancer.

Key Reference

Vogelzang N. Prostate cancer: Enhancing screening and improving local therapy. Report from the 35th annual meeting of the American Society of Clinical Oncology; May 17, 1999.

• Spectroscopic MRI may be useful in helping to determine tumor aggressivity. The chemical pattern is different in Gleason 6 or less tumors and in Gleason 7 or higher cancers. The prognostic accuracy of spectroscopic MRI was highly significant in a study of 26 cases of cancer proven by subsequent biopsy.

The combined use of endorectal MRI and spectroscopic

MRI will, in my opinion, become a standard part of the diagnostic evaluation. The latest erMRI statistics report a staging accuracy of between 75% and 90%. erMRI is 96% accurate in determining seminal vesicle involvement and 81% accurate in predicting extra-capsular extension.

Key Reference

Wood P, Durhanewicz J et al. The role of combined MRI and MRSI in treating prostate cancer. *PCRInsights* 2000, 3: 1-5.

• Future improvements in diagnosis and evaluation of cancer aggressiveness may include measuring a protein called "thymosin beta 15 (TB 15)" in prostate biopsy samples. This may prove helpful in determining which tumors are more likely to metastasize to bone, allowing for more intense early treatment in these men.

Dr. Arnab Chakravarti of Harvard Medical School and his associates observed that 62% of men with high levels of this protein in their biopsy tissue had their cancer spread to bone. Only 13% of men with the least amount of this protein developed bone metastases over an average (median) time of six years. Additionally, 83% of men with the lowest levels had no rise in PSA over this time period while only 25% of men with the greatest amounts of TB 15 were free from cancer as determined by PSA measurements.

Key Reference

Proceedings of the 91st Annual Meeting of the American Association for Cancer Research, as reported by Kevin Singer at the Oncology.com Web site.

• Finally, lasers are being developed to identify proteins in prostate cancer cells, BPH cells, and normal prostate cells. Early work points to a different pattern of proteins in each of these three cell types. Although still in its infancy, this technology, known as the "Protein Chip System," may prove useful in differentiating cancer, BPH, and normal prostates.

Watchful Waiting

A new study out of the University or California-San Francisco Medical Center followed 329 men who chose this conservative path. These men tended to be older (51% over age 75), have Gleason scores of 6 or less, and have organ-confined disease (97%). Fifty-two percent of the men who chose watchful waiting resorted to more aggressive therapy, usually hormones, within 5 years.

Ninety men with a median PSA of 5.0 who chose watchful waiting were followed at Johns Hopkins and monitored for about two years. Twenty-five selected other treatment during this period. Of the remaining 65 men, 24 progressed and 41 did not over a 2-year period. Urologist Dr. H. Ballentine Carter recommends that men who choose conservative management monitor their progress with prostate biopsies annually. In this study he found PSA was not a useful tool in predicting which men were progressing. Biopsy was much more reliable.

Key Reference

Proceedings of the 95th Annual Meeting of the American Urological Association, Atlanta, Georgia as reported by Kevin Singer at the Oncology.com Web site.

Surgery

• A new surgical procedure developed at the Mayo Clinic removes tissue surrounding the prostate more extensively. Removing the soft tissue surrounding the prostate right down to the wall of the rectum decreases the probability of positive surgical margins in men with extracapsular extension. While this sounds promising, it is not yet known how this will affect survival; also, the procedure has more side effects.

• Dr. Gerald Chodak, a urologist and professor at the University of Chicago, has developed a protocol that gets men out of the hospital 24 hours after radical prostatectomy. Using a combination of epidural anesthesia that blocks all pain during surgery, methadone for pain control after surgery, and extensive counseling, Dr. Chodak was able to send 74% of 252 patients home the day after surgery. It appears that this approach is safe and doesn't significantly add to post-surgery complications. Only three of the 187 men discharged one day after surgery were readmitted to the hospital for surgery-related complications.

• A multi-institutional trial is currently underway to test a new treatment for incontinence due to prostate surgery. Called "Extracorporeal Magnetic Innervation" or ExMI™ for short, it uses magnetic pulses to strengthen the pelvic muscles that provide bladder control by stimulating contractions. Treatments, using a machine that delivers painless magnetic pulses, are done in the doctor's office. This treatment is already being successfully used by gynecologists in women who leak urine. Participating in the study on male incontinence after prostate surgery are the University of Washington, the Mayo Clinic, the University of Pennsylvania, the Cleveland Clinic, Eastern Virginia Medical School, and Emory University Medical School.

External Beam Radiation Therapy (EBRT)

Big news here. Dr. Gerald Hanks reported at the 2000 meeting of the American Society of Clinical Oncology (ASCO) on a multi-center randomized study of more than 1,500 men with stage T3 or T4 prostate cancer. The study compared four months of complete androgen blockade combined with EBRT with the same regimen, but with an additional two years of CAB. Notably, there was a significant overall survival advantage in men with Gleason 8-10 tumors receiving the extra two years of hormones—80% survival compared with 69% in the men who got only four months of hormones. No survival advantage was detected at five years in men with Gleason 6 or less tumors.

According to Dr. D'Amico at Harvard, by the time you read this book another study will have been released on men with clinical stage T3 or T4 and Gleason 6 or less cancers. It will show that men who received four months of hormones and EBRT have a 5% survival advantage over men with comparable disease who received EBRT without hormonal blockade.

Increasing the dose of EBRT in men with high-risk cancers (Gleason 8-10) increases life expectancy and five-year freedom from cancer as determined by PSA testing, reports a multi-center group that pooled their data. Five-year overall survival improved from just under 60% in men receiving less than 70 Gy to just over 70% in men getting 70-75 Gy, and over 80% in men who received 75-80 Gy. Although this was a retrospective study, it confirms the results of other investigators. These results compare favorably, according to the authors of this study (led by Dr. Hanks), with published surgical data that report a 28% to 46% overall five-year survival in men with Gleason 8-10 cancers. IMRT should also be used, when available, in this high-risk group.

Conclusion: Although men with Gleason 6 or less tumors and clinical stage T3-T4 need to be studied longer, as of five years after treatment, there is no significant difference between four months of completed androgen blockade (CAB) and 28 months of CAB, in the ability to extend life when combined with EBRT. However, four months of CAB is significantly better than none.

Men with stage T3-T4 and Gleason 8-10 cancers need long-term hormone treatment combined with EBRT. A minimum of 28-36 months of hormones increases life expectancy. Depending on the situation, lifetime hormonal therapy may be the best course in extending survival in this group.

According to Dr. D'Amico, men with Gleason 7 tumors should be grouped with the Gleason 8-10 class. Gleason 4+3 cancers should be treated more aggressively with hormones than Gleason 3+4 tumors.

As discussed in the section on radiation, men with high-risk cancer (Gleason 8-10) should receive high-dose EBRT (at least 78 Gy), preferably combined with IMRT, along with hormonal therapy.

Radiation Sensitizers and Combination Therapies

One of the areas being developed in radiation therapy involves methods that increase the sensitivity of prostate cancer cells to the effects of radiation. Some of these agents are injected directly into the tumor, others are injected intravenously.

Combining radiation with chemo is one area under study. 5-fluorouracil (5-FU) is one such sensitizing agent. It's currently being evaluated in combination with radiation in breast cancer. It is unknown whether 5-FU sensitizes prostate cancer cells to radiation, but in the future investigations involving the combination of chemo and radiation are likely to proceed. Other "radiosensitizers" are also being investigated.

Future combination therapies besides chemo and, of course, hormones may include therapies designed to stimulate the immune system or to increase the expression of anti-tumor genes, like p53 or PTEN (see "Genetic Medicine" below).

Brachytherapy

Investigations are in progress using seeds combined with p53 gene therapy in men who have had a recurrence after radiation.

Interstitial Microwave Thermoablation

This experimental technique is being studied by Dr. John Trachtenberg at Princess Margaret Hospital in Toronto,

Canada. Going through the skin, this technique uses heat to kill cancer cells. It's being tested on men who have had a recurrence after radiation. One patient also received this treatment as primary therapy; after 18 months, his PSA was undetectable. This procedure is still highly experimental, but warrants further exploration.

Key Reference

Lancaster C, Toi A, and Trachtenberg J. Interstitial microwave thermoablation for localized prostate cancer. *Urology* 1999; 53: 828-831.

In the future, brachytherapy may include heat combined with seeds. Pre-clinical testing has begun at the University of California-San Francisco using microwave-focused heat. According to radiation oncologist Dr. Mack Roach, thermotherapy (heat) can double the effectiveness of radiation, provided the heat reaches the cancer cells.

Endorectal MRI is also being developed for use in combination with seeds. One of the current limitations of seeds is that they only cover 85%-95% of the prostate. Obviously, if cancer happens to be present in the 5% to 15% of the gland the radiation from the seeds misses, then some cancer cells survive. Using erMRI to guide seed placement, the minimum coverage can be increased to 97% of the prostate. In addition, more accurate seed placement improves the quality of life by reducing urinary and sexual complications. This technique is now being used by Dr. D'Amico at Harvard's Brigham and Women's Hospital.

Hormones

New developments in hormonal therapy include the forthcoming release of Viadur, a one-year depot LH-RH agonist. It was approved by the FDA in the summer of 2000 after successful clinical trials. Men on long-term hormonal therapy will only need to have Viadur, delivered via a titanium implant about the size of a toothpick, inserted annually. It provides constant daily hormone release.

A new hormone known as an LH-RH antagonist (as opposed to agonist) is far along in clinical testing. Sparing you the physiology, this drug reduces the risk of osteoporosis associated with long-term hormonal therapy. Removing this potentially serious side effect of hormones is an important advancement in hormonal therapy.

The use of 150 mg of Casodex daily, as a replacement for either medical or surgical castration, is provocative. To date, there has been only one study and it showed no significant difference in life expectancy between this high dose of Casodex and castration. However, experts I've talked to explain that this study was "underpowered," meaning that it consisted of too few subjects. Also, 150 mg of Casodex has not been tested in combination with radiation or as intermittent hormonal therapy. High-dose Casodex used alone will be closely studied. It has significant potential advantages due to fewer side effects than castration. With Casodex testosterone levels remain normal, while blocking its stimulating effect on the androgen receptor. Libido, potency, testicular size, and muscle mass remain normal. Also, there's less osteoporosis with long-term Casodex therapy. If it checks out, this treatment might replace castration or LH-RH agonists and antagonists as the best way to eliminate the effects of androgens on prostate cancer with the fewest side effects.

New Treatments For Men When Hormones No Longer Work

Vitamin D Analogues

Vitamin D analogues are closely related to vitamin D, but they're designed in such a way that calcium levels in the blood and urine are reduced. This lessens potentially serious side effects of high doses of vitamin D.

Receptors for active vitamin D metabolites are found in the nucleus of both hormone-dependent and hormone-independent prostate cancer cells. Vitamin D acts by attaching to this receptor, thereby slowing growth, reducing invasiveness, and increasing differentiation by returning prostate cancer cells to a more normal state.

One vitamin D analog, which binds strongly to this nuclear receptor and is now being tested in clinical trials, is l-alphahydroxy vitamin D2 (doxercalciferol). This produces five times less rise in blood-calcium levels than the standard active form of vitamin D, 1,25-dihydroxy vitamin-D3 (calcitriol).

Preliminary results from clinical trials with doxercalciferol are encouraging. Two out of 16 patients showed objective improvement in their bone scans after 12 weeks of treatment and nine had stable disease. Larger studies are in progress. It's important not to use PSA to measure the effects of vitamin D and its analogues on prostate cancer. PSA levels may actually *increase* during vitamin D therapy, at the same time objective tumor responses are seen on X-ray and cancer-related symptoms are decreasing.

The future for vitamin D analogues is most likely to be in combination with other anti-cancer agents or therapies. According to Dr. Snuffy Myers, analogues improve the efficacy of several chemo agents. Dr. George Wilding at the University of Wisconsin will be doing a clinical trial on the combination of doxercalciferol with Taxotere, a chemotherapy agent with known effectiveness against prostate cancer. Dr. Wilding will also be studying the effect of this drug in combination with hormones and bisphosphonates in men with androgen-independent cancer. Additionally, he'll be looking to see if doxercalciferol makes a difference in outcome when given prior to a radical prostatetomy in newly diagnosed cases of prostate cancer.

Dr. Donald Trump and his team at the University of Pittsburgh Medical School will be conducting clinical trials on calcitriol with each of the following drugs: Carboplatin, a platinum-containing chemotherapeutic agent; Taxol, a taxane related to Taxotere (the effect of Taxol or Taxotere combined with calcitriol is greater than either drug used alone); and Dexamethasone, a steroid that increases the effects of calcitriol.

If you're interested in participating in a clinical trial using doxercalciferol either alone or in combination with other agents, contact George Wilding, M.D., Professor of Medicine at the University of Wisconsin Comprehensive Cancer Center.

For participation in a calcitriol trial, contact Donald Trump, M.D. Professor of Medicine, Roswell Park Medical Center, Rochester, New York.

In the Physicians' Health Study at Harvard, June Chan, Sc.D., found that in a group of about 20,000 doctors, those who drank six glasses of milk or more per week had lower blood levels of the active form of vitamin D than those who drank two or fewer glasses weekly. It still remains to be determined, however, whether it's calcium's effect in lowering vitamin D levels that accounts for calcium's association with an increased risk of fatal prostate cancer or a direct effect of calcium. Calcium is known to play an important role in binding cells together, including cancer cells. It's possible this helps cancer cells to form tumors. The relationships between calcium, vitamin D, and prostate cancer will continue to be studied to unravel their interrelationship.

Key Reference

Presentations at the seventh annual Prostate Cancer Foundation Retreat, Lake Tahoe, Nevada, September, 2000.

Chemotherapy

Significant advances continue to be made in chemotherapy. Here are some key points to remember.

Although it now appears that certain chemotherapeutic regimens, such as Taxotere and Emcyt, prolong life in cases of androgen-independent prostate cancer, they probably cannot cure the disease when used as the sole treatment.

In the future it's likely that chemotherapy will be combined with other treatments, such as those that interfere with the tumor's blood supply, to increase the possibility of cure or long-term remission.

It's also likely that chemotherapy may be used early in the disease in combination with surgery, radiation, and/or hormones, as it's currently used in breast cancer. Recent data showing that hormones stop cancer-cell growth, but don't kill the cells, increases the likelihood that chemo will be used more "up-front," since chemo kills cancer cells.

New Developments in Chemo

Dr. Dan Petrylak reports that the median survival for a regimen of Taxotere and Emcyt is now 30 months and counting, compared to less than a year with conventional therapy.

A multi-center Phase III trial is commencing, which will compare Taxotere and Emcyt with mitoxantrone and prednisone in cases of androgen-independent prostate cancer. Six hundred and twenty men will be enrolled in this study. A Phase III trial is the final step before FDA approval.

A caveat: Although Taxotere and Emcyt are likely candidates for being the most effective chemo regimen for men with advanced prostate cancer, this has yet to be conclusively proven. Other candidates include the combination of Taxol, Emcyt, and carboplatin (TEC) being investigated by Dr. Scher and his team at Sloan Kettering, and the Logothetis Protocol being used by Chris Logothetis' group at M.D. Anderson. Having said this, experts in the field, like Dr. Mario

Eisenberger and Dan Petrylak, believe that the taxanes (Taxotere and Taxol) appear to be the most active single chemotherapeutic agents in the fight against advanced prostate cancer.

Apoptosis-Inducing Drugs

As you'll recall, the built-in suicide program (apoptosis) in all normal prostate cells is over-ridden in prostate cancer cells. Restoring apoptosis to cancer cells is a fertile target for prostate cancer researchers. A number of pro-apoptotic drugs are in various stages of development and testing.

MGI 114

Dr. Neil Senzer of the Sammons Cancer Center in Dallas, Texas, presented evidence at the 1999 American Society for Clinical Oncology (ASCO) meeting on the anti-tumor effects of a mushroom derivative dubbed MGI 114. This novel product is part of a group of agents called "acylfulvenes." It binds to DNA in the prostate cancer cells and induces apoptosis and death of cancer cells.

In a clinical trial of 21 men at the Sammons Center, 16 showed stable or decreased PSA levels. More extensive trials are now underway. MGI 114 has few side effects and can be administered multiple times.

Beta-Lapachone

This agent comes from a South American tree. It has been shown in the lab to cause apoptosis in both androgen-dependent and androgen-independent prostate cancer cells.

It works by interfering with the way cancer cells reproduce by disrupting the unwinding of the DNA in cancer cells, a necessary part of reproduction. Laboratory results indicate that beta-lapachone works independent of the p53 cancer-suppressor gene. It may, therefore, prove to be of use in men with a defective p53 gene, a common finding in men with advanced prostate cancer.

Key References

Planchon S et al. Beta-lapachone-mediated apoptosis in human promyelocytic leukemia (HL-60) and human prostate cancer cells. *Cancer Research* 1995; 55: 3706-3711.

Manna S et al. Suppression of tumor necrosis factor-activated nuclear transcription factor-kappaB, activator protein-1, c-Jun N-terminal kinase, and apoptosis by beta-lapachone. *Biochem Pharmacology* 1999; 57:763- 774.

Li Y et al. Release of mitochondrial cytochrome C in both apoptosis and necrosis induced by beta-lapachone in human carcinoma cells. *Molecular Medicine* 1999; 5:232-239.

Ansamycins

These natural products work on so-called "chaperone proteins" in prostate cancer cells. Chaperone proteins carry substances from the cell surface to the cell center (nucleus) where they are used for growth and proliferation. Ansamycins, by interfering with a key chaperone protein called HSP-90, block cancer cells from dividing. Ansamycins also work on cell pathways that inhibit apoptosis, restoring mortality to cancer cells. Ansamycins are not very toxic, so they have the potential to be combined with other treatments. More and more it seems as though the future for the treatment of advanced prostate cancer will involve a combination of anti-cancer agents. Clinical trials on ansamycins are under way at Sloan Kettering in New York.

Telomerase Inhibitors

What makes cancer cells immortal? To answer this question, it's important to understand how normal cells divide and eventually die. In order to replicate, normal cells must copy their DNA. During this process, small pieces of DNA are lost at the end of the DNA strand. These bits of DNA at the end of the strand are called "telomeres." Each time the cell divides, another bit of DNA is lost from the telomere, causing it to become shorter and shorter. When they become sufficiently short, the DNA strand no longer functions properly and the cells die.

Cancer cells have an enzyme called "telomerase" that stops the loss of bits of DNA from the telomeres. Without telomere shortening, cancer cells continue to survive and divide. Only cancer cells have telomerase. This makes telomerase an excellent target for diagnostic tests for cancer and anti-cancer therapies.

At the University of Texas Southwestern Medical School, Dr. Jerry Shay and his colleagues have designed telomerase inhibitors using an "antisense" approach. What's antisense? The genetic message from DNA is carried by RNA (ribonucleic acid) to form a specific protein. (Remember: one gene, one protein.) Antisense works to change the genetic message by binding with the RNA. In the case of telomerase, telomerase antisense binds with its RNA so that it no longer produces the protein (telomerase) that protects the telomere from shortening. Interestingly, the growth rate of the cancer cell is unaffected, but the telomere now shortens normally as bits of DNA are again broken off as the cell divides and apoptosis is re-established. Cancer cells are once again mortal and eventually die.

Since it takes time for cancer cells to go through the process of multiple divisions, leading to ultimate apoptosis, experts think that telomerase inhibitors will work best when combined with another treatment that reduces the cancer burden, such as surgery, radiation, or chemo. Another attractive potential combination is with anti-angiogenesis drugs, giving the cancer cells time to die while the tumor is stopped from growing due to insufficient nutrients.

Phase II trials are now in progress testing telomerase antisense in prostate cancer patients. Contact Jerry Shay, Ph.D., at the University of Texas Southwestern Medical School.

CN 706

Some of the new therapies under development sound like science fiction. CN 706, produced by Calydon, Inc., in Sunnyvale, Calif., is one of these. It's a type of virus called an "adenovirus" that replicates itself only in prostate cancer cells, not normal prostate cells. It attaches to the cancer cells and "instructs" the cancer cell's DNA to copy the viral DNA instead of its own. Not only is apoptosis induced by this cancer-cell-specific viral infection, the cancer cells actually explode. This produces an inflammatory response and T-cells rush to the involved areas. The result is that a man's immune system is stimulated to fight other cancer cells, a synergistic effect. Pre-clinical trials have shown this in mice, and Phase I clinical trials are now underway at Johns Hopkins.

In this trial, small doses of CN 706 are being injected directly into the prostate in a pattern similar to the way radioactive seeds are distributed. Side effects appear to be minor even at high doses. Some men get a slight fever or flu-like symptoms. Preliminary results in men with three consecutive rises in PSA after radiation or surgery show a substantial drop in PSA levels and a lengthening of the time it takes for the PSA level to double. CN 706 appears to be synergistic with radiation or chemotherapy with the taxanes Taxol and Taxotere. This is the next area to be investigated.

A new virus, called CV 787, is being developed for treating metastatic disease. Contact David Karpf, M.D., at Calydon, Inc., for information on upcoming clinical trials.

Therapies That Decrease Bcl-2

As we've discussed, some genes suppress cancer-cell growth and other genes stimulate cancer-cell proliferation. The latter often work by interfering with apoptosis. Bcl-2 is one of these. Methods to attack Bcl-2 are a hot field of scientific investigation. Vitamin D can down regulate (reduce) Bcl-2. So can PC-SPES. Small molecules are also being developed to work against Bcl-2. One such Bcl-2 antagonist is called BH-3. It is a peptide (part of a protein) that inhibits the effects of Bcl-2.

An antisense to Bcl-2 RNA is also in the works. By binding to the RNA generated from Bcl-2's DNA, it stops the production of the Bcl-2 protein. Since Bcl-2 is so common in advanced prostate cancer, reducing its production should prove effective in prolonging life by increasing apoptosis in cancer cells. As with other prostate cancer therapies, Bcl-2 inhibitors may be combined with other treatments, like angiogenesis inhibitors, in the future treatment of advanced prostate cancer.

Parthenolide—A Novel Drug From the Herb Feverfew

One of the many substances that operate at the cellular level in prostate cancer is "nuclear factor kappa B" (NFkB). Its effect is to markedly increase the amount of a protein similar to the Bcl-2 protein, called Bcl-xl. Like Bcl-2, Bcl-xl interferes with normal apoptosis. Parthenolide, an extract from feverfew, inhibits NFkB activity (as does beta-lapachone, discussed previously). In the lab, parthenolide inhibits the proliferation of both androgen-dependent and androgen-independent prostate cancer cells. Of interest to researchers is the fact that androgen-independent prostate cancer cells seem to be more affected than androgen-dependent cells. Phase I clinical trials have begun at Indiana University Medical School. Contact Dr. Christopher Sweeney.

Epithelial Growth Factor Receptor (EGFR) Blocking Agents

Epithelial growth factor (EGF) is a protein in prostate cancer cells that interferes with apoptosis. It has its anti-apoptotic effect when it binds with its receptor in the cell (EGFR). Two exciting drugs that block the ability of EGF to attach to EGFR are currently in clinical trials. One drug, produced by Genentech, is called 2C4; the other is Iressa (also called ZD1839), made by Astra Zeneca. They both work on androgen-dependent and androgen-independent prostate cancer cells. Iressa can be taken orally. Phase II clinical trials are now in progress at M.D. Anderson Cancer Center using Taxotere, Emcyt, and Iressa.

Another interesting promoter of apoptosis in prostate cancer cells is a medical mouthful called "TNF receptor apoptosis-inducing ligand," mercifully shortened to "TRAIL." TRAIL induces apoptosis in prostate cancer cells, but has little effect on normal prostate cells.

In animals TRAIL has potent anti-tumor activity and also increases the sensitivity of prostate cancer cells to chemo. Human trials will commence shortly.

Another related drug is called Tarceva. Tarceva, also developed by Genentech, is a chemically unique drug. Also known as OSI-774, Tarceva is mechanistically similar to Iressa and acts as an EGFR antagonist. It's a promising drug and clinical trials are now underway.

Injections Into the Prostate

Besides CN 706, other agents are being tested to control prostate cancer that are also injected directly into the prostate. Delivering drugs directly into the prostate may kill tumors selectively without harming other tissues.

Investigators at M.D. Anderson Cancer Center in Houston, Texas, are excited about two different preparations that can be injected directly into the prostate. As you know, p53 is an important cancer-suppressor gene. Researchers at M.D. Anderson are injecting p53 protein directly into the prostate gland prior to radical prostatectomy. They're also testing p53 in combination with EBRT. A clinical trial is also commencing comparing seeds alone with seeds plus intraprostatic p53.

The second injection treatment being pioneered at M.D. Anderson is called "PS-341." This compound, produced by Millennium Pharmaceuticals, is classified as a proteosome inhibitor. Without boring you with the science, its net effect is to stabilize p53 and decrease the amount of a harmful substance called interleukin-6. The combined effect is toxic to prostate cancer cells. Dr. Chris Logothetis is enthusiastic about the potential of PS-341. "Ultimately, it may be possible to explode prostate cancer cells selectively by injecting PS-341 into the prostate at an early stage in prostate cancer," Dr. Logothetis told me at the September 2000 Prostate Cancer Foundation Retreat. Phases I trials are also commencing at M. D. Anderson using PS-341 in combination with the chemotherapeutic agent Adriamycin.

Treatment Aimed At Stopping Metastases

As you know, by far the favorite "home away from home" for prostate cancer cells is bone. One approach to prevent cancer cells from going to bone is to keep them from escaping the prostate. Another is to change the bone environment, so it's considerably less hospitable to newly arrived prostate cancer cells.

Matthew Smith, M.D., Ph.D., at Massachusetts General Hospital in Boston is one of the most knowledgeable people on the interaction of prostate cancer cells with bone. I spoke with him at the 2000 Prostate Cancer Foundation Retreat. He told me that prostate cancer cells are a lot like bone cells, so when they lodge in bone, they act like bone cells. A positive feedback loop is established between the cancer and bone cells, each stimulating proliferation of the other.

The parallels between bone and prostate are striking. As Dr. Smith puts it, "The microenvironment between bone and the prostate are very similar. Prostate cancer cells are happy in the bone environment. This makes bone an excellent target for prostate cancer therapy." Dr. Smith thinks it's possible that an increase in bone turnover, as occurs in osteoporosis, may stimulate prostate cancer cells in the bone marrow. An increase of bone resorption occurs when bone is lost in osteoporosis. This bone loss stimulates new bone formation. The loss occurs faster than the formation, resulting in osteoporosis. The process results in an increase in bone activity, especially cell turnover. It is conceivable, according to Dr. Smith, that this increased turnover may stimulate prostate cancer cells to proliferate, leading to bone metastases. If this is true, reducing bone turnover might be helpful. This could be a rationale for the use of bisphosphonates, which might slow bone resorption, reducing overall bone activity. Dr. Smith is conducting clinical trials on Aredia, an intravenously administered bisphosphonate.

Testosterone, estrogen, vitamin D, and calcium are active in both bone and prostate. IGF-1 is thought to be important in maintaining bone integrity and has also been implicated in the development and progression of prostate cancer.

Reducing IGF-1 levels may also slow bone turnover. PSA has the ability to cleave IGF-1 from its binding proteins (IGFBPs). Potential therapeutic targets include antibodies to IGF-1 and methods to increase IGFBPs to bind and inactivate IGF-1. It's believed that one of the ways consuming fewer calories is effective against prostate cancer is by reducing IGF-1 levels.

(A vegan diet lowers IGF-1 levels an average of 9% compared to meat eaters and 7% compared to egg- and milk-consuming vegetarians, according to a British study presented in the July 2000 issue of the *British Journal of Cancer*. Since elevated IGF-1 levels are associated with an increased risk of the development of prostate cancer, reducing IGF-1 levels might reduce the risk, concludes Tim Key, Ph.D., the study's lead author.)

Another compound that reduces bone turnover is called "Atrasentan (ABT-627)." Produced by Abbott Laboratories, Atrasentan blocks a bone protein known as endothelin-1. Discovered in Japan in 1988, this protein is classified as a "sarafotoxin." Related to snake venom, it's a potent vasoconstrictor (contracts blood vessels). Prostate cancer cells have receptors for endothlin-1 on their surface. When endothelin-1 binds with this receptor, it causes pain. This may be a major source of the pain associated with bone metastases. Endothelin-1 also inhibits apoptosis of prostate cancer cells in bone and increases their division rate.

In studies done by Dr. Michael Carducci, Dr. Joel Nelson, and their group at Johns Hopkins, Atrasentan was found to block the binding of endothelin-1 with its receptor on the prostate cancer cell. In the first randomized placebo-controlled double-blind trial, Atrasentan reduced pain, but didn't demonstrate significant activity in preventing new cancer spots from appearing on bone scans. The end-point of this trial was at least two new spots on the bone scan. Using this end-point, Atrasentan showed no significant activity. It's quite possible that these "new" spots were there prior to Atrasentan administration, but were too small to see. Bone scans are notoriously tough to read. Atrasentan is based on a brilliant hypothesis and is being developed by top-flight investigators. Additional trials by Abbott Laboratories and others of this well-conceived drug are underway.

Atrasentan can be taken orally and has only modest side effects (headache, runny nose, and an increase in viral infections). About 30% of the men have some swelling in their arms or legs.

Interestingly, Atrasentan reduces bone turnover by slowing the rate of bone breakdown. This fact dovetails nicely with Dr. Smith's view that reducing bone turnover may be beneficial in men with advanced prostate cancer.

Lowering Blood IGF-1 Levels

In October 2000, I got back the results of my first-ever IGF-1 blood test. I was surprised and dismayed to discover that it was 65% higher than the upper limit of the normal range. As you know, an elevated IGF-1 level is associated with an increased risk of developing prostate cancer, especially if IGF-binding protein-3 (IGFBP-3) levels are low. But I don't believe this is the whole story. There's also a growing body of evidence that may implicate high IGF-1 with the recurrence and progression, not only the initial development, of prostate cancer. Although this has not yet been proven, enough data currently exists for me to be sufficiently concerned to take steps to lower my IGF-1 levels.

In the laboratory IGF-1 stimulates cell division in cancer cells. This "mitogenic" effect increases the proliferation and invasive potential of prostate cancer cells. As you read earlier, IGF-1 is also known to stimulate activity in bone. It is likely, though unproven, that prostate cancer cells lodged in bone grow and proliferate more vigorously in the presence of IGF-1. The protective effect of IGFBP-3 on the progression of cancer in the face of high levels of IGF-1 has not yet been determined.

What really got my attention, though, when I researched this subject was information on the effect of elevated IGF-1 levels on prostate cancer's sister disease, breast cancer. Dr. Vadgama and his team at UCLA reported in the November 1999 issue of the journal *Oncology* on 130 women with breast cancer. They measured plasma IGF-1 levels and found that IGF-1 levels were higher in women whose cancer recurred, and that IGF-1 levels increased with tumor size.

Tamoxifen, a weak estrogenic compound used in the prevention and treatment of breast cancer, significantly reduces IGF-1 levels and the risk of recurrence of breast cancer, according to these UCLA investigators. Women with plasma IGF-1 levels of less than 120 ng/ml were found to have an increased probability of surviving. The investigators drew the following conclusions: "Lowering plasma IGF-1 may offer the following benefits.

• Reduce the risk of developing breast cancer in high-risk groups.

• Slow the progression of breast cancer in patients at early stages of the disease.

• Increase the probability of survival."

Although unproven and a leap of faith, I think it's logical to extrapolate that IGF-1 is likely to have similar effects in prostate cancer as in breast cancer. To my way of thinking, it makes sense to take all reasonable steps to lower my IGF-1 level and raise my IGFBP-3 level, probably reducing the chances of my disease progressing.

I already eat a vegan diet that reduces IGF-1 by about 9%. Without this, my IGF-1 level would have been even higher.

Studies in rodents show that restricting calorie intake by 20% reduces IGF-1 levels by an average of 24%. Studies in humans, who go out to eat and attend many more parties than laboratory mice and whose caloric intake is difficult to control and monitor, have not yet been done. Its logical to conclude that they would parallel the reduction in IGF-1 levels that comes with calorie restriction in mice. Although I admit that reducing calorie consumption is not an easy task, I have embarked on a calorie-reduction effort. Reducing calories also increases IGFBPs, but the effect of this has not yet been evaluated in prostate cancer. However, a recent study seems to indicate higher levels of the IGFBPs-1 and 2 decrease the risk of colon cancer. IGFBP-3 is the key IGF-binding protein in prostate cancer.

Although the amount of sugar intake makes a difference in insulin levels, it doesn't seem to affect IGF-1 levels, according to a Danish study. It's calories, not sugar, that seem to affect IGF-1.

Increased exercise, especially moderately strenuous aerobic exercise, also reduces IGF-1 levels and increases IGFBP-3. I've started working with a physical trainer. This way, reasons not to exercise will diminish in importance, since I now have an exercise appointment to keep three times per week.

Since the test, I've reduced my IGF-1 level by 30% by reducing calories and exercising more vigorously.

Dr. Nelson's IGF-1 Reduction

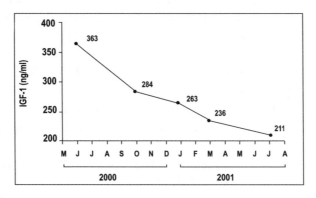

Some preliminary evidence indicates that silibinin, an active compound from Silybum marianum (milk thistle) discussed in the "Nutrition" section of the book, may increase IGFBP-3 levels. Although it is far too soon to draw a definitive conclusion about this, I don't know of any significant side effects from silibinin consumption. According to Dr. Giovannucci, the only food source with significant amounts of silibinin is artichokes. Fortunately, silibinin is available as a supplement, in the form of silymarin, or milk thistle extract. I've doubled my intake of Life Extension's 100 mg silymarin (35 mg silibinin) to two capsules three times a day. A new silibinin formula containing 266 mg silibinin per capsule is now available from Life Extension. I will switch to this more potent preparation. Silymarin has also been linked to increased expression of the p21 cancer-suppressor gene. I also eat more artichokes. In summer they are readily available. Cooked hearts can be frozen and eaten regularly all year long. Bottled artichoke hearts are also available any time of year.

Late Note: By January 2003 my IGF-1 level had decreased further to 190 ng/ml, just over half of my initial reading of 368 ng/ml in June 2000. This further drop may be due to silibinin and/or lycopene supplements, both of which have been associated with (but not yet proven to cause) a decrease in IGF-1 levels.

Some drugs also lower IGF-1. One of the most interesting classes of drugs are the SERMs (Selective Estrogen Receptor Modulators), discussed later in this chapter. SERMs, like tamoxifen and arzoxifene, decrease the growth of transplanted androgen-sensitive prostate tumors in animals. Tamoxifen significantly decreases IGF-1 levels and reduces the risk of recurrence in women with breast cancer. Since its also active in prostate cancer and is likely to reduce IGF-1 levels in men as well as women, it may prove to be useful for cancer control in men with prostate cancer. Side effects are generally not serious and the anti-tumor effect in prostate cancer approaches that of surgical or medical castration. Clinical trials are warranted.

Scientists at Tulane University School of Medicine in New Orleans, led by Andrew Schally M.D., Ph.D., have been experimenting with an antagonist to growth-hormone-releasing hormone (GH-RH) called MZ-4-71, using rats implanted with prostate cancer. After treating the animals for six weeks with MZ-4-71, they observed a significant size reduction in a variety of androgen-independent tumors. Blood levels of growth hormone and IGF-1 were significantly decreased in the MZ-4-71-treated animals. The investigators conclude that, "the GH-RH antagonist MZ-4-71 suppresses growth of PC-3, DU-145 and Dunning AT-1 androgen-independent prostate cancer. They postulate a potential mechanism for the cancer cell suppression involves a reduction in IGF-1 levels, either by reducing secretion in the liver or by diminishing IGF-1 production in prostate cancer cells.

Human trials are required to test the efficacy of this agent in men with prostate cancer, especially after relapse.

Recommendations For Men With High IGF-1 Levels
• Have your IGF-1 and IGFBP-3 level checked. Normal IGFBP-3 may be helpful in protecting against the potential harmful effects of elevated IGF-1, but this has not been proven.

• A vegan diet reduces IGF-1 plasma levels by an average of about 9%.

• Reducing calories by 20% (from normal levels) will likely reduce IGF-1 levels by as much as 25%, and may increase IGFBP-3.

• Moderately strenuous exercise will also help lower IGF-1 and may increase IGFBP-3.

• Eat lots of artichokes. Consider taking milk thistle or silibinin supplements (I now prefer silibinin).

• If you have elevated IGF-1 levels, I suggest you closely follow developments in clinical trials of SERMs, such as tamoxifen, and trials of GH-RH antagonists, such as MZ-4-71.

• Antibodies to IGF-1 are being developed. In the future, gene therapy that increases the amount of IGFBP-3 and reduces the amount of free-circulating IGF-1 is also feasible using current available technology.

• Newly released data indicate that lycopene may lower IGF-1 levels. Eat lots of tomato products or consider taking lycopene supplements.

Key References

Vadgama J et al. Plasma insulin-like growth factor-I and serum IGF-binding protein-3 can be associated with the progression of breast cancer, and predict the risk of recurrence and the probability of survival in African-American and Hispanic women. *Oncology* 1999; 57: 330-340.

Dun S et al. Dietary restriction reduces insulin-like growth factor I levels, which modulates apoptosis, cell proliferation, and tumor progression in p53-deficient mice. *Cancer Research* 1997; 57: 4667-4672.

Frystyk J et al. The effect of oral glucose on serum-free insulin-like growth factor-I and II in healthy adults. *J Clin Endocrinol Metab* 1997; 82: 3124-3127.

Bergan R et al. A Phase II study of high-dose tamoxifen in patients with hormone-refractory prostate cancer. *Clin Cancer Res* 1999; 5: 2366-2373.

Jungwirth A, Schally A, et al. Inhibition of in vivo proliferation of androgen-independent prostate cancer by an antagonist of growth hormone- releasing hormone. *British Journal of Cancer* 1997; 75: 1585-1592.

Prostate-Cancer-Specific "Smart Bombs"

One of the most promising new technologies for prostate cancer uses antibodies found exclusively in prostate cells. Because these antibodies recognize a single specific protein or antigen, they are called "monoclonal antibodies" or MABs. A toxic radioactive isotope can then be attached to the antibody, resulting in a kind of "magic bullet" or "smart bomb" that homes in on prostate and prostate cancer cells specifically without affecting other organs. Prostate and prostate cancer cells are selectively killed. Since normal prostate cells are expendable, this selectivity is ideal.

Currently, the leading agent in this field is called "J591." Developed by Dr. Neal Bander, Professor of Urology at New York Presbyterian Hospital, J591 shows excellent targeting for prostate cancer metastases. It attaches to a protein on the surface of prostate cancer cells called "prostate-specific membrane antigen" (PSMA). In a test on 32 men, 81% showed excellent targeting anywhere the PSMA happened to be. What's more, 83% of the men tested had bone metastases. This antibody seems capable of going on "search-and-destroy" missions against distant prostate cancer cell colonies in bone. When the radioactive isotope Indium-111 is attached to this antibody, its uptake correlates well with a bone scan, proving the excellent targeting.

In a Phase I/II clinical trial started in the summer of 2000, not only was excellent targeting shown in both bone and soft-tissue metastases (lymph nodes, etc.), but the antibody was well-tolerated by the men who received it, with no significant side effects.

Indium-111 is not the most potent radioisotope. There is much excitement among researchers about using a radioisotope called "Bismuth-213 (Bi-213)." Bi-213 emits alpha particles that are highly toxic to prostate cancer cells. Clinical trials of J591 with Bi-213 attached will be starting at Sloan Kettering in New York very soon.

Large quantities of J591 antibody suitable for use in humans have been engineered by Biovation, Ltd. J591 has been approved by the FDA for use in humans.

Studies will also soon be commencing on the combined use of J591 with chemotherapeutic agents.

For men with advanced metastatic disease, J591 therapies are among the most promising approaches to selectively killing prostate cancer cells in areas where they have metastasized with minimal toxicity to unaffected organs. The quality of life can be preserved while the cancer is treated.

Another kind of smart bomb is being developed at the Imperial College in London, England. A team of scientists led by Dr. Mahendra Deonarain is working with a natural enzyme found in cassava plants, almond trees, and hydrangeas. This enzyme produces cyanide, but only when it comes in contact with a particular sugar molecule. Otherwise, it's inert and harmless.

In nature this enzyme and reactive sugar molecules are normally kept apart. But British scientists saw an opportunity to attach this enzyme to a tumor-specific antibody, such as PSMA. The enzyme is thus selectively bound only to the targeted cancer cells.

Next, a second drug containing only the sugar that activates the release of the cyanide is introduced. As the sugar circulates in the bloodstream, it triggers the release of minute quantities of cyanide directly into the cancer cells, killing them.

Because of the agents used, cancer cells can't develop resistance to this treatment. Changing form by mutating, one of a cancer cell's best defense mechanisms against chemotherapeutic agents, is useless against the killing effects of the cyanide. For this reason, the cyanide can, theoretically, continue to be used until all the cancer cells are killed.

Clinical trials involving a number of different cancers are currently being organized.

Smart Bombs With Chemo

The future of chemo will be to specifically target prostate cancer cells. This way, the toxic effects of chemo on normal cells and organs will be avoided. How close are we to cancer cell-targeted chemo? Closer than you might imagine.

The November 2000 issue of *Nature Medicine* reports on animal studies of such a product being tested by Merck Research Laboratories in West Point, Pennsylvania. Merck scientists have attached the potent chemo agent Adriamycin (doxorubicin) to a small seven-amino-acid peptide that splits off from the doxorubicin only in the presence of PSA. Since PSA is produced virtually exclusively by prostate cancer cells in men who have failed surgery or radiation, this peptide-chemo smart bomb selectively targets prostate cancer cells.

According to Dr. Raymond Jones at Merck, L-377, 202, as this preparation is called, is "15 times more effective than conventional doxorubicin—when both drugs are used at their maximally tolerated doses."

Human trials are next.

Key Reference

Internet site medscape.com Doxorubicin-peptide conjugate targets PSA-producing prostate cancer in mice. Reuters Medical News, November 1, 2000. As reported in *Nature Medicine* 2000; 6: 1248-1252.

Anti-Angiogenesis Therapies

Developing treatments that interfere with a tumor's ability to make new blood vessels is another hot area of cancer research. Attacking the tumor's blood supply is an attractive approach, because it also side-steps the ability of cancer cells to mutate. Without an ever-increasing web of blood vessels to support them, colonies of tumor cells can't continue to grow.

Tumor cells produce substances that stimulate the development of blood vessels. These "pro-angiogenic" factors include vascular endothelial growth factor (VEGF), basic fibroblast growth factor (bFGF), and interleukin 8 (IL-8). Interestingly and enigmatically, cancer cells also produce "anti-angiogenic" substances that slow blood-vessel growth. The two major ones are angiostatin and endostatin. In people with cancer, the balance between pro-angiogenic and anti-angiogenic factors is somehow tipped in favor of the pro-angiogenic factors; thus, new blood vessels are formed.

Thanks to the pioneering work by Dr. Judah Folkman of Children's Hospital and Harvard Medical School in Boston, potent anti-angiogenesis endostatin and angiostatin are now being developed for use in a variety of cancers, including breast, lung, colon, and prostate.

Phase I clinical trials of endostatin are currently under way at the University of Wisconsin and M. D. Anderson. Trials of angiostatin should commence soon.

All in all, about 20 angiogenesis inhibitors are currently being tested in clinical trials. One of these is thalidomide. Yes, this is the same drug that was banned for causing birth defects in newborns. In prostate cancer, thalidomide inhibits angiogenesis. In a Phase II trial of 18 men, all 18 had drops in their PSA levels and stabilization of their disease. Larger trials are in progress at the National Institutes of Health (NIH) Clinical Center in Bethesda, Maryland.

New Potent Angiogenesis Inhibitors

Three new compounds appear to be more potent inhibitors of angiogenesis than endostatin and angiostatin. One comes from Dr. Folkman's lab. It's called "antithrombin III (aaAT III)." It works like its predecessors, but requires lesser amounts and less frequent dosing to get the same effects (more potent). The other two, known as METH-1 and METH-2, come from combining work done by researchers at UCLA with genetic information provided by Human Genome Sciences. The two proteins were found by searching Human Genome Sciences' database of genes from the human genome project. Both of these newly discovered proteins appear to be more potent than endostatin and angiostatin in preventing the development of new blood vessels, according to Dr. Luisa Iruela-Arispe of UCLA's Jonsson Cancer Center.

Other angiogenesis inhibitors include genistein, Linomide (roquinimex), pentoxifylline, and a variety of new antisense agents to growth factors for tumor blood vessels, like VEGF and bFGF. As you'll recall, antisense works like an antibody by attacking the RNA messenger that converts the DNA code to a protein. Attack the messenger and you inhibit production of the protein VEGF or bFGF. This cuts off the production of new cancer-feeding blood vessels.

Note that angiogenesis inhibitors can also interfere with normal blood-vessel formation. Fortunately, in adults, requirements for new blood-vessel formation are low. One area of potential concern, however, is the new blood vessels formed after a myocardial infarction (heart attack). This potential side effect is being examined. Another concern is that these drugs might interfere with wound healing. Men who have heart conditions or have had recent surgery should proceed with caution in trials of anti-angiogenesis agents.

A Future Approach to Disrupting Prostate Cancer Blood Vessels

Some of the approaches for treating prostate cancer currently under development are truly awe-inspiring.

One of the most intriguing was recently described to me by Professor Avigdor Scherz, Ph.D., of the Weizmann Institute of Science in Israel. Dr. Scherz observed that it takes considerably longer for blood to travel through blood vessels servicing tumors than it does through normal blood vessels. He also noticed that tumor capillaries are fragile, leak easily, and are not readily repaired when damaged. Dr. Scherz ingeniously used chlorophyll from bacteria to develop a drug that works on tumor blood vessels. The drug is inactive until it is exposed to light. About 20 minutes of direct stimulation by light activates the drug, causing the cancer-supporting capillaries to break and the tumor to die from lack of sufficient oxygen and nutrients. In prostate cancer, photo-stimulation might be accomplished by direct fiber optics inserted into the rectum.

Not only does this drug have the potential to destroy the primary prostate tumor, but it also precipitates an inflammation in the area. This stimulates an immune-system response that may fight distant micrometastases (microscopic areas of tumor cells). In the future a drug like this may become an option for the initial treatment of primary prostate cancer instead of surgery or radiation. It's clear to me that at some point in the future, a therapy will be devised that destroys the entire prostate gland in men over 40, eliminating the risk of prostate cancer.

I want to mention one final drug that inhibits angiogenesis. It's called SU6668 and it's made by the Sugen Corporation of South San Francisco, California. It's of special interest because it inhibits a variety of tumor-generated growth factors, including VEGF, bFGF, and platelet-derived growth factor (PDGF). Inhibiting more than one growth factor may be necessary to stop new blood-vessel growth.

It's been tested in mice on a variety of tumors. The tumors decreased in size in every mouse and disappeared completely in the majority.

Phase I human trials on a variety of cancers are now under way at UCLA. SU6668 was well-tolerated in mice and is expected to be non-toxic to people as well.

Sugen also has another angiogenesis inhibitor called SU5416, which blocks the receptor that VEGF attaches to on endothelial (lining) cells to stimulate blood-vessel growth. It's currently in Phase I/II clinical trials.

Targeting the Androgen and Estrogen Receptors

The dynamics and the interrelationship between the cellular receptors for circulating androgens and estrogens is the subject of intense investigation. The gene sequence that comprises these receptors is now being researched.

Molecular differences between the androgen receptor in normal prostate cells and in cancer cells are being studied.

Dr. Chawnshang Chang at the University of Rochester has found a protein dubbed ARA-70 that increases the activity of the androgen receptor. Surprisingly, the activity of ARA-70 is greatly enhanced by estrogen rather than testosterone. It's conceivable that this discovery relates to the ultimate progression of prostate cancer in the absence of male hormones during androgen blockade. It may also tie in with Dr. Coffey's theory that estrogens may be more of a culprit in the development of prostate cancer than has been appreciated so far.

Selective Estrogen Receptor Modulators (SERMs)

In breast cancer, SERMs, such as tamoxifen, have been effective in reducing the effects of estrogen on the estrogen receptor. SERMs decrease breast cancer growth in animals and have been effective in Phase I and Phase II trials on women with breast cancer.

Interestingly, SERMs are also active against prostate cancer. Tamoxifen inhibits the growth of prostate cancer cells in the laboratory and induces the production of the cancer-suppressing protein p21.

A related SERM called Arzoxifene, a weak estrogen, has been shown to have an anti-tumor effect in prostate cancer. Arzoxifene inhibits the effects of both androgens and estrogens on the proliferation of androgen-dependent prostate cancer cells. In animals it reduces tumor growth.

It can be taken orally, has low toxicity, and does not reduce testicular weight as do testosterone-blocking hormones. Clinical trials of Arzoxifene will begin shortly.

Key References

Rohlff C et al. Prostate cancer cell growth inhibition by tamoxifen is associated with inhibition of protein kinase C and induction of p21 (waf 1/cip1). *Prostate* 1998; 37: 51-59.

Presentation by Blake Neuberger, Ph. D., Senior Research Scientist at Lilly Research Laboratories at the 7th Annual Prostate Cancer Foundation Retreat, Lake Tahoe, Nevada, September 2000.

Non-Steroidal Anti-Inflammatory Drugs (NSAIDS)

Perhaps the hottest story in prostate cancer is the role that NSAIDs seem to play in both prevention and proliferation of the disease. This is a rapidly unfolding story and should be closely monitored by all men reading this book.

NSAIDs are anti-inflammatory drugs, such as aspirin, ibuprofen, and the newer drugs like Celebrex and Vioxx. In the "Nutrition" section of this chapter, we discussed Dr. Giovannucci's recent finding of a reduced risk of prostate cancer in a large group of doctors who consumed aspirin regularly. This finding was recently confirmed by researchers at the Ohio State University Comprehensive Cancer Center, where Drs. Nelson and Harris found a highly significant 66% reduction in the risk of prostate cancer in men who consumed NSAIDs daily. These drugs also seem to play an important role in inhibiting angiogenesis. Scientists are now beginning to understand how NSAIDs may work. Here's what they're finding.

Earlier in this book we discussed the detrimental effects of arachadonic acid, which promotes the proliferation of prostate cancer. We made recommendations on ways to reduce arachadonic acid levels, like adopting a vegan diet.

Arachadonic acid is converted to substances called eicosanoids by the action of two enzymes: cyclooxygenases (COXs) and lipooxygenases (LOXs; not to be confused with salt-preserved salmon). Recent studies at George Washington University in Washington, D.C. indicate that COX induces invasiveness of prostate cancer cells. This invasiveness is blocked by COX inhibitors, but not LOX inhibitors, indicating that COX is the enzyme most related to cancer invasiveness and metastasis.

There are two kinds of COX: COX-1 and COX-2. COX-1 is found in many normal cells, including those lining the stomach and in cancer cells as well. COX-2 is found in much greater quantities in cancer cells than in normal cells. In fact, British researchers reported in the September 2000 edition of the *British Journal of Urology* that prostate cancer cells have four times as much cancer-spreading COX-2 as normal prostate cells. If the action of COX-2 could be blocked, this would logically reduce the chances of prostate cancer invasion and metastasis.

New COX-2 inhibiting drugs are now available. Celebrex and Vioxx are the two best known. They're available only by prescription. COX-2 inhibitors selectively inhibit COX-2 without affecting COX-1. For this reason, their long-term use won't affect the COX-1 needed for the function of normal cells, including those lining the stomach. Gastric irritation is not usually a problem with COX-2 inhibitors as it can be with medications like aspirin or ibuprofen, which inhibit both COX-1 and COX-2.

New studies show that COX-2 inhibitors not only reduce the potential for cancer cells to spread, they also reduce new blood-vessel formation by tumors and induce apoptosis in both androgen-dependent and androgen-independent prostate cancer cells. The cells that form new blood vessels for prostate cancer, it turns out, also have high levels of COX-2.

By using a COX-2 inhibitor like Celebrex, a man with prostate cancer appears to be getting at least a triple whammy: apoptosis of cancer cells; a potent anti-angiogenic effect; and a reduction in invasive potential of the cancer cells. Add to this the benefit of effective pain reduction and the reduced risk of colon cancer and probably other cancers. A Swiss study reported a 60% reduction in all cancers verified at autopsy in people who used large quantities of analgesics for long periods prior to death. When urinary-tract tumors, known to be increased by large quantities of analgesics, were removed from the mix, the incidence of cancer was reduced by 78%!

You can see why NSAIDs, especially COX-2 inhibitors, have so much potential in assisting in both the prevention and spread of prostate cancer. It will be quite a while, however, before prospective, placebo-controlled, double-blind studies, the *sine qua non* of medical trials, prove this effectiveness, as well as evaluate the side effects in men with prostate cancer. One known side effect is that the combination of a COX-2 inhibitor with aspirin may cause gastric (stomach) bleeding. This is not true for very low-dose aspirin, such as a daily baby aspirin (used to prevent heart disease), but it is a risk with higher doses. Blood-thinning supplements, such as vitamin E, Gingko biloba, and curcumin, could conceivably have similar unwanted effects.

What have I decided to do personally in light of this new but as yet unproven information? I've decided to take 200 mg of Celebrex twice daily. I will also continue to take a baby aspirin each day. However, I've discontinued Gingko biloba and curcumin and limited my vitamin E intake to 400 IU daily.

I suggest that each man weigh the risk/reward ratio and consult with his team of doctors on whether a COX-2 inhibitor is warranted in his particular case. Men at high risk should be especially vigilant for developments in this area. At the time of this writing, conclusive proof of efficacy is not in hand, but the science, epidemiologic studies, and animal studies done to date certainly have the halls of prostate academia buzzing.

Key References

Attiga F et al. Inhibitors of prostaglandin synthesis inhibit human prostate cell invasiveness and reduce the release of matrix metalloproteinases. *Cancer Research* 2000; 60: 4629-4637.

Masferrer J et al. Antiangiogenesis and antitumor activities of cyclooxygenase-2 inhibitors. *Cancer Research* 2000; 60: 1306-1311.

Hsu A et al. The cyclooxygenase-2 inhibitor celecoxib induces apoptosis by blocking Akt activation in human prostate cancer cells independently of Bcl.-2. *J Biol Chem* 2000; 275: 11397-11403. Note: celecoxib is the scientific name of Celebrex.

Bucher C et al. Relative risk of malignant tumors in analgesic abusers. Effects of long-term intake of aspirin. *Clinical Nephrology* 1999; 51: 67-72.

Nelson J and Harris R. Inverse association of prostate cancer and non-steroidal anti-inflammatory drugs (NSAIDs): results of a case-controlled study. *Oncol Rep* 2000; 7: 169-170.

Lord Winston of Hammersmith Hospital, London, England, September 2000 *British Journal of Urology,* as reported by intellihealth.com

Exisulind

A new class of drugs called "selective apoptotic antineoplastic drugs (SAANDs)" has the remarkable ability to induce apoptosis in cancer cells, but not in normal cells. Exisulind is a metabolite of sulindac, a NSAID. But unlike the NSAIDs, exisulind inhibits neither COX-1 nor COX-2. It works by inhibiting a substance known as "cyclic GMP phosphodiesterase." Blocking this substance kills cancer cells by apoptosis. It works on both androgen-dependent and androgen-independent prostate cancer cells. Exisulind is safe, well-tolerated, and can be taken orally.

A Phase II/III, multi-center, placebo-controlled trial was conducted on 96 men who had rising PSAs after radical prostatectomy and hadn't received hormonal therapy. A rising PSA after surgery, as you know, means that cancer cells still exist and that there are micrometastases, although no tumor can yet be detected either locally or in distant sites. The men in this trial who were given exisulind had a significantly slower rise in their PSA level than men who were given the placebo.

Exisulind has several other interesting properties. It induces apoptosis in cancer cells that are deficient in p53, and those that overexpress bcl-2. In other words, it can overcome these genetic defects that interfere with apoptosis. This is an important point because many men with advanced disease have defects in one or both of these genes.

Exisulind works synergistically with the taxanes, Taxol and Taxotere. It also works together with retinoids and platinum-containing chemotherapy agents, making it potentially useful in combination therapy.

Due to its lack of side effects, exisulind may prove to be beneficial in the prevention of prostate cancer. Who knows? Perhaps in the near future men over 50 may take daily exisulind and Celebrex to prevent prostate cancer. Although it's far too soon to make such a recommendation, it's certainly not beyond the realm of possibility.

Key References

Goluboff E et al. Exisulind (suldinac sulfone) suppresses growth of human prostate cancer in a nude mouse xenograft model by increasing apoptosis. *Urology* 1999; 53: 440-445.

Lim J et al. Suldinac derivatives inhibit growth and induce apoptosis in human prostate cancer cells lines. *Biochem Pharmacol* 1999; 58: 1097-1107.

Pamucku R. Aptosyn (exisulind) A cGMP PDE inhibitor with potential utility in prostate cancer. Presentation at the 7th Annual Prostate Cancer Foundation Retreat. September, 2000. Lake Tahoe, Nevada.

Using Viruses to Destroy Prostate Cancer

Dr. Robert Martuza and his colleagues at Massachusetts General Hospital in Boston are working on developing a herpes virus designed to kill prostate cancer cells.

The virus is injected directly into the prostate right after radiation. Its effects are thought to add to those of radiation. There is no viral toxicity to nerves with this engineered herpes virus. Pre-clinical work has shown the virus to be very effective in eradicating hormone-dependent prostate cancer cells. A single injection in mice with transplanted prostate cancer resulted in a reduction in size or disappearance of the tumor in 40% of the mice. This virus is also being developed to attack metastatic prostate cancer by intravenous injection.

CN 706, a preparation that uses a different engineered virus to attack prostate cancer cells when injected directly into the prostate, was discussed earlier in this chapter.

Another virus, called "KD3 adenovirus," is being engineered to selectively attack cancer cells by Dr. William Wold of St. Louis University Medical School. Dr. Wold is working on a cancer-cell-specific virus (it only attacks cancer cells). It can be used in combination with radiation. KD3 and radiation used together do a better job of killing prostate cancer cells than either used separately.

Gene Therapy (Genetic Medicine)

Prostate cancer can be thought of as a disease in which cellular "on-off" growth signaling is out of whack due to a variety of genetic abnormalities. Cancer-causing genes may be inappropriately switched on; cancer-suppressing genes may be switched off due to defects in cancer-suppressor genes such as p53, p21, p27, and PTEN.

With the genetic revolution now in full swing, thanks to the mapping of the human genome, scientists now have the ability to isolate genes, clone them, and change (engineer) them into more healthful versions. The object is to introduce a gene into a cancer cell that either returns its function to normal or kills it by restoring apoptosis.

Scientists can use whole genes or portions thereof to change cancer cell function. How do these genes get inside cancer cells? They're "packaged" inside viruses. Viruses carry DNA that instructs the cells they attack to replicate the virus. Usually harmless viruses are selected as carriers. In the engineered carrier viruses, the viral DNA is replaced with the genetic material that the doctors want to introduce into the prostate cancer cells.

Targets for gene therapy include introducing p53, p21, p27, and PTEN cancer-suppressor genes. Antisense that inhibits the action of Bcl-2 (discussed earlier) is another example of genetic medicine.

Proteins, the end product of genes, can also be delivered into cancer cells by an ingenious technique developed by Dr. Steven Dowdy and collaborators at the Howard Hughes Medical Institute of St. Louis, Missouri. Proteins are normally too large to enter cells. But Dr. Dowdy's team has found a way to get them in: They attach the desired protein to a minute piece of another protein they've isolated from the HIV virus. This bit of protein is harmless (it doesn't cause AIDS). It's composed of a tiny 11-amino-acid sequence known as "TAT," to which the much larger desired protein is attached. This reacts with lipids (fats) on the cell surface, causing a minute opening in the lipid layer of the cell membrane. The desired protein then passes into the cell. The way this is engineered, proteins can pass into the cell, but nothing can leak out of it—one-way traffic. This amazing delivery system can be used to introduce large proteins, such as those that come from tumor suppressor genes, to prostate cancer cells anywhere in the body, including the prostate, bone, and bone marrow.

The p27 tumor-suppressor gene has been hooked up to TAT (TAT-p27) and tested in mice. A limited dose prevented tumor growth for an extended period of time. Human studies should commence soon.

Another use of genetic technology is in the development of vaccines and other immune-system stimulators. This application is called "immunotherapy."

Researchers at Johns Hopkins Oncology Center, led by Dr. Jonathan Simons, are using a man's own prostate cells, removed at the time of radical prostatectomy. These cells are implanted with a potent immune-system-stimulating gene called GM-CSF. This gene stimulates the immune system when the patient's genetically engineered prostate cells are re-introduced as a vaccine. Clinical trials currently in progress show an increase in T-cell immune response to this vaccine. Twenty percent of the men getting the vaccine had at least a 50% decrease in PSA. Other vaccines are also being tested. One advantage to vaccines is the absence of side effects.

A compound that uses DNA bound to a lipid also stimulates the immune system. It's in Phase II trials at UCLA and the Cleveland Clinic. Called "Leuvectin," it slowed or stopped the rise of PSA in 33% of patients in a small preliminary trial.

Stimulating a man's T-cells to attack cancer cells is also the object of work being done by Dr. Gerald Murphy at the Pacific Northwest Cancer Foundation in Seattle, Washington. Dr. Murphy and his group take immune system cells called "dendritic cells" from a man's own blood by a process that separates them from other cells. He allows them to multiply, then infuses them with a protein specific to prostate cancer cells. Dendritic cells are designed to present unwanted foreign antigens to T-cells, directing the T-cells as to which invaders to attack. Dr. Murphy then injects these concentrated, protein-infused dendritic cells back into the man. T-cells now rush to the injection site. They receive the message to attack and kill any cell that contains that protein, e.g., prostate cancer cells. The T-cells then circulate, killing prostate cancer cells wherever they may be.

Anti-CTLA-4

As with most body processes, the immune system has an on-off switch. The "switch" that turns the immune system off is called CTLA-4. After the T-cells attack cancer cells for a time, CTLA-4 works to shut down the immune response. For this reason repeated T-cell stimulation is often necessary in immunotherapy. But what if CTLA-4 could somehow be inhibited? Then the T-cells would continue to attack unfettered.

James Allison, Ph.D., Professor of Immunology and Director of the Cancer Research Laboratory at the University of California-Berkeley, has developed an anti-CTLA-4 antibody. When anti-CTLA-4 antibodies are injected into mice, their immune systems don't shut off. The on-switch, called "CD-28," keeps stimulating the immune system, uninhibited by CTLA-4.

Human anti-CTLA-4 has now been developed. Trials combining it with the GM-CSF vaccine are now being organized. CTLA-4 will also be tested in combination with anti-angiogenesis drugs. An immune system "stuck" in the on position, in combination with stimulated T-cells and/or drugs that interfere with the tumor's blood supply, is intriguing and holds great promise. These clinical trials will be closely watched.

Yet another novel approach to immune therapy was presented at the 2000 Prostate Cancer Foundation Retreat by professor Laurie Glimcher, M.D., of Harvard University. Dr. Glimcher is working on a different way to destroy cancer cells. During an immune response, the immune system produces small hormone-like molecules called "cytokines." Cytokines are produced by T-cells and are responsible for inflammation and immunity. Some are helpful and some are harmful. The helpful cancer-fighting cyokines are produced by a cell called Th-1. One critical cytokine for cancer-cell rejection produced by Th-1 cells is known as interferon-gamma (IFG). Th-2 cells produce a harmful cytokine called interleukin-4.

It turns out that another form of T-cell, called T-helper cells, have the ability to become either Th-1 or Th-2 cells. Dr. Glimcher and her collaborators looked for methods to induce T-helper cells to become Th-1 cells instead of Th-2 cells in order that the immune system would make more interferon-gamma and less interleukin-4. And she succeeded! She isolated a molecule called "T-Bet," a master regulator of Th-1 cell production. In the presence of T-Bet, T-helper cells become Th-1 cells. In the laboratory, 72% of T-helper cells exposed to T-Bet produced IFG. Only 3% of T-helper cells not exposed to T-Bet produced IFG. Additionally, T-Bet can convert mature Th-2 cells into Th-1 cells, resulting in more IFG production.

Natural killer cells have high levels of T-Bet. Investigators

are developing methods for men with prostate cancer to produce more T-Bet, increasing their cancer-rejecting IFG levels.

Late-Breaking News

A landmark study on the prevention of prostate cancer
was reported in the July 17, 2003, edition of the *New England Journal of Medicine*. This large-scale trial sponsored
by the National Cancer Institute (NCI) involved 18,882 men
55 years of age or more. These men, all of whom initially
had normal digital-rectal exams (DRE) and PSAs of 3.0 ng/
ml or less, were randomly assigned to receive either a placebo or 5 mg of finasteride (Proscar) daily. The men were
followed for 7 years and the end point of the study was biopsy-proven prostate cancer. All men who had either an abnormal DRE or who had an annual PSA of 4.0 or more, adjusted for Proscar's effect on PSA, were biopsied.

The results were so remarkable that the NCI decided to
close the study 15 months early. The men who got the Proscar
had a 24.8% reduction in the risk of getting prostate cancer.
This is a huge decrease in risk for a group of this size. Additionally, the men who received Proscar had a reduced number of urinary symptoms than the men getting the placebo,
presumably due to a shrinking of the size of the prostate.

However, there were a few glitches. The number of men
with aggressive cancers (Gleason score 7-10) was higher in
the Proscar-treated group, 6.4% versus 5.1%. This is a statistically significant difference. Also, the men who took
Proscar had more sexual side effects than the placebo group.

The increase in aggressive cancers in the Proscar-treated
group is open to some speculation. It was seen only during the
first year and didn't increase over time. Additionally, there is
evidence that hormonal therapy changes the structure of prostate cancer cells, making them appear to be more aggressive
than they are. Dr. I.M. Thompson, lead author of the original

study on Proscar prevention, has suggested that the apparent increase in Gleason 7-10 tumors in the finasteride-treated group may, indeed, be an artifact rather than a source of concern.

I'm certain more studies will examine the pros and cons of the use of Proscar as a prostate cancer preventative. Meanwhile, it seems to me that Proscar is likely to become an important part of a prostate cancer prevention program.

What course should men take? Dr. Thompson suggests this guideline: "Men should be presented with the benefits and risks of taking finasteride and be assisted in integrating their sexual and urinary symptoms into their decision-making process."

In other words, it may be right for some, but not for others.

Key References:

Thompson IM et al. The influence of finasteride on the development of prostate cancer. *New Eng J Med* 2003; 349: 215-224.

Thompson IM et al. Prevention of prostate cancer with finastride: US/European perspective. *Eur Urol* 2003; 44: 650-655.

That's All, Folks

Well, there you have it. In the interest of space I've had to exclude a number of promising therapies. The message, however, is clear. There are now more reasons than ever to be hopeful of being able to control and cure prostate cancer in the foreseeable future. Though we still have a long way to go, great strides are being made.

I want again to thank the Prostate Cancer Foundation, especially Dr. Howard Soule, for inviting me to the Prostate Cancer Foundation Retreats from which much of the information in this final chapter has been derived. Forty percent of the profits from this book are being donated to the Prostate Cancer Foundation. If this book has been helpful, the Prostate Cancer Foundation is the organization to thank.

APPENDIX I

The TNM Staging System for Prostate Cancer

T1-a: An incidental tumor found during a transurethral resection of the prostate (TURP), the cancer comprising less than 5% of the removed tissue.

T1-b: The same as T1-a, but with the tumor comprising 5% or more of the removed tissue.

T1-c: A tumor detected by biopsy based on an elevated PSA. The tumor can't be felt by DRE.

T2-a: A tumor felt by DRE that comprises less than half of one side of the prostate.

T2-b: A tumor felt by DRE that comprises 50% or more of one side of the prostate.

T2-c: A tumor felt by DRE that involves both sides of the prostate.

T3: A tumor that can be felt by DRE that involves the seminal vesicles.

T4: A tumor that can be felt by DRE that has spread beyond the prostate into the surrounding tissues.

N0: No detectable cancer in the lymph nodes.

N+: Cancer is detectable in the lymph nodes.

M0: No detectable cancer in the bone or other distant sites.

M+: Detectable distant metastases usually to bone.

My cancer involved only one lobe of the prostate and occupied about 50% of the lobe. Its TNM grade, therefore, was T2 NOMO, since no lymph-node or bone metastases were found. Since the cancer occupied about 50% of one lobe, some doctors classified it as T2-a, others as T2-b.

APPENDIX II

Thanks to the Johns Hopkins Brady Urological Institute for the 2002 upgraded Partin Tables, available on the Internet at:

www.urology.jhu.edu/Partin_tables/

Besides providing complete risk assessment tables for organ-confined disease, extraprostatic extension, seminal vesicle involvement, and lymph node metastases stratified by initial PSA measurements, this Web site includes a program that *automatically* calculates the probabilities of each of the above circumstances. Simply enter your PSA, Gleason score, and clinical stage in the designated spaces, and your entire risk-profile will automatically be calculated. I commend the Brady Urological Institute for providing this useful service to men with prostate cancer.

APPENDIX III

Functional Foods and What They Provide

Chart 1

Top antioxidant foods based on their ability to absorb oxygen radicals (in descending order of potency, assuming equal quantities (by weight) of each food:

Prunes
Raisins
Blueberries
Kale
Strawberries
Spinach
Raspberries
Brussels sprouts
Plums
Broccoli
Beets
Oranges
Red grapes
Red bell peppers
Cherries
Yellow corn

Eggplant
Carrots
Source: University of California, Berkeley Wellness Letter;
November 1999; 16: 2.

Chart 2
Foods High In Selenium:
Brazil nuts (highest by far)
Tuna
Flounder
Sole
Oysters
Turkey

Chart 3
Foods High In Lycopene:
Tomato paste
Tomato sauce
Tomato juice
Ketchup
Barbecue sauce
V-8 juice
Fresh tomatoes
Watermelon
Pink grapefruit
Guavas

Chart 4
Foods And Supplements That Reduce Inflammation:
Fish
Fish oil supplements
Green tea
Soy
Curcumin
Allium vegetables (garlic, scallions, onions)
Red wine

Chart 5
Foods And Supplements Associated With Cholesterol Reduction:
Fish
Fish oil supplements
Lycopene-rich food and lycopene supplements
Olive oil
Nuts
Green tea

Chart 6
Foods Rich In Polyphenols:
Chocolate
Grapes (red and purple)
Red wine
Green tea
Olive oil

Chart 7
Foods That May Stimulate The Immune System:
Maitake mushrooms and maitake extract supplements
Shiitake mushrooms
Fish oil
Olive Oil
Astragulus (Chinese herb)
Reishi (Chinese herb)

Chart 8
Non-dairy Sources Of Dietary Calcium:
Green leafy vegetables (spinach, bok-choi, Chinese broccoli, chard, kale)
Seaweed
Almonds

Chart 9
Sources Of Lutein:
Chard (silverbeet)

Avocados
Spinach
Chinese Greens (bok choi, Chinese broccoli, choi sum, etc.)
Choi sum, etc.

Chart 10
High Fiber Foods:
Beans
Lentils
Berries
Prunes
Figs
Grains (whole)
Cereals
Bran
Peas

Chart 11
Foods Rich In Gamma-tocopherol:
Sesame seeds (best source)
Almonds
Walnuts
Macadamia nuts
Cashews
Hazelnuts

Chart 12
Foods And Supplements Associated With An Up-regulation Of P21 And/Or P27 Cancer-suppressor Genes:
Artichokes
Silymarin or silibinin supplements
Quercetin (from fruits and vegetables)
Selenium-containing foods (see chart 2)
Crucifers (broccoli, cauliflower, cabbage, Brussels sprouts, etc.)
The class of prescription drugs known as SERMs (tamoxifen, Arzoxifene) also up-regulate p21.

Chart 13

Foods High In Soy Protein:
    Tofu
    Natto (fermented soy beans)
    Miso
    Soy protein isolate supplements
    Soy milk (low-fat or non-fat)
    Edamame (boiled fresh soybeans)

Chart 14

Foods Rich In Sulforathane; Glucosinolates, And Isothiocyanates (Crucifers):
    Cabbage
    Broccoli
    Brussels sprouts
    Cauliflower
    Arugula
    Radishes
    Kale
    Chard (silverbeet)
    Watercress
    Broccoli sprouts
    Collard greens
    Horseradish
    Mustard greens

Chart 15

Foods Rich In Beta-carotene:
    Papayas
    Mangos
    Apricots
    Pumpkins
    Carrots
    Cantaloupe

Chart 16
Foods Rich In Anthocyanins:
    Blueberries
    Raspberries
    Apples (red)
    Red wine
    Red grape juice
    Red or purple grapes

Chart 17
Foods Rich In Citrus Bioflavonoids And Limonene:
    Grapefruit (but beware of interaction with some medications)
    Lemons
    Tangelos
    Oranges
    Tangerines
    Limes
    Citrus rind (zest)

Note—The rind from each of these (preferably organically grown) can be widely used in everything from rice pudding to spaghetti sauce. Citrus rind is particularly high in citrus bioflavonoids and limonene.

Chart 18
Nutrients And Lifestyles Changes That Lower IGF-1 And/Or Raise IGFBP-3 Blood Levels:
    Vegan diet
    Artichokes
    Silymarin supplements or silibinin supplements
    Lycopene
    Vitamin D from sunlight
    Calcitriol (Rocaltrol) capsules (by prescription)
    Celebrex (blocks the action of IGF-1; available by prescription)
    Calorie reduction
    Increased exercise
    Soy

APPENDIX IV

Sources Of Supply

Chocolate (might as well do the most pleasurable first)
Dolfin S.A. (88% cocoa)
B-1440 Wauthier-Braine
Belgium
Tel: 32-2-3662424
Web site: www.dolfin.be

Michel Cluizel (this 85%-cocoa chocolate is my favorite)
Chocolatier
201 Rue Saint-Honore
75001 Paris
France

Greer & Blacks (70% cocoa organic dark chocolate)
P.O. Box 1937
London, W11 1ZU
England

Supplements
Life Extension Foundation
Ft. Lauderdale, FL
Tel: 800/544-4440
Web site: www.lef.org

Selenium, gamma-tocopherol, silymarin, silibinin, curcumin, vitamin D-3, conjugated linoleic acid, lightly caffeinated green tea, decaffeinated green tea, soy genistein isoflavone extract, lycopene.

Nature's Way Products, Inc.
Springvale, UT 84663
Thisilyn, standardized milk-thistle extract

Twin Laboratories
Ronkonkoma, NY 11779
Vege Fuel soy protein isolate—30 mg of soy protein per serving

Fish Oil
Nordic Naturals (Highly purified lemon-flavored capsules that have no objectionable fishy aftertaste)
Web site: www.nordicnaturals.com

Blackmores Ltd.
23 Rosebery Street
Balgowlah
New South Wales 2093
Australia (widely available throughout Australia and New Zealand)

Soy Protein Bar
GeniSoy Products Co.
Fairfield, CA 94533
Tel: 888/GENISOY
Web site: www.genisoy.com
non-fat chocolate-flavored soy protein bar

BroccoSprouts®
Tel: 410/837-9244
Johns Hopkins' patented broccoli sprouts

Meditation Tapes
Synchronicity
Tel: 800/962-2033

Cookbooks
The Taste for Living World Cookbook by Beth Ginsberg and Michael Milken, 1999; a Prostate Cancer Foundation publication (formerly CaP CURE).

The Taste for Living Cookbook: Michael Milken's Favorite Recipes for Fighting Cancer, by Beth Ginsberg and Michael Milken, 1998; a Prostate Cancer Foundation publication.

Eating Your Way to Better Health by C.E. Myers Jr., M.D. 2000, Rivanna Health Publications.

Qi Gong and Traditional Chinese Medicine
Dr. Daoshing Ni
1131 Wilshire Blvd. Suite 300
Santa Monica, CA 90401
Tel: 310/917-2204
Web site: www.taoofwellness.com
acupuncture and Chinese herbs

Massage
For a standardized, tension-releasing, *chi*-generating shiatsu massage in Australia, New Zealand, London, and selected locations in the United States, contact Tao Shiatsu at: www.taoshiatsu.com.

Support Groups, Web Sites, and Resources

Us Too! International, Inc.
930 North York Road, Suite 50
Hinsdale, IL 60521
Tel: 800/808-7866
Web site: www.ustoo.com

An international support group to help men with prostate cancer make treatment choices and deal with both physical and emotional issues. Us Too also publishes a newsletter.

National Cancer Institute (NCI)
Tel: 800/422-6237

NCI's "hotline" for information on new drugs and clinical trials.

Prostate Cancer Foundation (formerly CaP CURE)
1250 Fourth Street, Suite 360
Santa Monica, CA 90401
Tel: 310/458-2873
Web site: www.capcure.org

The Prostate Cancer Foundation's Web site has valuable information on nutrition and new therapies. Audio copies of the annual Prostate Cancer Foundation prostate cancer retreat are also available.

Prostate Forum
P.O. Box 6696
Charlottsville, VA 22906
Web site: www.prostateforum.com

Dr. Charles (Snuffy) Myers' highly informative and up-to-date monthly newsletter for men with prostate cancer.

UC Berkeley Wellness Letter
P.O. Box 420148
Palm Coast, FL 32142

Balanced reporting on issues of general wellness, nutrition, and supplements.

The Johns Hopkins Medical Institutions
White Papers Prostate Bulletin
P.O. Box 420875
Palm Coast, FL 32142

A quarterly bulletin on prostate problems, including cancer and BPH.

New Medicines in Development for Cancer Pharmaceutical Research and Manufacturers of America
1100 Fifteenth Street, NW
Washington, D.C. 20005
Web site: www.phrma.org

A detailed breakdown of clinical trials and the drug companies behind them for many kinds of cancer, including prostate.

KEY REFERENCE
ABBREVIATIONS

Adv Exp Med Biol — Advances in Experimental Medicine and Biology

Adv Neuroimmunol — Advances in Neuroimmunology

Am J Clin Nutr — American Journal of Clinical Nutrition

Am J Epidemiol — American Journal of Epidemiology

Am J Surg Pathol — American Journal of Surgical Pathology

Ann Intern Med — Annals of Internal Medicine

Ann Surg Oncol — Annals of Surgical Oncology

Anticancer Res — Anticancer Research Journal of Urology

Behav Med — Behavioral Medicine

Biochem Pharmacol — Biochemical Pharmacology

Biochem Mol Biol Int — Biochemistry and Molecular Biology International

Br J Cancer — British Journal of Cancer

Br (or Brit) J Urology — British Journal of Urology

CA Cancer J Clin — California Cancer Journal for Clinicians

CMAJ — Canadian Medical Association Journal

Cancer Invest — Cancer Investigation

Cancer J — Cancer Journal

Cancer Lett — Cancer Letters

Cancer Res — Cancer Research

Cancer Epidemiol Biomarkers Prev — "Cancer, Epidemiology, Biomarkers, and Prevention"

Clin Cancer Res — Clinical Cancer Research

Epidemiol Reviews — Epidemiologic Reviews

Eur Urol — European Urology

Exp Biol Med — Experimental Biology and Medicine

Exp Cell Res	Experimental Cell Research
Health Psych	Health Psychology
Hematol Oncol Clin North Am	Hematology/Oncology Clinics of North America J Urology
Infect Urology	Infectious Urology
Int J Obes Relat Metab Disord	International Journal of Obesity and Related Metabolic Disorders
Int J Oncol	International Journal of Oncology
Int J Radiat Oncol Biol Phys	"International Journal of Radiation Oncology, Biology, Physics"
J Cell Biochem	Journal of Cellular Biochemistry
J Clin Oncol	Journal of Clinical Oncology
J Clin Endocrin Metab	Journal of Clinincal Endocrinology and Metabolism
J Nutr	Journal of Nutrition
J Radiology	Journal of Radiology
JAMA	Journal of the American Medical Association
J Natl Cancer Instit	Journal of the National Cancer Institute
Med Hypotheses	Medical Hypotheses
New Engl J Med	New England Journal of Medicine
Nutr and Cancer	Nutrition and Cancer
Nutr Today	Nutrition Today
Nutr Metab Cardiovasc Dis	"Nutrition, Metabolism, and Cardiovascular Disease"
Oncol	Oncology
Oncol Rep	Oncology Reports
Pharmacol Biochem Behav	"Pharmacology, Biochemistry, and Behavior"
Proc Natl Acad Sci USA	Proceedings of the National Academy of Sciences of the United States of America
Prostaglandins Leukot Essent Fatty Acids	"Prostaglandins, Leukotrines, and Essential Fatty Acids"
Radiol Clin North Am	Radiologic Clinics of North America
Regul Toxicol Pharmacol	Regulatory Toxicology and Pharmacology
Semin Radiat Oncol	Seminars in Radiation Oncology
Semin Urol Oncol	Seminars in Urological Oncology
J Biol Chem	The Journal of Biological Chemistry
Urol Clin North Am	The Urologic Clinics of North America

Index

Symbols

A

E

G

M

O

W

Y

Z

About the Author

Many books on prostate cancer have been written either by medical doctors who are experts in the field or by patients who've gone through the difficult emotions and decisions. *Prostate Cancer—Prevention and Cure* is written by a doctor who also had prostate cancer. The combination provides a unique perspective on this common disease.

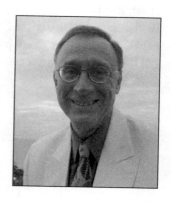

Lee Nelson, M.D., has kept abreast of the medical benefits of nutrition and its effect on disease for more than 20 years. The importance of nutrition in reducing heart disease and cancer is now well-established. But Dr. Nelson doesn't believe that nutrition alone is likely to cure cancer, although it may go a long way toward preventing it. In *Prostate Cancer—Prevention and Cure*, Dr. Nelson shows you how conventional medicine and complementary therapies working in concert are a much more potent combination than is either independently.

In writing this book, Dr. Nelson reviewed more than 2,000 medical papers and abstracts. He interviewed many of the top experts in the field. He also made extensive use of his experiences fighting and recovering from prostate cancer. Doctors' opinions have not been accepted on blind faith, but have been rigorously examined and questioned in light of the current medical literature. As Dr. Nelson says, "If I had been aware of the contents of this book at the time of my diagnosis of prostate cancer, I would have done a number of things quite differently. My hope is that the reader will reap the benefits of my learning curve and get the very best diagnosis, treatment, and nutritional support available."

Since being diagnosed with prostate cancer, Dr. Nelson has dedicated himself to educating men about the disease. He lives in New Zealand, where he consults with men about their medical situations, helps them through the complex decisions, and provides advice on nutrition, exercise, and other complementary lifestyle and attitudinal approaches to curing prostate cancer.